THE ZONE COLLECTION

THE ZONE
COLLECTION

Dr. Barry Sears

ReganBooks
An Imprint of HarperCollins*Publishers*

This book is not intended to replace medical advice or be a substitute for a physician. If you are sick or suspect you are sick, you should see a physician. If you are taking a prescription medication, you should never change diet (for better or worse) without consulting your physician, because any dietary change will affect the metabolism of that prescription drug.

Prevention will always be the best medicine. However, prevention can only be undertaken by the individual, and that includes eating correctly. This is the foundation of a healthy lifestyle. You have to eat, so you might as well eat wisely.

Although this book is about food, the author and publisher expressly disclaim responsibility for any adverse effects arising from the use of nutritional supplements to your diet without appropriate medical supervision.

INTRODUCTION

The Zone remains a controversial nutritional breakthrough because it requires you to think of food as if it were a drug. In fact, food may well be the most powerful drug you will ever take because of its almost immediate effects on hormones, which are hundreds of times more powerful than any drug. The goal of the Zone dietary plan is to keep these hormones controlled by your diet within zones that are neither too high nor too low. In the Zone, life becomes much easier. Outside the Zone, life becomes more difficult. The choice is yours.

The Zone is not some mystical place, but a real physiological state in your body that can be measured in the blood. But you don't need constant blood tests to follow this program; simply follow the easy-to-prepare meals described in this book. Considering the powerful medical and health benefits associated with the Zone, reaching it is fairly simple—but it depends on two words most Americans hate to hear: balance and moderation. You balance your plate at each meal with protein and carbohydrate, and you keep the calories you consume to a moderate level by eating primarily fruits and vegetables—instead of starches and grains—when you choose your carbohydrates. If you practice these simple principles, then the Zone dietary plan becomes your most powerful "drug"— one that will help you to attain a longer and better life.

The primary hormone affected by the Zone dietary plan is called insulin. Your body must have some insulin, otherwise you will die. But excess insulin is just as harmful as too little insulin, for the following reasons:

Excess insulin makes you fat and keeps you fat.
Excess insulin increases your risk for heart disease.
Excess insulin shortens your lifespan.

These are three pretty powerful reasons to keep your insulin levels in a Zone that is neither too high nor too low. A high-protein diet pushes insulin too low. A high-carbohydrate diet pushes insulin too high. The Zone dietary program maintains the balance of insulin you need.

What can you expect if you follow the principles of the Zone dietary plan? Here's my promise to you. Within one week you will be:

Thinking better

You are now controlling blood sugar that the brain needs for efficient functioning.

Performing better

By lowering insulin, you can access your own stored body fat for an unlimited supply of energy.

Looking better

You are losing fat (especially the medically dangerous fat around your waist), that makes your clothes fit better.

We are in the midst of an obesity epidemic that threatens our health care system. This epidemic has not been caused by dietary fat, since we are consuming the lowest level of fat in our diet in the past fifty years. What has caused this epidemic is the over-production of insulin caused by the over-consumption of excess carbohydrates.

Losing excess weight is simply a matter of controlling your insulin levels. It doesn't require hunger or deprivation. The Zone dietary program is a proven approach that you can learn quickly and easily and follow for a lifetime, and this book provides you with the meals to do exactly that. All you have to do is use them and make food the central part of your life, as it should be.

A WEEK IN
THE
ZONE

Also by Barry Sears, Ph.D.

The Zone

Mastering the Zone

Zone-Perfect Meals in Minutes

Zone Food Blocks

The Anti-Aging Zone

The Soy Zone

The Top 100 Zone Foods

Coming Soon in Hardcover

The Omega RX Zone

A WEEK IN
THE
ZONE

Barry Sears, Ph.D.

ReganBooks
An Imprint of HarperCollins*Publishers*

This book is not intended to replace medical advice or be a substitute for a physician. If you are sick or suspect you are sick, you should see a physician. If you are taking a prescription medication, you should never change diet (for better or worse) without consulting your physician, because any dietary change will affect the metabolism of that prescription drug.

Prevention will always be the best medicine. However, prevention can only be undertaken by the individual, and that includes eating correctly. This is the foundation of a healthy lifestyle. You have to eat, so you might as well eat wisely.

Although this book is about food, the author and publisher expressly disclaim responsibility for any adverse effects arising from the use of nutritional supplements to your diet without appropriate medical supervision.

Library of Congress Cataloging-in-Publication Data has been applied for.

ISBN 0-06-103083-X

CONTENTS

ACKNOWLEDGMENTS

The success of the Zone books that I have written during the past five years is primarily due to my support team, which is comprised of not only my coworkers, but also my closest friends. These include my wife, Lynn Sears, who does much of the editing of my books, and my brother, Doug Sears, who has a very clear insight and understanding of how to translate cutting-edge science into easily understood terms for the general public. In addition, I wish to especially thank Deborah Kotz for her excellent advice and input in helping develop this book.

At the same time, I also have a team at ReganBooks that consistently does an outstanding job of fine-tuning my books for the general public. For this particular book, I want to give special thanks to Vanessa Stich and Cassie Jones for their excellent editing.

Of course, my greatest thanks always goes to Judith Regan, who had the courage and foresight to support the Zone, and in the process helped improve the lives of millions of people.

INTRODUCTION

Since the publication of *The Zone* in 1995, more than 3 million Zone books have been sold in America. Furthermore, these books have been translated into 14 languages, making the Zone a worldwide phenomenon. The concept that hormones can be controlled by the diet is quickly becoming recognized as one of the key medical breakthroughs that will be the centerpiece for twenty-first-century health care.

Even with this growing recognition, the Zone remains misunderstood by many. Some think of the Zone as a high-protein diet, which it is not. Many more consider the Zone too difficult to follow, which it is not. What the Zone is is a powerful, yet simple to use dietary program that will allow you to lose excess body fat, reduce the likelihood of chronic disease, and enable you to live a longer and better life. All of these benefits come from your ability to use food to lower excess insulin levels.

This book represents the condensation of many of the themes that I have explored in greater detail in my previous five Zone books. It is written in such a form that makes it extraordinarily simple for you to spend a week in the Zone. Within that short time span you will experience the power of improved insulin control. That power can be yours on a lifetime basis as long as you follow the simple how-to instructions in this book.

This book answers many questions people have asked me over the past five years of how and why the Zone works. For more detailed information on various components of the Zone, I strongly refer you back to the appropriate Zone book that describes in more detail the science behind the Zone or in-depth discussions of how to cook in the Zone. At the same time, I also present here some of the newest published research that validates the Zone as your key to a better and healthier life in the new millennium. All that I ask is you try the Zone for a week. I promise you it will change your life forever.

1

WHAT IS THE ZONE?

For generations, every male on my father's side of my family suffered from a similar fate: a premature heart attack that cut their life short decades too early. After my father died in 1972 at the age of 54, I realized that I had a genetic time bomb ticking away inside me. I knew I couldn't change my genes, but I was determined to find a way to lead a normal, healthy life span.

My quest to save myself has led me to a surprisingly simple conclusion. As it turns out, the key to a longer, better life is not some magic pill or potion. It is a powerful hormone produced by your diet called insulin. My research showed that if you were able to keep insulin levels within a certain zone—not too high and not too low—you could dramatically improve your health and prevent a wide range of diseases. What's more, you could also make your body start using fat for energy, thus allowing you to lose excess body fat without feeling hungry!

So how do you begin to regulate your insulin levels and begin the journey to better health? Again, I found that the answer was simple: by eating the right combination of foods at every meal. Essentially, you need to start treating the Zone diet as a drug. Once you start taking this drug, you will automatically achieve:

- Permanent loss of excess body fat
- Dramatic reduction in the risk of chronic diseases like heart disease, diabetes, and cancer
- Improved mental and physical performance
- A longer life

The first person to recognize food as a wonder drug was Hippocrates, the father of medicine, who instructed us to "let food be your medicine, and let medicine be your food." Now some twenty- five hundred years later, we are just beginning to understand the importance of his words.

Make no mistake about it; food is a powerful drug. In fact, it may be the most powerful drug you will ever take. However, like any drug, food can help you or harm you depending on how you use it. Used correctly, food can make you more energized and healthier with the guarantee of a longer and more active life. Used incorrectly, food can become your worst enemy, robbing you of a healthy body, healthy weight, and a healthy mind, as millions of Americans are quickly finding out for themselves. Most important, if food is used improperly, it can also shorten your life.

You may think you already know how to properly use food by avoiding fat, and eating plenty of carbohydrates like pasta, bagels, bread, and rice. If you've been following these dietary guidelines, however, you may be puzzled as to why you're *gaining* rather than losing weight. Truth is, you have it backward. If you're like most Americans, you're probably eating far too many carbohydrates. This is why more than 50 percent of Americans are overweight today compared to 33 percent twenty years ago—even though we're now eating less fat than ever before. This is called the American paradox. If fat were the enemy, then we should have declared victory over obesity many years ago. The fact is that dietary fat was never the real enemy. **The real cause of our growing epidemic of obesity is excess production of the hormone insulin. It is excess insulin that makes you fat and keeps you fat.**

You are constantly reminded that a calorie is a calorie, and that weight gain is simply more calories coming in than calories going out. Since fat contains more calories per gram than does protein or carbohydrate, simple logic would dictate that removing fat from the diet should make us thinner. Such caloric thinking can be summarized as follows "if no fat touches my lips, then no fat reaches my hips." Well, it doesn't take a rocket scientist to walk on the streets of America and realize that statement simply isn't true. On the hormonal level, all calories are not created equal. The hormonal effect of a calorie of carbohydrate is different than the hormonal effect of a calorie of protein, and is still different from the hormonal effect of a calorie of fat. Each of these three nutrients has its own unique effects on your body's hormones. In the proper balance, these three nutrients are exactly what your body needs to remain healthy by keeping insulin within the Zone. When these nutrients are out of balance and insulin levels surge too high, they can wreak havoc on your body's hormonal equilibrium, resulting in weight gain, an increased likelihood of chronic disease, and acceleration of the aging process. On the other hand, if insulin levels are too low, your cells begin to starve because a certain amount of insulin is required to drive life-sustaining nutrients into your cells.

The Zone is like the story of Goldilocks and the Three Bears. One bowl of porridge was too hot (too much insulin), one bowl was too cold (too little insulin), and one was just right (the Zone).

ZONE BENEFITS

In the Zone, almost magical metabolic changes occur. Only in the Zone can you release excess fat from your fat cells to be used as fuel by your body twenty-four hours a day, allowing you to lose weight and enjoy more energy simultaneously. Only in the Zone can you reduce the likelihood of chronic disease. Only in the Zone can you live a longer life. It's as easy as eating the right combination of protein, carbohydrates, and fat at every meal and snack.

The benefits of maintaining insulin in the Zone are almost immediate, because your blood sugar is also automatically stabilized. As a result, you feel less hungry, you are more mentally alert and more energized throughout the day. Carbohydrate cravings become a thing of the past so that you can free your body from its slavery to food. How long does it take to see these benefits if you follow the basic guidelines presented in this book? No more than seven days.

With one week in the Zone, you will feel more alert, less fatigued, and never be hungry. And you will lose excess body fat at the fastest possible rate. Most important, you'll be doing everything in your power to keep yourself healthy and reduce the likelihood of developing such killers as heart disease, diabetes, and cancer. The end result is that you will live longer.

THE BASIC ZONE RULES

Although the next chapters will give you more details of the Zone program and additional tools you need to get yourself into the Zone, here is the basic starter package. To get your feet wet, read these basic Zone rules. You may even want to make a copy of this page and keep it in your wallet for reference when you're eating on the road.

Make sure every meal and snack gets you to the Zone by eating the right combination of low-fat protein, the appropriate type carbohydrate (preferably fruits and vegetables), and a little dash of "good" fat (like a sprinkling of nuts or olive oil).

1. Always eat a Zone meal within one hour after waking.
2. Try to eat five times per day: three Zone meals and two Zone snacks.
3. Never let more than five hours go by without eating a Zone meal or snack—regardless of whether you are hungry or not. In fact, the best time to eat is when you aren't hungry because that means you have stabilized your insulin levels. Afternoon and late evening snacks (which are really mini-Zone meals) are important to keep you in the Zone throughout the day.
4. Eat more fruits and vegetables (yes, these are carbohydrates) and ease off the bread, pasta, grains, and other starches. Treat breads, pasta, grains, and other starches like condiments.
5. Drink at least eight 8-ounce glasses of water every day. That's about a gallon of water.
6. If you make a mistake at a meal, don't worry about it. There's no guilt in the Zone. Just make your next meal a Zone meal to get you back where you (and your hormones) belong.

Now that wasn't so hard. In fact, you are probably telling yourself, "I can do that." If you want to jump right into the Zone, then go immediately to Chapter 5, in which you'll find a week of Zone meals for males and females. If you want a little more information about the Zone, continue to Chapter 2, and I'll show you why living in the Zone is controlled by the hormones and how those hormones are generated by the food you eat.

2

FOOD AND HORMONES: YOUR KEYS TO ENTERING THE ZONE

Entering the Zone is simply learning how to maintain the hormones generated by the food you eat within zones (not too high, not too low) from meal to meal. It's like riding a hormonal bicycle. If you can maintain your balance, you have unlimited freedom to go almost anywhere. However, if you can't balance your bicycle, you will always be falling down, never reaching your final destination—a longer and better life.

The Zone is not some mystical place or clever marketing phrase. The Zone has precise medical definitions that can be measured by simple blood tests. But the easiest test to determine whether or not you are in the Zone is to take off your clothes and take a look at yourself in front of a mirror. If you are fat and shaped like an apple, you are definitely *not* in the Zone. As you can quickly see, most Americans are not in the Zone. But even if you are thin, you can still be out of the Zone, as indicated by constant fatigue, low stamina, and persistent hunger. A quick blood test to measure your insulin levels will tell you for sure. And if they are too high, getting into the Zone will lower them.

Just because the Zone is based on treating food with the same respect that you would treat any prescription drug doesn't mean food has to taste like a drug. In fact, this book will show how incredibly easy it is to take the foods you like to eat, make a few minor adjustments, and get into the Zone on a lifetime basis.

To enter the Zone, you need to begin thinking of food in terms of three categories: protein, carbohydrates, and fats. All foods are composed of these three "macronutrients" to varying degrees: most foods contain a bulk of one group, and trace amounts of the others. Just to make sure we are talking the same language, I often tell people that "protein moves around, and carbohydrates grow in the ground." Obviously, fish and chicken are both proteins, since they move around. But what about carbohydrates? Well, pasta is a carbohydrate because it comes from wheat and that grows in the ground. What about broccoli? It grows in the ground, so it also must be a carbohydrate. And apples? They come from apple trees, which grow in the ground. That also makes an apple a carbohydrate. The fact that fruits and vegetables are carbohydrates comes as a major revelation to most Americans. One reason people are so confused about what to eat is that they often don't fully understand what they are eating.

Protein, carbohydrates, and fats all have unique hormonal impacts. Carbohydrates stimulate insulin, protein affects the hormone glucagon, and fats affect still another group of hormones called eicosanoids. How these three hormone systems impact your life is the science behind the Zone.

Let's take insulin first. Insulin is a "storage hormone." It tells the body to store incoming nutrients. Without adequate insulin, your cells starve to death and you die. On the other hand, too much insulin will make you fat, and accelerates the aging process. There are two ways to increase insulin and drive yourself out of the Zone. The first is to eat too many carbohydrates at any one meal. Carbohydrates are powerful stimulators of insulin secretion. The other is to eat too many calories at any one meal. Excess calories (especially carbohydrates) increase insulin levels because they must be stored somewhere in the body, and that demands more insulin. Furthermore, any excess calories the body cannot immediately store will be converted to fat and sent straight to your hips, stomach, or other problem areas for storage. Unfortunately, the same high levels of insulin that cause you to store fat will also block the release of any stored body fat for energy. This is why excess insulin makes you fat and keeps you fat.

On the other hand, dietary protein stimulates the release of glucagon, which has the opposite hormonal effect of insulin. Glucagon is a "mobilization hormone." It tells the body to release stored carbohydrate in the liver to replenish blood sugar levels for the brain. Without adequate levels of glucagon, you will always feel hungry and mentally fatigued because the brain is not getting enough of its primary fuel—blood sugar.

Insulin and glucagon are constantly performing this balancing act. If one hormone goes up, then the other hormone goes down. This is why the balance of protein to carbohydrate at *every* meal and snack is critical for maintaining insulin within the Zone.

Finally, there is fat. Fat has no direct effect on insulin. Nor does it have any effect on glucagon. So why not simply take all fat out of the diet? The reason is that fat has an effect on another group of hormones called eicosanoids, and these hormones also help control insulin levels. In many ways, eicosanoids are master hormones that orchestrate the functions of a vast array of other hormonal systems in your body. In a way, eicosanoids are analogous to a computer. Each of these hormones is shown below in a cartoon-like format.

The Zone is about how these three hormonal systems (insulin, glucagon, and eicosanoids) are controlled by the food you eat. The Zone is about hormonal thinking, not caloric thinking. It's a new way of looking at the food we eat, and that's what makes the Zone controversial, even though it is ultimately based on balance and moderation.

Hormones Affected by Your Diet

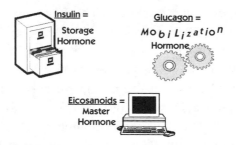

More than three million Americans have entered the Zone, and they can attest that the Zone works. More important, in the last year numerous scientific studies (see Chapter 15) by independent investigators have validated the Zone. Yet how could our government and all the nutritional "experts" have missed the boat? Because they are still thinking calorically, not hormonally.

Before you can fully understand the revolutionary implications of the Zone and all the vast benefits of being in the Zone, you need to clear your mind of many misconceptions about nutrition.

All too frequently, the dietary advice you read about in news-papers or magazines is totally conflicting, if not downright danger-ous to your health. Yet the more you hear something, the more you read about it, the more you're likely to believe it. With all the news reports and TV commercials touting the wonders of bagels, pasta, and breakfast cereals, you have more than likely been piling on these fat-free carbohydrates at the expense of protein and fat. Nutritional mantras like "eat no fat," "avoid protein," and "use pasta as the main course" dance around in your head at every meal. What passes as nutritional "wisdom" can sabotage your weight and health unless you understand some Zone facts that are based on hormon-al thinking. These facts upset much of this nutritional mythology that currently pervades America.

ZONE FACT #1: IT IS EXCESS INSULIN THAT MAKES YOU FAT AND KEEPS YOU FAT

You can't get fat by eating dietary fat alone—although none of us could live on only olive oil and vegetable shortening anyway. This is because dietary fat has no direct effect on insulin. So what does make you fat? It's excess levels of insulin. There are two ways to increase insulin levels in your body. The first is by eating too many fat-free carbohydrates at any one meal. The other is by eating too many calories at any one meal. In the past 15 years, Americans have done both simultaneously. This is why we have become the fattest people on the face of the earth, even though we are eating less fat than we were 15 years ago. Think of it this way: the best way to fatten cattle is to raise their insulin levels by feeding them excessive amounts of low-fat grain. By the same token, the best way to fatten humans is to raise their insulin levels by feeding them excessive amounts of low-fat grain, but now in the form of pasta and bagels.

ZONE FACT #2: YOUR STOMACH IS POLITICALLY INCORRECT

Your stomach is one giant vat of acid that can't tell one carbohydrate from another. From that perspective, one Snickers bar will be broken down by the stomach into the same amount of carbohydrate as found in 2 ounces of pasta. Now, you probably wouldn't eat four Snickers bars at one sitting, but it's very easy to eat 8 ounces of pasta. And that 8 ounces of pasta will send your insulin levels soaring. The more insulin you produce, the fatter you become.

ZONE FACT #3: EVERYONE IS NOT GENETICALLY THE SAME

Life just isn't fair. Genetically, some of us are luckier than others when it comes to handling dietary carbohydrates. For some, it seems as if just looking at a potato will make us fat. Others can eat all the potato chips they want without gaining an ounce because they don't make very much insulin when they eat carbohydrates. You know who these people are, and they probably aren't your closest friends. Unfortunately, about 75 percent of us have a relatively strong insulin response to carbohydrates, which means that our bodies make too much insulin if they overconsume carbohydrates. Excess insulin production makes our blood sugar fall too quickly, which makes us tired, fatigued, and hungry for more carbohydrates. (This is the biochemical reason that you crave carbohydrates all day long.) The amount of carbohydrates your body can handle properly without an excessive insulin response depends on your own genetic makeup. How can you tell if you're sensitive to carbohydrates? Eat a big pasta meal at noon, and then see how you feel three hours later. If you are hungry and having trouble staying awake, then you fall into the 75 percent of the population who are not so genetically lucky.

ZONE FACT #4: UNTIL 10,000 YEARS AGO, THERE WERE NO GRAINS ON EARTH

We are told that bread is the staff of life. The fact is that modern man has not changed, to any great extent, genetically for the past 100,000 years. For most of the time that humans have lived on the planet, we ate only two food groups: low-fat protein, and fruits and vegetables. The Zone is the diet that we were genetically designed to eat. Grains were simply not part of the diet that modern man evolved from. When grains were introduced 10,000 years ago, three things happened immediately:

1. Mankind shrank in size due to the lack of adequate protein.
2. Diseases of "modern civilization," such as heart attacks and arthritis, first appeared and were routinely reported in the medical textbooks of ancient Egypt.
3. Obesity became prevalent. In fact, it is estimated that the ancient Egyptians—with their grain-based diets—had about the same rate of obesity as Americans do today.

Since our genes haven't changed much in the past 100,000 years, don't expect them to change much in the next 100,000 years.

ZONE FACT #5: IT TAKES FAT TO BURN FAT

If you are thinking calorically, this statement makes no sense because fat contains calories. On the other hand, if you are thinking hormonally, this statement makes perfect sense, because fat has no effect on insulin. However, the right types of fat do play an indirect role in helping lower the insulin response to carbohydrates. First, fat slows down the entry rate of carbohydrates into the bloodstream, thereby decreasing the production of insulin. Second, fat sends a hormonal signal to the brain that says, "Stop eating," and the fewer calories you eat, the less insulin you make. Third, fat makes food taste better (just ask the French). So by taking fat (which has no effect on insulin) out of the diet and replacing it with carbohydrates (which have a strong stimulatory effect on insulin), you are virtually guaranteeing that you will become fatter. However, not all fats are created equal. The best type of fat to add back into your diet is heart-healthy monounsaturated fat, found in such foods as olive oil, avocados, almonds, and macadamia nuts, and long-chain omega-3 fats, found in fish and fish oils.

ZONE FACT #6: THE PRIMARY PREDICTOR OF HEART DISEASE IS HIGH LEVELS OF INSULIN

Heart disease is the number-one killer of both men and women in America. However, the best predictor of heart disease is not high cholesterol, not high blood pressure, but elevated levels of insulin. How can you tell if you have elevated insulin? Look in the mirror. If you're fat and shaped like an apple, you have elevated insulin. However, you can be thin and still have elevated insulin. How can you tell? Have a blood test to measure your lipid levels. If you have high triglycerides (more than 150 mg idl) and low HDL cholesterol (less than 35 mg idl), you are producing too much insulin and are at increased risk for heart disease. This is why high-carbohydrate, low-fat diets can be extremely dangerous for cardiovascular patients. They may lose weight if they're eating fewer calories, but they often experience an increase in triglycerides and a decrease in HDL cholesterol, which dramatically increases cardiac risk.

ZONE FACT #7: CARBOHYDRATES ARE DRUGS THAT CAN ACCELERATE AGING

Carbohydrates are not manna from heaven. You need some carbohydrates at every meal for optimal brain function, but like any drug, excess carbohydrates at meal will have a toxic side effect: the overproduction of insulin. The primary cause of aging is due to the continued production of excess insulin and its ability to accelerate the development of chronic disease.

ZONE FACT #8: THE ZONE IS NOT A HIGH-PROTEIN DIET

A high-protein diet is exactly that: you are eating excessive amounts of protein, often rich in saturated fat. In the Zone, you never eat more than 3 to 4 ounces of low-fat protein at any one meal. This is exactly what virtually every nutritionist recommends. Furthermore, you are always eating more carbohydrates than protein in the Zone, so it's impossible for the Zone to be considered a high-protein diet. As I explain in greater detail in Chapter 14, although high-protein diets are currently popular, they are virtually guaranteed to fail to provide permanent weight loss. And if followed for any extended period of time, high-protein diets will most likely increase your risk for heart disease.

WHAT THE ZONE CAN DO FOR YOU

With this quick primer on food and hormones, let's explore what the Zone can do for you in both the short term and the long term. If you're following the Zone, here are some of the immediate benefits you will observe during your first week. You will:

Think Better

By keeping your blood sugar levels stable throughout the day, your brain is constantly being supplied with energy. You'll find that you have a better ability to concentrate, and won't suffer from that mental haziness that can occur two to three hours (if not sooner) after eating a high-carbohydrate meal. You will feel more refreshed in the morning and more energized throughout the day. Afternoon slumps will be a thing of the past, as will be carbohydrate cravings.

Perform Better

By stabilizing insulin levels, you will be able to access stored body fat as a virtually unlimited supply of energy throughout the day. (Remember that excess insulin prevents the release of stored body fat.)

Look Better

Don't expect a lot of immediate weight loss on the Zone during the first week of the program, because it's physically impossible to lose more than 1 to 1½ pounds of body fat per week. However, all of the weight you will lose in the Zone will be pure fat, as opposed to water and muscle. Your body composition will change, and as a consequence, your clothes will start fitting better even though your scale isn't moving that much.

Feel Better

You'll feel less cranky and moody in between meals because you won't experience those sugar lows that make you tired, hungry, and irritable. Overall, you'll feel like your life is on an even keel— a sign that your hormones are, too.

Experience Fewer Carbohydrate Cravings and Become Totally Satisfied with Fewer Calories

Carbohydrate cravings are not an indication that you are a weak-willed person. They are simply a consequence of making a poor hormonal choice at your last meal. Once you learn to make Zone meals, the underlying cause of carbohydrate cravings will disappear. As an added benefit of being in the Zone, you'll be eating fewer calories than you're used to, but won't feel as hungry because your blood sugar levels are stabilized. Recent studies at Harvard Medical School have confirmed this.

While these are great short-term benefits, the real reason you want to make the Zone an integral part of your life is because it can result in a vast number of long-term health benefits that come with better insulin control. These include:

1. **You will achieve permanent fat loss.** The only way to control your weight is to control your insulin levels. In the Zone, you will begin shedding all the excess body fat you need to lose: Many readers who have followed the plan have lost 20, 40, or even in some cases, more than 100 pounds. More important, they have kept those pounds off.
2. **You will reduce the risk of heart disease.** As you decrease insulin levels, your risk of heart disease plummets. This was demonstrated in a study published in the *Journal of the American Medical Association* that found that insulin levels are far more predictive for the development of heart disease than any other risk factor.
3. **You will be less likely to develop adult-onset (Type 2) diabetes.** We usually think of diabetes as a disease in which you make no insulin. This is called Type 1 diabetes. However,

more than 90 percent of all diabetics have the opposite problem: they make too much insulin. They are known as Type 2
diabetics, and now number some 15 million Americans.
Clinical studies have shown that the Zone lowers excess
insulin levels in Type 2 diabetics within four days.

4. **You will be protected from arthritis and osteoporosis.**
Lowering insulin can alleviate tissue inflammation, because
reduced insulin levels also mean reduced levels of the building
blocks of pain-producing eicosanoids. By decreasing these
eicosanoids, you relieve the pain and inflammation associated
with arthritis. Essentially, the Zone works in much the same way
as aspirin: both control pain by controlling eicosanoids. It has
also been shown that increased protein consumption actually
decreases the number of hip fractures in post-menopausal
women.

5. **You may reduce the risk of developing breast cancer.** A
number of studies have found an association between high
insulin levels and the increased risk of breast cancer. This is coupled with new research from Harvard Medical School demon-
strating that the more protein (and less carbohydrates) a woman
consumes, the better her survival rate after breast cancer.

6. **You'll get fewer infections.** Adequate protein ensures proper
functioning of the immune system, the body's natural defense
mechanism against disease. Many people on high-carbohydrate
diets have suppressed immune systems and are more suscepti-
ble to infection because of excess insulin levels. They're more
likely to get sick (not to mention catching more colds and the
flu) than people getting adequate protein throughout the day.

Bottom line, if you want to live a longer and better life, entering the Zone is your best and safest drug. But like any drug, it only
works if you take the recommended dose at the right time.

3

GETTING STARTED
IN THE ZONE

Now that you understand how protein, carbohydrates, and fats work together to control your hormone levels, your body fat composition, and your overall health, you can begin making Zone-perfect meals. These meals will be your passport to the Zone.

GETTING READY TO MAKE ZONE MEALS

Ironically, the Zone is based on two terms your grandmother told you: balance and moderation. You balance your plate at every meal, and never eat too many calories at a meal. The only tools you need are the palm of your hand and your eye.

START WITH PROTEIN

Every Zone meal starts with making sure that you have an adequate serving of low-fat protein. There are several reasons for this. The first is that your body needs a constant supply of dietary protein to replace the protein that is constantly lost from your body on a daily basis. Without adequate incoming protein, your muscles weaken and your immune system becomes far less effective. Second, protein stimulates the release of glucagon. Recall that glucagon is a mobilization hormone that tells the body to release stored carbohydrates from the liver to maintain adequate blood sugar levels for the brain. Without adequate protein in a meal, hunger (due to the inability to maintain blood sugar levels) will result in two to three hours after a meal. Finally, glucagon acts as a brake on excess insulin secretion. If glucagon levels increase, then insulin levels decrease. By stimulating the release of enough glucagon with adequate levels of protein, you now have an ideal control mechanism to prevent too much insulin from being released.

Finally, you always want to use low-fat protein. Why? Because you will always be adding a dash of monounsaturated fat to a Zone meal, and using low-fat protein means you can control the composition of your fat instead of overconsuming saturated fat.

A very common misconception about the Zone is that you have to eat animal protein. That's simply not true. You do have to consume adequate protein, but for a vegetarian that is very easy to achieve eating egg whites, low-fat dairy products, tofu, or soy meat substitutes. As I will explain in Chapter 8, using soy products as your primary protein source may actually be the healthiest version of the Zone for a longer life.

The first step of Zone meal preparation is to *never* consume any more low-fat protein at a meal than you can fit on the palm of your hand. And before you get too excited, that amount also means the thickness of your hand. For most American females, this is 3 ounces of low-fat protein, and for most American males this is about 4 ounces of low-fat protein. Unless you are very active, your body can't utilize any more protein than that at a single sitting: any excess protein will be converted to fat. You always want to use low-fat protein for Zone meals to keep the amount of saturated fat to a minimum (since it can indirectly increase insulin levels). What are some good sources of low-fat protein? Many of your best choices follow.

Best Protein Choices

- Skinless chicken
- Turkey
- Fish
- Very lean cuts of meat
- Egg whites

- Low-fat dairy products
- Tofu
- Soy meat substitutes

BALANCE WITH CARBOHYDRATES

Now that you have your protein portion for your Zone meal, you must balance the protein with carbohydrates. Unfortunately, most Americans have no idea what carbohydrates actually are. Many people think of them as only pasta and sweets, whereas in reality they also include fruits and vegetables. The fact that a fruit or vegetable is also a carbohydrate is a major revelation to most Americans. However, not all carbohydrates are equal in their ability to stimulate insulin. Some are "favorable" carbohydrates that have a low capacity to stimulate insulin, and others are "favorable" carbohydrates that have a high capacity to stimulate insulin. Since the name of the game is insulin control, you want to make sure that most of your carbohydrate choices come from favorable carbohydrates (primarily fruits and vegetables), and treat unfavorable carbohydrates (such as grains and starches) like condiments.

This definition of favorable and unfavorable is based on the concept of the *glycemic load*. That is calculated from the combination of both the density of the carbohydrate in a given volume, and the rate at which it will enter the bloodstream. More details about glycemic load are found in my book *The Zone*, but for now all you need to know is that the higher the glycemic load of a given volume of carbohydrate, the greater its ability to stimulate insulin.

Vegetables (except for corn and carrots) always have a low glycemic load, whereas fruits (except for bananas and raisins) will usually have an intermediate glycemic load. Starches and grains (except for oatmeal and barley, which are very rich in soluble fiber) have very high glycemic loads. Therefore, as you balance the protein on your plate, do so with a lot of vegetables, some fruits, and just a small amount of grains and starches. Below are listed some of the favorable and unfavorable carbohydrates.

Favorable and Unfavorable Carbohydrates

Favorable (have a lower effect on insulin)
Most vegetables (except corn and carrots)
Most fruits (except bananas and raisins)
Selected grains (oatmeal and barley)

Unfavorable (have a greater effect on insulin)
Grains and starches (pasta, bread, bagels, cereals, potatoes, etc.)
Selected fruits (bananas, raisins, etc.)
Selected vegetables (corn and carrots)

As you can readily see, a good portion of your current diet is probably heavy on large amounts of unfavorable carbohydrates without adequate levels of low-fat protein. That's a surefire prescription for elevated insulin, which means you are getting fatter and less healthy with each meal.

ADD FAT

Once you have balanced your plate with low-fat protein and favorable carbohydrates, there is one more thing to add before it's truly a Zone meal—fat. Remember, it takes fat to burn fat. But like carbohydrates, all fats are not equal.

There are two types of fats that fall into the category of "good" fats. These are monounsaturated fats and long-chain omega-3 fats. You get monounsaturated fats from olive oil, selected nuts, and avocados. Long-chain omega-3 fats come from fish and fish oils (like the cod liver oil your grandmother told you to take). These are exceptionally powerful allies in your quest for a longer life, as described in greater detail in my other books. But for the moment, just think of them as good fats.

However, there are some fats you want to restrict in your diet. These are saturated fats, trans fats, and arachidonic acid. I consider these to be really "bad" fats. You find saturated fats in fatty cuts of red meat and high-fat dairy products. Another type of fat to avoid is trans fats. These artificial fats were created by the food industry and are found in virtually all processed foods. Any time you see the words "partially hydrogenated vegetable oil," you know that food contains trans fats. These alien fats make processed food more stable (why do you think your Twinkie is still good after a year in your pocket?). Furthermore, Harvard Medical School has shown that the more trans fats you eat, the more at risk you are for heart disease. Finally, there is arachidonic acid, which is found primarily in fatty red meats, egg yolks, and organ meats. This particular polyunsaturated fat may be the most dangerous fat known when consumed in excess. In fact, you can inject virtually every type of fat (even saturated fat and cholesterol) into rabbits, and nothing happens. However, if you inject arachidonic acid into the same rabbits, they are dead within three minutes. The human body needs some arachidonic acid, but too much can be toxic. Ironically, the higher your insulin levels, the more your body is stimulated to make increased levels of arachidonic acid.

Listed below are both the "good" and "bad" fats for the Zone.

"GOOD" AND "BAD" FATS

Good Fats (monounsaturated fats and long-chain omega-3 fats)
Olive oil
Almonds
Avocados
Fish oils

Bad fats (saturated fats, trans fats, and arachidonic acid)
Fatty red meat
Egg yolks
Organ meats
Processed foods (rich in trans fats)

LET'S GET STARTED

Now that you have an idea of what types of protein, carbohydrate, and fat you will be using to make Zone meals, let me show you how easy it really is.

First, take your plate and divide it into three sections. On one-third of the plate put some low-fat protein that is no bigger or thicker than the palm of your hand. Then fill the other two-thirds of the plate until it is overflowing with fruits and vegetables. Then add a dash (that's a small amount) of monounsaturated fat, like olive oil, slivered almonds, or even guacamole. There you have it: a Zone meal.

I hope you can see that putting together a Zone meal isn't rocket science. But the key is consistency, since the hormonal benefits of each meal will only last four to six hours. You have to eat, so you might as well get the best hormonal bang for the buck out of each meal.

This means always balancing protein and carbohydrate at every meal and snack. For example, you can't have all of your protein in one meal and all of your carbohydrate in the next meal, because your insulin levels will swing all over the place. Consider your food like a medication. You have to take the right dose at the right time. Would you take a week's worth of drugs on Saturday afternoon? Of course not. And if you are taking your drug every day, would you take 5 mg in the morning, 500 mg at noon, and 28 mg in the evening? Of course not. You would try the best you could to take the same amount of the drug each time. Why? You want to keep the drug within a Zone; not too high (where it's toxic), nor too low (where it doesn't work). Treat food the same way. Your goal is to maintain insulin in a similar Zone by balancing protein and carbohydrate and using only your eye and the palm of your hand to do it.

A DAY IN THE ZONE

So now that we know the basic rules, let's see what a typical day in the Zone for a typical American female might look like, using the Zone rules discussed in Chapter 1:

Breakfast

A 6-egg-white omelet mixed with some asparagus and 2 teaspoons of olive oil. The breakfast would also include ⅔ cup of slow-cooked oatmeal and a cup of strawberries.

Lunch

A grilled chicken salad with 3 ounces of chicken breast, some olive oil and vinegar dressing, and fresh fruit for dessert.

Late-afternoon snack

2 hard-boiled eggs in which the yolks have been removed and replaced with hummus (mashed chickpeas and olive oil).

Dinner

5 ounces of salmon covered with a tablespoon of slivered almonds, two cups of steamed vegetables, and a cup of mixed berries for dessert.

Late-night snack

1 ounce of soft cheese and a glass of wine (or a small piece of fruit if you don't drink).

The first thing you notice is that this is real food. The second thing is that it's also a lot of food, which means you'll never be hungry. The third thing is that it's exceptionally rich in vegetables and fruits. And the final thing, which is not so obvious, is that the total calorie content for your day in the Zone is about 1,200 calories. This is what I call the Zone paradox. **You'll eat a lot of food without hunger, fatigue, or deprivation and without consuming a lot of calories.** Most important, if you eat all the food, you are greatly increasing your chance for a longer life by keeping your overall calorie count at the level consistent with maximum longevity (see Chapter 8 for more details). Keep in mind that the typical American male would eat similar foods, only each meal should be 25 percent larger to supply the 1,500 calories he would need on a daily basis.

ZONE MEAL TIMING

Meal timing is critically important for staying in the Zone, just like taking a drug. Following the Zone, you try to eat five times per day (three meals and two snacks). Plan your day accordingly, just like you schedule appointments, so you never let more than five waking hours go by without eating a Zone meal or snack. A typical meal schedule might be as follows: if you wake up at 6:00, then eat a Zone breakfast by 7:00 (as you will see from the recipes in this book, this is a big breakfast). Five hours later, it's noon, and time for lunch, which will be another big meal. Most people won't eat dinner before 7:00, which is more than five hours after lunch, so have a snack in the late afternoon. After eating your dinner at 7:00, make sure you have one final late-night snack before you go to bed, because your brain stills needs blood sugar during your eight hours of sleep. That's a typical day in the Zone.

TIMING OF ZONE MEALS

Meal	Timing	Approximate Time
Breakfast	Within 1 hour after waking	7:00 A.M.
Lunch	Within 5 hours after breakfast	12:00 P.M.
Late-afternoon snack	Within 5 hours after lunch	5:00 P.M.
Dinner	Within 2–3 hours after snack	7:00 P.M.
Late-night snack	Before bed	11:00 P.M.

Following this program, at the end of a day in the Zone you have consumed adequate amounts of high quality protein, extraordinary levels of vitamins and minerals from vegetables and fruits, and the same absolute amount of fat usually consumed in most vegetarian diets. You weren't hungry or fatigued because you controlled blood sugar and thus the brain was constantly supplied with the only fuel source (blood glucose) it can use. Furthermore, you didn't feel deprived because each of the meals contained large volumes of food. In fact, the size of each Zone meal can be very intimidating, because when you replace grains and starches with carbohydrates such as fruits and vegetables, the carbohydrate volumes on your plate quickly increase in size.

THE BATTLE OF THE FOOD PYRAMIDS

Now that you know what Zone meals look like, we can put this into graphic form by constructing the Zone Food Pyramid, as shown on the following page.

As you can quickly see, using the Zone Food Pyramid, you are consuming a lot of vegetables and fruits. In fact, you would be consuming about 10 to 15 servings per day. The U.S. government recommends three to five servings per day, and virtually no one in America eats that amount. The next level in the Zone Food Pyramid is adequate amounts of low-fat protein. Notice I didn't say animal protein, because low-fat protein can also include tofu, soy protein meat substitutes, and isolated protein powder. Further up the Zone Food Pyramid is the addition of monounsaturated fats. Finally, at the top of the Zone Food Pyramid, are grains and starches, used only in moderation. As you can see, nothing is ever forbidden in the Zone; you just have to eat unfavorable foods in moderation.

So now we can compare the Zone Food Pyramid with the USDA Food Pyramid.

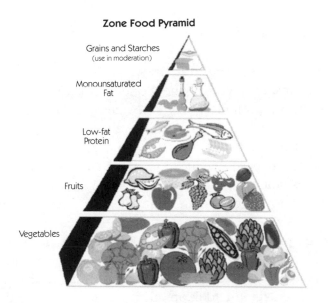

Zone Food Pyramid

Grains and Starches (use in moderation)

Monounsaturated Fat

Low-fat Protein

Fruits

Vegetables

Comparison of the Food Pyramids

When you look at carbohydrates from the Zone Pyramid per-spective, it becomes very clear why the USDA Food Pyramid is vir-tually guaranteed to increase insulin levels. The government rec-ommends eating 6 to 11 servings each day of unfavorable carbohy-drates, such as grains and starches. Using the Zone Food Pyramid, you might consume 2 servings. The government also recommends a minimum of 3 to 5 small servings of fruits and vegetables per day. Following the Zone Food Pyramid, you would eat 10 to 15 servings per day. Even though you are eating more *servings* of carbohydrates in the Zone, you are reducing your total *carbohydrate intake* by about 50 percent at the same time, because of the lower carbohy-drate content of vegetables and fruits. This 50 percent reduction in carbohydrate consumption also represents a 50 percent reduction of insulin secretion, with a corresponding increase in your chances of living a longer and healthier life at your ideal body weight.

WHY GRANDMOTHER WAS RIGHT

Now that I have gone into how to eat in the Zone in more detail, you begin to understand that your grandmother's dietary advice was based on hormonal thinking. Remember the four nutritional pearls of wisdom she told you.

1. **Eat small meals throughout the day.** One of the best ways to maintain insulin levels in the Zone is not to eat too much carbohydrate or protein at any one meal. Although carbohy-drate has a strong effect on insulin release, protein is also a weak stimulator of its release (however, protein has a strong impact on the release of glucagon, which inhibits insulin). By not overconsuming either protein or carbohydrate, you are well on your way to better insulin control as long as your meal is moderate in size.
2. **Have some protein at every meal.** The primary hormonal role of protein is to stimulate the release of glucagon, which mobi-lizes the release of stored carbohydrates so that your brain can use them for energy. In addition, glucagon also reduces the out-

put of insulin. Using the palm of your hand (and its thickness) is a good indicator of the maximum amount of protein you should consume at any meal.

3. **Always eat your vegetables and fruits.** Now you know these carbohydrates will have a lower impact on insulin release because these are more favorable carbohydrates with a decreased glycemic load compared to grains and starches. This is also good common sense, since most of your vitamins and minerals come from vegetables and fruits. By eating primarily vegetables and fruits, you're automatically controlling the amount of carbohydrates you eat at any given meal. What's more, the fiber in these low-density carbohydrates slows digestion and lowers the rate of insulin secretion.

4. **Take your cod liver oil.** I know nothing is higher on the "yecch" scale than cod liver oil. However, it does contain long-chain omega-3 fatty acids that do a great job of keeping insulin under control and are critically important for your cardiovascular and immune function. Furthermore, they are also critically important for your brain (that's why they call fish and fish oil "brain food"). You can still hold your nose and take your cod liver oil like your grandmother did, or you can opt for a more palatable choice in the form of salmon, which is rich in the same fatty acids, or a new generation of almost tasteless fish oils.

I hope you now realize that your grandmother was actually describing how to reach the Zone. In fact, she was at the cutting edge of twenty-first-century biotechnology when it came to insulin control.

At this point, you are probably again saying that magical phrase, "I can do that." All you have to do is use the palm of your hand and be able to tell time. If you can, then living in the Zone on a lifetime basis is going to be incredibly easy.

4

A ZONE MAKEOVER FOR YOUR KITCHEN

You're about to start your week in the Zone, but first you need the proper preparation. That's what this chapter is all about: readying your kitchen to become a food pharmacy.

During the first week that you're in the Zone, you should try to make your kitchen as Zone-friendly as possible. That means taking certain "Zone-hostile" foods out of your pantry, refrigerator, and freezer and replacing them with foods that fit into your new Zone eating plan.

This way, every time you open the refrigerator door you'll be pulling out a drug as powerful as any that your doctor can prescribe. You'll be using these Zone-friendly foods to lose weight and ward off illness. You'll get a powerful burst of energy from better insulin control that will keep you mentally and physically alert throughout the day. Follow these simple steps and you'll be on your way to a lifetime of better health.

Note: These rules apply to the first week that you're in the Zone. I'm trying to make your first experience with the Zone easier by taking away all foods that are considered high-density carbohydrates—meaning they have a lot of carbohydrates packed into a small amount of space. You don't need to banish Zone-hostile foods forever. After the first week, you can add them back in small amounts and still stay in the Zone.

THE BIG CLEAR-AWAY

The first thing you want to do is temporarily remove all the potentially dangerous foods from your kitchen that will drive you out of the Zone. Take all unfavorable carbohydrates like pasta, rice, dry cereal, pancake and cookie mixes, breads, and bagels and put them in a bag. I'd also like you to do the same with any dried fruit you might have, since these also are concentrated sources of carbohydrates. Then store them in a taped box in a dark corner of your basement where you aren't likely to venture in the next week. Do the same for any breadmakers, pasta machines, and juicers you own.

MAKE A FAT SWITCH

Get rid of vegetable oil, vegetable shortening, butter, whole-milk dairy products, and any other foods that contain high amounts of saturated and omega-6 polyunsaturated fats. Replace the vegetable oils and shortenings with olive oil and nut butters (almond is the best) that are rich in monounsaturated fat. Replace the whole-milk dairy products with low-fat cottage cheese, low-fat milk, and part-skim ricotta cheese. Replace bologna and bacon with low-fat sources of protein like chicken, turkey, and fish. Also, stock up on soybean-based food products like meatless ground beef, soy hamburgers, and soy sausages. The key is to use low-fat protein sources so you can add back the small amounts of monounsaturated fat.

BE PICKY ABOUT PRODUCE

Even when it comes to fruits and vegetables, you need to be selective. Certain fruits and vegetables are high-density carbohydrates, which means they can raise your insulin levels as much as a cookie or candy bar. Again, I'd like you to get rid of all fruit juices and dried fruit, since they are concentrated sources of sugar. I'd also like you to avoid these Zone-hostile fruits: bananas, cranberries, dates, figs, guavas, kumquats, mangos, papayas, dried prunes, and raisins. The best choices for fruit include apples, apricots, pears, oranges, raspberries, plums, blueberries, strawberries, grapes, and grapefruit. Starchy vegetables are the most Zone-hostile and include acorn squash, beets, butternut squash, carrots, corn, French fries, parsnips, peas, and potatoes. The best choices for vegetables include dark green leafy vegetables, tomatoes, celery, mushrooms, and peppers. For a complete list, see Appendixes B and C for Zone Food Choices.

If the thought of cutting up fresh vegetables several times a day sounds too time-consuming, then stock up on frozen vegetables or purchase pre-cut vegetables. Frozen fruits and vegetables are picked when at their ripest and then quick-frozen—often within hours after harvesting. The end result is that frozen produce often has a higher vitamin content than fresh fruits and vegetables, which can sit around at distribution centers and supermarkets for days or weeks before you actually buy them. The longer fresh produce sits around, the more nutrition (especially vitamins) is lost. If you don't mind the taste of frozen produce, by all means, stock it in your freezer. Canned produce, on the other hand, will have fewer vitamins and minerals than fresh or frozen produce because it is more processed and loaded with preservatives. It's okay in a pinch if you haven't had time to get to the supermarket.

RESTOCK YOUR KITCHEN WITH ZONE STAPLES

Keeping certain staples around the house will make Zone cooking and snacking incredibly easy. Since Zone staples have a long shelf life, measured in months, you won't have to buy these as often. Slow-cooking oatmeal is one staple you should definitely have on hand, since it's one of the few grains I readily recommend on the Zone. Why is oatmeal so Zone-friendly? It's rich in soluble fiber that slows down the absorption of carbohydrate and contains an essential fatty acid that is found in mother's breast milk. The best kinds of oatmeal are called Scottish oats or Irish oatmeal, made from thick, coarse oats that take about 30 minutes to cook. The next best choice is old-fashioned oats, which take about five minutes to cook and still retain their chewy texture. (Avoid instant oatmeal, since it is more processed to make it cook faster and thus enters your bloodstream quickly, causing an insulin surge.)

One protein source that can be considered a Zone staple

because of its very long shelf life is isolated protein powder. Protein powder can be added to fresh fruit shakes or vegetable soups and stews to fortify them with protein to turn them into Zone meals. Hormonally speaking, the best type of protein powder is soybean isolate, since it has the least effect on insulin and the greatest effect on glucagon. Unfortunately, this type of protein powder doesn't taste as good as other isolated protein sources such as whey, milk, or egg proteins. My suggestion is to use various combinations with the maximum amount of soy protein until you find a balance that meets your taste requirements.

Another vital Zone staple is nuts. Thousands of years ago, people ate nuts for fat before they were able to extract oil from olives and seeds. I prefer that you choose nuts that are rich in monounsaturated fats, like macadamia nuts, almonds, cashews, and pistachios. Peanuts are a good source of monounsaturated fat—though not as good as other kinds of nuts. Remember, nuts, including peanut butter, are primarily a source of fat. And you only need to eat a relatively small amount of nuts or nut butter to get a good dose of the monounsaturated fat that your body needs.

When you're stocking up on staples, don't leave out the spices. Spices make food taste better, and the more you use, the greater the taste sensation. Spices have no effect on insulin, so feel free to indulge your taste buds.

SHOPPING LIST FOR YOUR WEEK IN THE ZONE

Now it's time to take a trip to the supermarket. During your week in the Zone, you'll probably need to go shopping two or three times to ensure that you have the freshest fruits, vegetables, and protein. For instance, you can only keep fresh fish, chicken, and meat for two or three days at most in your refrigerator before they spoil, although you can freeze and rethaw them.

As you find yourself perusing through aisles of gleaming apples and stacked broccoli bunches, you'll probably notice that you're spending most of your time on the periphery of the supermarket, rather than in the inner aisles. This is no accident. The periphery usually contains fresh and frozen produce and perishable items like milk, cheese, poultry and fish, while the inner aisles contain processed foods like breakfast cereal, pasta, flour, and snack products. A good rule of thumb to follow whenever you're supermarket shopping is to spend most of your time on the periphery of the supermarket and very little time in the aisles that hold the greatest temptations. (Remember, if you don't buy it, you won't have any Zone no-no's beckoning you in the kitchen.)

The following shopping list for your week in the Zone is divided into two parts, which means you'll need to go shopping at the beginning of the week and then again in the middle of the week. The list is divided into categories to help you stay organized while you shop and to help you avoid forgetting any items.

SHOPPING LIST #1: FOR DAYS 1, 2, 3, 4

Meat/Fish/Poultry

Turkey breast slices (deli-style)
Ham (deli-style)
Skinless chicken breast
Lean Canadian bacon (or turkey bacon strips or soy sausage links)
Tuna (canned albacore packed in water)
Flounder fillet
Lean ground beef (or ground turkey or soy burger patty)
Lean ground lamb

Vegetable Protein

Soy protein powder
Tofu (firm)

Fruits

Strawberries
Blueberries
Oranges
Apples
Seedless grapes
Cantaloupe

Reduced-sugar canned pineapple
Reduced-sugar canned mandarin oranges
Kiwi

Vegetables

Green-leaf lettuce
Mushrooms (white, brown, or button)
Tomatoes
Broccoli florets
Yellow onions
Celery
Lettuce leaves
Green beans
Green peppers
Scallions
Red onions

Beans and Legumes

Canned chickpeas
Snow peas

Dairy Products

Cottage cheese
Swiss cheese
Low-fat yogurt
Parmesan cheese
Reduced-fat American cheese
Reduced-fat smoked mozzarella
Egg whites (or egg substitute)
Low-fat milk (1%)

Grains

Hamburger rolls
Cooked brown rice

Spices

Cinnamon
Fresh ginger
Fresh garlic
Black pepper
Lemon juice
Dried basil
Dried oregano
Cilantro
Cumin
Coriander
Celery salt

Miscellaneous

Macadamia nuts
Almonds (slivered)
Olive oil
Red-wine vinegar
Cider vinegar
Soy sauce
Vegetable spray
Light mayonnaise
Dill pickles
Applesauce
Dry onion soup mix

SHOPPING LIST #2: FOR DAYS 5, 6, 7

Meat/Fish/Poultry

Lean Canadian bacon (or turkey bacon strips or soy sausage links)
Lean ground beef (or substitute ground turkey or vegetable protein
    crumbles)
Shrimp
Skinless chicken breast
Salmon steak

Turkey bacon (or lean Canadian bacon or soy sausage links)
Tuna (canned albacore packed in water)

Fruits

Unsweetened applesauce
Peaches
Oranges
Pears
Lemons
Apples
Mandarin oranges
Nectarines

Vegetables

Yellow onions
Asparagus spears
Red peppers
Green peppers
Green-leaf or romaine lettuce
Broccoli florets
Tomatoes
Zucchini
Button mushrooms
Celery
Onions
Green beans

Beans and Legumes

Canned kidney beans
Canned black beans
Canned chickpeas

Dairy Products

Cottage cheese
Low-fat Monterey Jack cheese

Egg whites (or egg substitute)
Low-fat milk (1%)
Mozzarella cheese (shredded)

Grains

Slow-cooked (steel-cut) oatmeal

Spices

Nutmeg
Cinnamon
Chili powder
Garlic powder
Black pepper
Fresh garlic
Lemon juice
Dried rosemary
Dried tarragon
Dried dill
Dried chives
Dried parsley
Dried basil

Miscellaneous

Almonds
Applesauce
Olive oil
Wine vinegar
Salsa or canned stewed tomatoes
Tomato sauce
Dry white wine
Vegetable spray
Light mayonnaise
Cider vinegar

Once you've completed your shopping trip, you can move on to the simple Zone meals outlined in Chapter 5. These meals, given separately for both males and females, will take you through your first seven days in the Zone. Take these "drugs" as directed, and you begin to change your life forever. They are designed to be simple and straightforward, with few ingredients and limited preparation and cooking time. Keep in mind that Chapter 5 is a very specific map that will guide you through your first week. Once you complete this week, you will find more Zone recipes in Chapter 6 and a sampling of some of the vegetarian meals from the Soy Zone in Chapter 8 that you can mix and match for all your meals and snacks for a lifetime in the Zone. Happy cooking, and Zone appetit!

5

RECIPES FOR A WEEK IN THE ZONE

Now that your kitchen is prepared and you understand the boundaries of the Zone, I want to show you what a typical week in the Zone looks like for both males and females. Each of these meals has the right balance of protein, carbohydrate, and fat, which means that each of these meals can be used like a drug to keep insulin within the Zone for the next four to six hours. More important, they're delicious, and quick and easy to prepare.

If you follow the simple (and great-tasting) meal planner outlined in the following pages, you'll have a surefire path straight into the Zone. Within one week, you'll be looking better, feeling better, and starting your body on a lifelong journey to optimum health.

TYPICAL FEMALE
Day 1

Breakfast: Fruit Salad

Ingredients
 ¾ cup low-fat cottage cheese
 1 cup fresh or reduced-sugar canned pineapple, cubed
 ⅓ cup reduced-sugar canned mandarin oranges, drained
 3 macadamia nuts, crushed

Instructions: Place cottage cheese in a bowl. Fold in pineapple, oranges, and nuts.

Lunch: Chef's Salad

Ingredients
1 cup green-leaf lettuce (substitute lettuce of your choice), washed, dried, and torn into large pieces
¼ cup canned chickpeas, drained and rinsed
½ cup button mushrooms, washed, dried, and coarsely chopped
½ cup celery, washed, dried, and coarsely chopped
1 tablespoon olive oil-and-vinegar dressing*

Zone oil-and-vinegar dressing contains 1 teaspoon olive oil and 2 teaspoons vinegar. Extra vinegar may be added to taste.
1½ ounces deli-style turkey breast, cut into strips
1½ ounces deli-style ham, cut into strips
1 ounce reduced-fat Swiss cheese (substitute any reduced-fat cheese), julienned

For Dessert
1 medium apple

Instructions: Toss lettuce with chickpeas, mushrooms, and celery. Dress, toss, and add meat and cheese. Serve apple for dessert.

Dinner: Ginger Chicken

Ingredients
1 teaspoon olive oil
3 ounces boneless, skinless chicken breast, cut lengthwise into thin strips
2 cups broccoli florets, washed
1½ cups snow peas, washed
¾ cup yellow onion, peeled and chopped
1 teaspoon fresh ginger, grated

For Dessert
½ cup seedless grapes

Instructions: In a wok or large nonstick pan, heat oil over medium high heat. Add chicken and sauté, turning frequently, until lightly browned, about 5 minutes. Add broccoli, snow peas, onion, ginger, and ¼ cup water. Continue cooking, stirring often, until the chicken is done, water is reduced to a glaze, and vegetables are tender, about 20 minutes. If the pan dries out during cooking, add water in tablespoon increments to keep moist. Serve grapes for dessert.

Day 2

Breakfast: Yogurt and Fruit

Ingredients
    1 ounce lean Canadian bacon (substitute 3 turkey bacon strips or
        2 soy sausage links)
    ½ cup fresh blueberries, rinsed and drained
    1 tablespoon slivered almonds
    1 cup plain low-fat yogurt

Instructions: Prepare bacon or soy patties, following package instructions. Stir fruit and nuts into yogurt, and serve with bacon or links on the side.

Lunch: Tuna Salad

Ingredients
    3 ounces albacore tuna packed in water, drained
    ¼ cup celery, washed, dried, and coarsely chopped
    1 tablespoon olive oil-and-vinegar dressing*
    1 or 2 lettuce leaves, washed and dried
    ½ cantaloupe, seeds scooped out
    ½ cup blueberries, rinsed and drained

Instructions: Mix tuna with celery and stir in dressing. Prepare a bed of the lettuce leaves and top with tuna mixture. Stuff cantaloupe with berries and serve for dessert.

*Zone oil-and-vinegar dressing contains 1 teaspoon olive oil and 2 teaspoons vinegar. Extra vinegar may be added to taste.

Dinner: Foiled Flounder with Green Beans

Ingredients
vegetable spray
4½ ounces boneless flounder fillet (substitute mild, flaky fish of
    your choice)
2 tablespoons yellow onion, peeled and chopped
sprinkling of Parmesan cheese
¼ teaspoon freshly ground pepper, or to taste
squirt lemon juice
1½ cups fresh green beans, washed, ends removed, and halved
1 tablespoon almonds, slivered

For Dessert
1 cup fresh or reduced-sugar canned pineapple

Instructions: Preheat oven to 425°. Tear off an 18-by-12-inch piece of foil. Spray the center lightly with vegetable spray, and place fish in the center of the foil. Top with onion and sprinkle with cheese, pepper, and lemon juice. Fold foil loosely over fish, leaving ample space for air. Carefully turn up and seal the ends and the middle so that juices won't leak out. Bake in the preheated oven 18 minutes. Meanwhile, steam the green beans: in a large pot fitted with a steaming basket, bring 1 inch water to boil. Add beans to the basket and steam until crisp-tender, 10 minutes. Drain, place in serving bowl, and fold in almonds. When fish is done, carefully open foil to prevent steam burns, and remove to a plate. Serve with green beans. Serve pineapple for dessert.

Day 3

Breakfast: Fruit Smoothie

Ingredients
20 grams protein powder
1 cup blueberries
1 cup strawberries

3 macadamia nuts
4 ice cubes

Instructions: Place all ingredients in a blender and blend at high speed until smooth, about 1 minute. Add a little water if smoothie is too thick. If you prefer, eat the nuts on the side.

Lunch: Cheeseburger

Ingredients

3 ounces lean (less than 10% fat) ground beef (substitute 3 ounces ground turkey or 1 soy burger patty)
1 ounce reduced-fat American cheese (substitute cheese of choice)
1 tablespoon light mayonnaise
½ hamburger roll
1 thick tomato slice, optional
1 large lettuce leaf, optional
1 dill pickle wedge, optional

For Dessert

⅔ cup unsweetened applesauce
sprinkling of cinnamon

Instructions: Preheat broiler. Place burger on foil or rack and broil 5 minutes. Flip and continue cooking another 5 minutes for medium rare. One minute before expected doneness, top with cheese, and remove when melted. Spread mayonnaise on the roll. Top with burger, tomato, and lettuce. Serve pickle on the side. Sprinkle applesauce with cinnamon and serve for dessert.

Dinner: Vegetarian Stir-fry

Ingredients

1 teaspoon olive oil
⅔ cup vegetable protein crumbles* (substitute 4 ounces firm tofu)
1½ cups yellow onions, peeled and chopped
2 cups broccoli florets, washed

2 cups button mushrooms, washed, dried, and thinly sliced
1 ounce reduced-fat Swiss cheese, shredded

For Dessert
½ cup grapes

Morningstar Farms makes Burger-Style Recipe Crumbles, which looks like ground beef and is a good vegetarian source of protein.

Instructions: Heat oil in a nonstick sauté pan or wok over medium-high heat. If using tofu, remove from wrapping, drain, and crumble. Add tofu or soy crumbles and stir until mixed with the oil. Add onions, broccoli, and mushrooms. Reduce heat to medium and stir-fry, stirring often, until vegetables are tender, about 15 minutes. Stir in cheese and heat until melted, about 1 minute. Serve grapes for dessert.

Day 4

Breakfast: Scrambled Eggs and Bacon

Ingredients
vegetable spray
4 egg whites (or ½ cup egg substitute)
1 teaspoon olive oil
1 tablespoon low-fat milk (optional)
1 ounce lean Canadian bacon (substitute 3 turkey bacon strips
    or 2 soy sausage links)

For Dessert
1 cup grapes
⅓ cup mandarin oranges

Instructions: Lightly coat a large nonstick pan with vegetable spray, and heat over medium flame. Beat egg whites with olive oil and milk, if desired. Pour into pan and cook, stirring often, until scrambled and fully set. Prepare bacon or soy links, following package instructions. Mix grapes and oranges and serve for dessert.

Lunch: Tofu Dip and Veggies

Ingredients
4 ounces firm tofu
1 ounce reduced-fat Swiss cheese, grated
¼ cup canned chickpeas, drained and rinsed
1 teaspoon olive oil
2 tablespoons fresh lemon juice
2 tablespoons Lipton's dry onion soup mix (substitute spices of
    your choice, to taste*)
1 medium green pepper, washed, cored, seeded, and cut in
    wedges
2 cups broccoli florets

For Dessert
Kiwi

Instructions: Drain tofu. Put tofu, cheese, chickpeas, olive oil,
lemon juice, and onion soup mix in a blender. Blend until smooth.
(For best flavor, refrigerate the dip at least 2 hours or overnight.)
Place dip in a bowl in the center of a large plate. Arrange pepper
strips and broccoli around bowl for dipping. Serve kiwi for dessert.

*If you don't want to use the packaged soup mix, experiment with
minced onions, garlic, or vegetable bouillon granules.*

Dinner: Spiced Lamb with Vegetables

Ingredients
4½ ounces lean ground lamb
1 teaspoon cider vinegar
1 teaspoon olive oil
½ cup scallions, finely chopped
¾ cup red onions, cut in chunks
2 cups mushrooms
1½ cups tomatoes, diced
½ cup green beans, diced
1 tablespoon cilantro

2 teaspoons fresh ginger, minced

¼ teaspoon cumin

¼ teaspoon coriander

⅛ teaspoon black pepper

½ teaspoon celery salt

⅛ teaspoon cinnamon

Instructions: In a small glass bowl, combine lamb, vinegar, and spices. Cover and refrigerate for 30 minutes. Heat the oil in a medium nonstick sauté pan. Add meat mixture and vegetables. Cook, breaking meat up as it cooks, until lamb is cooked through and vegetables are tender. Spoon onto plate and serve.

Day 5

Breakfast: Old-fashioned Oatmeal

Ingredients

⅔ cup slow-cooking (steel-cut) oatmeal*

2 ounces lean Canadian bacon (substitute 6 turkey bacon strips
    or 2 soy sausage links)

⅓ cup unsweetened applesauce

1 tablespoon almonds, slivered

sprinkling of nutmeg

sprinkling of cinnamon

¼ cup low-fat cottage cheese

Instructions: Bring 3 cups water to a brisk boil over high heat. Add oatmeal, stirring well. When smooth and beginning to thicken, reduce heat to low and simmer for 30 minutes, stirring occasionally. While oatmeal is cooking, prepare bacon or soy patties, following package instructions. Remove oatmeal from the heat. Stir in applesauce and almonds. Sprinkle with cinnamon and nutmeg. Serve bacon and cottage cheese on the side.

*By slow cooking, we mean slow cooking. Oatmeal that calls itself slow-cooking but takes only 5 minutes isn't the real McCoy (or per-

haps we should say the real McCann's, a popular brand). To shorten the morning cooking time, make a big batch during the weekend, freeze, and microwave the correct amount in the morning. You may also put the oatmeal in a wide-mouth thermos with 1⅓ cups boiling water, and let it cook overnight.

Lunch: Chili (Meat or Vegetarian)

Ingredients
   1 teaspoon olive oil
   4½ ounces lean (less than 10%) ground beef (substitute ground
      turkey or 1 cup vegetable protein crumbles*)
   ¼ cup yellow onions, peeled and minced
   1 teaspoon chili powder, or to taste
   ½ teaspoon garlic powder, or to taste
   ½ teaspoon freshly ground pepper, or to taste
   1 cup salsa or stewed tomatoes with liquid
   ¼ cup kidney beans, drained and rinsed
   Sprinkling of low-fat Monterey Jack cheese (optional)

Instructions: In a large nonstick sauté pan, heat oil over medium-high flame. Add meat and sauté, stirring often, until lightly browned, about 5 minutes. If using protein crumbles, heat until blended with oil, about 2 minutes. Add onions, chili powder, garlic powder, pepper, salsa, and kidney beans. Simmer, stirring occasionally, until onion is wilted and flavors are blended, about 20 minutes. Place in bowl and top with cheese, if desired.

Morningstar Farms makes Burger Style Recipe Crumbles, which look like ground beef and are a good vegetarian source of protein.

Dinner: Shrimp Scampi with Vegetables

Ingredients
   1 teaspoon olive oil
   1 cup asparagus spears, washed, woody bases discarded, and
      bias-sliced into 1-inch-long pieces
   ¾ cup yellow onions, peeled and finely chopped

1 medium green pepper, washed, cored, seeded, and roughly
chopped
2 cloves garlic, peeled and minced, or to taste
4½ ounces shrimp, shelled and deveined
¼ cup dry white wine (optional)
1–2 teaspoons lemon juice, or to taste
2 lemon wedges, optional

For Dessert
1 medium peach

Instructions: In a large nonstick pan, heat oil over medium-high heat. Sauté asparagus, onions, green pepper, and garlic, stirring often until tender, about 10 minutes. Add shrimp, white wine, and lemon juice. Lower heat to medium and cook 5 minutes, stirring often, until shrimp are pink. Place on plate and garnish with lemon wedges. Serve peach for dessert.

Day 6

Breakfast: Spanish Omelet

Ingredients
vegetable spray
2 tablespoons yellow onion, peeled and finely chopped*
2 tablespoons green pepper, cored, seeded, and roughly
chopped*
4 large egg whites (or ½ cup egg substitute)
1 tablespoon low-fat milk (optional)
1 teaspoon chili powder, or to taste (optional)
1 teaspoon olive oil
¼ cup canned black beans, drained
1 ounce low-fat Monterey Jack cheese, shredded
1 tablespoon salsa (optional)

For Dessert
1 medium orange

Instructions: Lightly coat a large nonstick sauté pan with vegetable spray, and heat over medium flame. Add onion and green pepper and sauté, stirring often, until tender, about 10 minutes. Remove and set aside. Meanwhile, beat egg whites with milk, if desired. Stir in chili powder. Heat olive oil in the large nonstick sauté pan over medium heat. Pour in the egg whites and cook until almost set, occasionally lifting edges so that uncooked portion flows underneath, 2 to 3 minutes. When eggs are set, place onions, green pepper, black beans, and cheese on top. Fold with a spatula and continue cooking until lightly browned, about 1 minute. Top with salsa. Serve orange for dessert.

No one wants to chop vegetables first thing in the morning. Buy a bag of frozen onions and green peppers and just pour out what you need. Return the rest to the freezer.

Lunch: Grilled Chicken Salad

Ingredients
1 cup green-leaf or romaine lettuce, washed, dried, and torn into
     large pieces
1 cup broccoli florets
½ green pepper, cored, seeded, and cut into thin strips
1 medium tomato, sliced
1 tablespoon olive oil-and-vinegar dressing*
1 tablespoon lemon juice

Zone oil-and-vinegar dressing contains 1 teaspoon olive oil and 2 teaspoons vinegar. Extra vinegar may be added to taste.
1 teaspoon Worcestershire sauce
½ teaspoon freshly ground pepper, or to taste
3 ounces precooked grilled skinless chicken breast, sliced into
     bite-sized chunks

For Dessert
1 medium pear

Instructions: Toss lettuce with broccoli, green pepper, and tomato. Combine dressing with the lemon juice, Worcestershire sauce, and pepper. Toss with vegetables until well combined, and top with chicken chunks. Serve pear for dessert.

Dinner: Broiled Salmon

Ingredients
    4½ ounces salmon steak, about 1 inch thick
    1 teaspoon olive oil
    ½ teaspoon dried rosemary, or to taste
    ½ teaspoon dried tarragon, or to taste
    ½ teaspoon dried dill, or to taste
    2 cups zucchini, washed, ends removed, and sliced into ¼-inch
        strips

For Dessert
    1 apple

Instructions: Preheat broiler. Brush salmon with oil and sprinkle with herbs. On a roasting pan or aluminum foil, broil for 4–5 minutes per side, depending on thickness, turning once. Meanwhile, steam the zucchini: in a large pot fitted with a steaming basket, bring 1 inch water to boil. Add zucchini to the basket and steam until crisp-tender, 4 to 6 minutes. Serve apple for dessert.

Day 7

Breakfast: Vegetable Omelet

Ingredients
    1 cup asparagus spears, woody bases discarded, bias-sliced into
        1-inch pieces
    1 teaspoon olive oil
    ¼ cup yellow onions, peeled and finely chopped
    ½ cup button mushrooms, washed, dried, and thinly sliced

4 egg whites (or ½ cup egg substitute)
1 tablespoon low-fat milk (optional) vegetable spray
3 strips turkey bacon (substitute 1 ounce lean Canadian bacon
    or 2 soy sausage links)
⅔ cup mandarin oranges

Instructions: In a large pot fitted with a steaming basket, bring 1 inch water to boil. Add asparagus to the basket and steam until crisp-tender, 5 minutes, and set aside. Heat olive oil in a large nonstick sauté pan over medium heat. Add onions and mushrooms and lightly sauté until onion is wilted, about 10 minutes. Remove from pan and set aside to cool. Meanwhile, beat egg whites with milk, if desired. Stir in cooled onions and mushrooms. Lightly coat the sauté pan with vegetable spray, and heat over medium flame. Pour in the egg mixture and cook until almost set, occasionally lifting edges so that uncooked portion flows underneath, 2 to 3 minutes. When eggs are set, top with asparagus tips and fold with a spatula. Continue cooking until lightly browned, about 1 minute. Prepare bacon or soy links, following package instructions, and serve on the side with oranges.

Lunch: Stuffed Tomatoes

Ingredients
3 ounces albacore tuna packed in water, drained
1 tablespoon light mayonnaise
¼ cup celery, washed and minced
1 tablespoon onion, peeled and minced
2 large tomatoes, washed, tops removed, and hulled

For Dessert
1 nectarine

Instructions: In a medium mixing bowl, combine tuna, mayonnaise, celery, and onion. Stuff into tomatoes and serve. Serve nectarine for dessert.

Dinner: Chicken Marinara with Three-Bean Salad*

Ingredients

1½ cups green beans, washed, ends removed, and cut in half
¼ cup canned chickpeas, drained
¼ cup canned kidney beans, drained
1 teaspoon olive oil
2 tablespoons cider vinegar, or to taste
1 teaspoon dried chives
1 teaspoon dried parsley
½ teaspoon freshly ground pepper, or to taste
1½ teaspoons dried basil
2 ounces boneless, skinless chicken breast cutlets
2 tablespoons prepared tomato sauce
¼ teaspoon garlic powder, or to taste
1 ounce low-fat mozzarella cheese, shredded

If possible, make three-bean salad ahead of time (up to 2 days) and store, tightly sealed, in the refrigerator.

Instructions: Preheat oven to 450°. In a large pot fitted with a steaming basket, bring 1 inch water to boil. Add green beans to the basket and steam until crisp-tender, 10 minutes. Remove from basket, drain, and combine with chickpeas and kidney beans. In a small mixing bowl, combine olive oil, vinegar, chives, parsley, pepper, and 1 teaspoon of the basil; experiment with the oil-vinegar ratio to taste. Toss with beans, cover, and refrigerate for 30 minutes. Place chicken in a large piece of foil. Top chicken with tomato sauce and sprinkle with the remaining ½ teaspoon basil, garlic powder, and cheese. Fold foil loosely over chicken, leaving ample space for air. Carefully turn up and seal the ends and the middle so that juices won't leak out. Bake in the preheated oven for 20 minutes. Remove from oven and carefully open foil to prevent steam burns. Serve with bean salad.

TYPICAL MALE
Day 1

Breakfast: Fruit Salad

Ingredients
   1 cup low-fat cottage cheese
   1 cup fresh or reduced-sugar canned pineapple, cubed
   ⅔ cup reduced-sugar canned mandarin oranges, drained
   4 macadamia nuts, crushed

Instructions: Place cottage cheese in a bowl. Fold in pineapple, oranges, and nuts.

Lunch: Chef's Salad

Ingredients
   1 cup green-leaf lettuce (substitute lettuce of your choice),
      washed, dried, and torn into large pieces
   ½ cup canned chickpeas, drained and rinsed
   ½ cup button mushrooms, washed, dried, and coarsely chopped
   ½ cup celery, washed, dried, and coarsely chopped
   4 teaspoons olive oil-and-vinegar dressing*
   3 ounces deli-style turkey breast, cut into strips
   1½ ounces deli-style ham, cut into strips
   1 ounce reduced-fat Swiss cheese (substitute any reduced-fat
      cheese), julienned

For Dessert
   1 medium apple

Instructions: Toss lettuce with chickpeas, mushrooms, and celery. Dress, toss, and add meat and cheese. Serve apple for dessert.

*Zone oil-and-vinegar dressing for this meal contains 1⅓ teaspoons olive oil and 2 teaspoons vinegar. Extra vinegar may be added to taste.

Dinner: Ginger Chicken

Ingredients
1⅓ teaspoons olive oil
4 ounces boneless, skinless chicken breast, cut lengthwise into
    thin strips
2 cups broccoli florets, washed
1½ cups snow peas, washed
¾ cup yellow onion, peeled and chopped
1 teaspoon fresh ginger, grated

For Dessert
1 cup seedless grapes

Instructions: In a wok or large nonstick pan, heat oil over medium-high heat. Add chicken and sauté, turning frequently, until lightly browned, about 5 minutes. Add broccoli, snow peas, onion, ginger, and ¼ cup water. Continue cooking, stirring often, until the chicken is done, water is reduced to a glaze, and vegetables are tender, about 20 minutes. If the pan dries out during cooking, add water in tablespoon increments to keep moist. Serve grapes for dessert.

Day 2

Breakfast: Yogurt and Fruit

Ingredients
1 ounce lean Canadian bacon (substitute 3 turkey bacon strips or
    2 soy sausage links)
½ cup fresh blueberries, rinsed and drained
4 teaspoons slivered almonds
1½ cups plain low-fat yogurt

Instructions: Prepare bacon or soy patties, following package instructions. Stir fruit and nuts into yogurt, and serve with bacon or links on the side.

Lunch: Tuna Salad

Ingredients
4 ounces albacore tuna packed in water, drained
¼ cup celery, washed, dried, and coarsely chopped
4 teaspoons olive oil-and-vinegar dressing*
1 or 2 lettuce leaves, washed and dried
½ cantaloupe, seeds scooped out
¾ cup blueberries, rinsed and drained

Instructions: Mix tuna with celery and stir in dressing. Prepare a bed of the lettuce, and top with tuna mixture. Stuff cantaloupe with berries and serve for dessert.

Zone oil-and-vinegar dressing for this meal contains 1⅓ teaspoons olive oil and 2 teaspoons vinegar. Extra vinegar may be added to taste.

Dinner: Foiled Flounder with Green Beans

Ingredients
vegetable spray
6 ounces boneless flounder fillet (substitute mild, flaky fish of
    your choice)
2 tablespoons yellow onion, peeled and chopped
sprinkling of Parmesan cheese
¼ teaspoon freshly ground pepper, or to taste
squirt lemon juice
3 cups fresh green beans, washed, ends removed, and halved
4 teaspoons almonds, slivered

For Dessert
pineapple

Instructions: Preheat oven to 425°. Tear off an 18-inch-by-12-inch piece of foil. Spray the center lightly with vegetable spray, and place fish in the center of the foil. Top with onion and sprinkle with cheese, pepper, and lemon juice. Fold foil loosely over fish, leaving ample space for air. Carefully turn up and seal the ends and the middle so that juices won't leak out. Bake in the preheated oven 18 minutes. Meanwhile, steam the green beans: in a large pot fitted with a steaming basket, bring 1 inch water to boil. Add beans to the basket and steam until crisp-tender, 10 minutes. Drain, place in serving bowl, and fold in almonds. When fish is done, carefully open foil to prevent steam burns, and remove to a plate. Serve with green beans. Serve pineapple for dessert.

Day 3

Breakfast: Fruit Smoothie

Ingredients
27 grams protein powder
1¼ cup blueberries
1½ cup strawberries
4 macadamia nuts
6 ice cubes

Instructions: Place all ingredients in a blender and blend at high speed until smooth, about 1 minute. Add a little water if smoothie is too thick. If you prefer, eat the nuts on the side.

Lunch: Cheeseburger

Ingredients
4½ ounces lean (less than 10%) ground beef (substitute 4½ ounces ground turkey or 1½ soy burger patties)
1 ounce reduced-fat American cheese (substitute cheese of choice)
1 tablespoon light mayonnaise
½ hamburger roll
1 thick tomato slice, optional
1 large lettuce leaf, optional
1 dill pickle wedge, optional
3 black olives

For Dessert
1 cup unsweetened applesauce
sprinkling of cinnamon

Instructions: Preheat broiler. Place burger on foil or rack and broil 5 minutes. Flip and continue cooking another 5 minutes for medium rare. One minute before expected doneness, top with cheese, and remove when melted. Spread mayonnaise on the roll. Top with burger, tomato, and lettuce. Serve pickle on the side. Either chop olives and place on top of cheeseburger or serve them on the side. Sprinkle applesauce with cinnamon and serve for dessert.

Dinner: Vegetarian Stir-fry

Ingredients
1⅓ teaspoons olive oil
1 cup vegetable protein crumbles* (substitute 6 ounces firm tofu)
1½ cups yellow onions, peeled chopped
2 cups broccoli florets, washed
2 cups button mushrooms, washed, dried, and thinly sliced
1 ounce reduced-fat Swiss cheese, shredded

Morningstar Farms makes Burger Style Recipe Crumbles, which looks like ground beef and is a good vegetarian source of protein.

For Dessert
1 cup grapes

Instructions: Heat oil in a nonstick sauté pan or wok over medium-high heat. If using tofu, remove from wrapping, drain, and crumble. Add tofu or soy crumbles and stir until mixed with the oil. Add onions, broccoli, and mushrooms. Reduce heat to medium and stir-fry, stirring often, until vegetables are tender, about 15 minutes. Stir in cheese and heat until melted, about 1 minute. Serve grapes for dessert.

Day 4

Breakfast: Scrambled Eggs and Bacon

Ingredients
vegetable spray
6 egg whites (or ¾ cup egg substitute)
1⅓ teaspoons olive oil
1 tablespoon low-fat milk (optional)
1 ounce lean Canadian bacon (substitute 3 turkey bacon strips
    or 2 soy sausage links)

For Dessert
1 cup grapes
⅔ cup mandarin oranges

Instructions: Lightly coat a large nonstick pan with vegetable spray, and heat over medium flame. Beat egg whites with olive oil and milk, if desired. Pour into pan and cook, stirring often, until scrambled and fully set. Prepare bacon or soy links, following package instructions. Mix grapes and oranges and serve for dessert.

Lunch: Tofu Dip and Veggies

Ingredients
6 ounces firm tofu
1 ounce reduced-fat Swiss cheese, grated
½ cup canned chickpeas, drained and rinsed
1⅓ teaspoons olive oil
2 tablespoons fresh lemon juice
2 tablespoons Lipton dry onion soup mix (substitute spices of
    your choice, to taste*)
1 medium green pepper, washed, cored, seeded, and cut in
    wedges
2 cups broccoli florets

For Dessert
    1 kiwi

Instructions: Drain tofu. Put tofu, cheese, chickpeas, olive oil, lemon juice, and onion soup mix in a blender. Blend until smooth. (For best flavor, refrigerate the dip at least 2 hours or overnight.) Place dip in a bowl in the center of a large plate. Arrange pepper strips and broccoli around bowl for dipping. Serve kiwi for dessert.

*If you don't want to use the packaged soup mix, experiment with minced onions, garlic, or vegetable bouillon granules.

Dinner: Spiced Lamb with Vegetables

Ingredients
    6 ounces lean ground lamb
    ⅓ cup brown rice
    1 teaspoon cider vinegar
    1⅓ teaspoons olive oil
    ½ cup scallions, finely chopped
    ¾ cup red onions, chunks
    2 cups mushrooms
    1½ cups tomatoes, diced
    ½ cup green beans, diced
    1 tablespoon cilantro
    2 teaspoons fresh ginger, minced
    ¼ teaspoon cumin
    ¼ teaspoon coriander
    ⅛ teaspoon black pepper
    ½ teaspoon celery salt
    ⅛ teaspoon cinnamon

Instructions: In a small glass bowl, combine lamb, rice, vinegar, and spices. Cover and refrigerate for 30 minutes. Heat the oil in a medium nonstick sauté pan. Add meat mixture and vegetables. Cook, breaking meat up as it cooks, until lamb is cooked through and vegetables are tender. Spoon onto plate and serve.

Day 5

Breakfast: Old-Fashioned Oatmeal

Ingredients
    1 cup slow-cooking (steel-cut) oatmeal*
    2 ounces lean Canadian bacon (substitute 6 turkey bacon strips
        or 1 soy sausage patty)
    ⅓ cup unsweetened applesauce
    1 tablespoon almonds, slivered
    sprinkling of nutmeg
    sprinkling of cinnamon
    ½ cup low-fat cottage cheese

Instructions: Bring 3 cups water to a brisk boil over high heat. Add oatmeal, stirring well. When smooth and beginning to thicken, reduce heat to low and simmer for 30 minutes, stirring occasionally. While oatmeal is cooking, prepare bacon or soy patties, following package instructions. Remove oatmeal from the heat. Stir in applesauce and almonds. Sprinkle with cinnamon and nutmeg. Serve bacon and cottage cheese on the side.

By slow cooking, we mean slow cooking. Oatmeal that calls itself slow-cooking but takes only 5 minutes isn't the real McCoy (or perhaps we should say the real McCann's, a popular brand). To shorten the morning cooking time, make a big batch during the weekend, freeze, and microwave the correct amount in the morning. You may also put the oatmeal in a wide-mouth thermos with 1⅓ cups boiling water, and let it cook overnight.

Lunch: Chili (Meat or Vegetarian)

Ingredients
    1⅓ teaspoons olive oil
    6 ounces lean (less than 10%) ground beef (substitute ground
        turkey or 1⅓ cups vegetable protein crumbles*)
    ¼ cup yellow onions, peeled and minced

1 teaspoon chili powder, or to taste

½ teaspoon garlic powder, or to taste

½ teaspoon freshly ground pepper, or to taste

1½ cups salsa or stewed tomatoes with liquid

¼ cup kidney beans, drained and rinsed sprinkling of low-fat
Monterey Jack cheese (optional)

Instructions: In a large nonstick sauté pan, heat oil over medium-high flame. Add meat and sauté, stirring often, until lightly browned, about 5 minutes. If using protein crumbles, heat until blended with oil, about 2 minutes. Add onions, chili powder, garlic powder, pepper, salsa, and kidney beans. Simmer, stirring occasionally, until onion is wilted and flavors are blended, about 20 minutes. Place in bowl and top with cheese, if desired.

*Morningstar Farms makes Burger Style Recipe Crumbles, which looks like ground beef and is a good vegetarian source of protein.

Dinner: Shrimp Scampi with Vegetables

Ingredients

1⅓ teaspoons olive oil

1½ cups asparagus spears, washed, woody bases discarded, and
bias-sliced into 1-inch-long pieces

1½ cups yellow onions, peeled and finely chopped

1 medium green pepper, washed, cored, seeded, and roughly
chopped

2 cloves garlic, peeled and minced, or to taste

6 ounces shrimp, shelled and deveined

¼ cup dry white wine (optional)

1–2 teaspoons lemon juice, or to taste

2 lemon wedges, optional

For Dessert

1 medium peach

Instructions: In a large nonstick pan, heat oil over medium-high heat. Sauté asparagus, onions, green pepper, and garlic, stirring often, until tender, about 10 minutes. Add shrimp, white wine, and lemon juice. Lower heat to medium and cook 5 minutes, stirring often, until shrimp are pink. Place on plate and garnish with lemon wedges. Serve peach for dessert.

Day 6

Breakfast: Spanish Omelet

Ingredients
vegetable spray
2 tablespoons yellow onion, peeled and finely chopped*
2 tablespoons green pepper, cored, seeded, and roughly
     chopped*
6 large egg whites (or ¾ cup egg substitute)
1 tablespoon low-fat milk (optional)
1 teaspoon chili powder, or to taste (optional)
1⅓ teaspoons olive oil
½ cup canned black beans, drained
1 ounce low-fat Monterey Jack cheese, shredded
1 tablespoon salsa (optional)

For Dessert
1 medium orange

Instructions: Lightly coat a large nonstick sauté pan with vegetable spray, and heat over medium flame. Add onion and green pepper and sauté, stirring often, until tender, about 10 minutes. Remove and set aside. Meanwhile, beat egg whites with milk, if desired. Stir in chili powder. Heat olive oil in the large nonstick sauté pan over medium heat. Pour in the egg whites and cook until almost set, occasionally lifting edges so that uncooked portion flows underneath, 2 to 3 minutes. When eggs are set, place onions, green pepper, black beans, and cheese on top. Fold with a spatula and continue cooking until lightly browned, about 1 minute. Top with salsa. Serve orange for dessert.

No one wants to chop vegetables first thing in the morning. Buy a bag of frozen onions and green peppers and just pour out what you need. Return the rest to the freezer.

Lunch: Grilled Chicken Salad

Ingredients
   2 cups green-leaf or romaine lettuce, washed, dried, and torn
      into large pieces
   1 cup broccoli florets
   ½ green pepper, cored, seeded, and cut into thin strips
   ¼ cup canned kidney beans, rinsed and drained
   1 medium tomato, sliced
   4 teaspoons olive oil-and-vinegar dressing*
   1 tablespoon lemon juice
   1 teaspoon Worcestershire sauce

*Zone oil-and-vinegar dressing for this meal contains 1⅓ teaspoons olive oil and 2 teaspoons vinegar. Extra vinegar may be added to taste.
   ½ teaspoon freshly ground pepper, or to taste
   4 ounces precooked grilled skinless chicken breast, sliced into
      bite-sized chunks

For Dessert
   1 medium pear

Instructions: Toss lettuce with broccoli, green pepper, kidney beans, and tomato. Combine dressing with the lemon juice, Worcestershire sauce, and pepper. Toss with vegetables until well combined, and top with chicken chunks. Serve pear for dessert.

Dinner: Broiled Salmon

Ingredients
   6 ounces salmon steak, about 1 inch thick
   1⅓ teaspoons olive oil
   ½ teaspoon dried rosemary, or to taste
   ½ teaspoon dried tarragon, or to taste

½ teaspoon dried dill, or to taste

2 cups zucchini, washed, ends removed, and sliced into ¼-inch
  strips

For Dessert
  1 apple
  1 plum

Instructions: Preheat broiler. Brush salmon with olive oil and sprinkle with herbs. On a roasting pan or aluminum foil, broil for 4–5 minutes per side, depending on thickness, turning once. Meanwhile, steam the zucchini: in a large pot fitted with a steaming basket, bring 1 inch water to boil. Add zucchini to the basket and steam until crisp-tender, 4 to 6 minutes. Serve apple and plum for dessert.

Day 7

Breakfast: Vegetable Omelet

Ingredients
  1 cup asparagus spears, woody bases discarded, bias-sliced into
    1-inch pieces
  1⅓ teaspoons olive oil
  ¼ cup yellow onions, peeled and finely chopped
  ½ cup button mushrooms, washed, dried, and thinly sliced
  6 egg whites (or ¾ cup egg substitute)
  1 tablespoon low-fat milk (optional)
  vegetable spray
  3 strips turkey bacon (substitute 1 ounce lean Canadian bacon
    or 2 soy sausage links)
  1 cup mandarin oranges

Instructions: In a large pot fitted with a steaming basket, bring 1 inch water to boil. Add asparagus to the basket and steam until crisp-tender, 5 minutes, and set aside. Heat olive oil in a large non-stick sauté pan over medium heat. Add onions and mushrooms and lightly sauté until onion is wilted, about 10 minutes. Remove from pan and set aside to cool. Meanwhile, beat egg whites with milk, if desired. Stir in cooled onions and mushrooms. Lightly coat the sauté pan with vegetable spray, and heat over medium flame. Pour in the egg mixture and cook until almost set, occasionally lifting edges so that uncooked portion flows underneath, 2 to 3 minutes. When eggs are set, top with asparagus tips and fold with a spatula. Continue cooking until lightly browned, about 1 minute. Prepare bacon or soy links, following package instructions, and serve on the side with oranges.

Lunch: Stuffed Tomatoes

Ingredients
    4 ounces albacore tuna packed in water, drained
    4 teaspoons light mayonnaise
    ¼ cup celery, washed and minced
    1 tablespoon onion, peeled and minced
    2 large tomatoes, washed, tops removed, and hulled
    1 small bread stick

For Dessert
    1 nectarine

Instructions: In a medium mixing bowl, combine tuna, mayonnaise, celery, and onion. Stuff into tomatoes and serve. Serve bread stick on the side. Serve nectarine for dessert.

Dinner: Chicken Marinara with Three-Bean Salad*

Ingredients
    1½ cups green beans, washed, ends removed, and cut in half
    ¼ cup canned chickpeas, drained
    ¼ cup canned kidney beans, drained
    1⅓ teaspoons olive oil

If possible, make the three-bean salad ahead of time (up to 2 days) and store, tightly sealed, in refrigerator.

2 tablespoons cider vinegar, or to taste
1 teaspoon dried chives
1 teaspoon dried parsley
½ teaspoon freshly ground pepper, or to taste
1½ teaspoons dried basil
3 ounces boneless, skinless chicken breast cutlets
2 tablespoons prepared tomato sauce
¼ teaspoon garlic powder, or to taste
1 ounce low-fat mozzarella cheese, shredded

For Dessert
1 peach

Instructions: Preheat oven to 450°. In a large pot fitted with a steaming basket, bring 1 inch water to boil. Add green beans to the basket and steam until crisp-tender, 10 minutes. Remove from basket, drain, and combine with chickpeas and kidney beans. In a small mixing bowl, combine olive oil, vinegar, chives, parsley, pepper, and 1 teaspoon of the basil; experiment with the oil-vinegar ratio to taste. Toss with beans, cover, and refrigerate for 30 minutes. Place chicken in a large piece of foil. Top chicken with tomato sauce and sprinkle with the remaining ½ teaspoon basil, garlic powder, and cheese. Fold foil loosely over chicken, leaving ample space for air. Carefully turn up and seal the ends and the middle so that juices won't leak out. Bake in the preheated oven for 20 minutes. Remove from oven and carefully open foil to prevent steam burns. Serve with bean salad. Serve peach for dessert.

6

MORE QUICK AND EASY ZONE BREAKFASTS, LUNCHES, DINNERS, AND SNACKS

Once you have spent a week in the Zone enjoying the meals provided in Chapter 5, I'm confident that you'll want to continue improving your health and appearance by eating more Zone meals. However, I also realize that finding the time to prepare healthy, appetizing meals can be something of a challenge. Therefore, all the recipes in this chapter are not only guaranteed to keep up in the Zone, they are also designed to minimize your time and effort in the kitchen. By combining these meals with those already offered in Chapter 5, you'll have a great set of breakfasts, lunches, dinners, and snacks to choose from every day.

Whereas all of the recipes in Chapter 5 were broken down into recipes for men and recipes for women, in this section, all of the recipes are calculated to fit into the male requirements. Does this mean you can't eat the recipes if you're a woman? Of course not— simply prepare the recipe as directed, then set aside ¼ of the finished dish, and save it as a snack for later. Better yet, simply reduce the recipe by ¼ before cooking. This may seem complicated, but remember that the Zone does not need to be an exact science. Take away a bit of the protein, carbohydrates, and fat, and you'll have a meal that fits perfectly into your unique eating plan.

All recipes make one serving.

BREAKFASTS

Blueberry Pancakes

Ingredients
  1 whole egg
  1⅓ cups soy flour*
  1 cup 1% milk
  ½ teaspoon vanilla
  ½ teaspoon cinnamon
  ½ cup blueberries
  1⅓ teaspoons olive oil

Instructions: In a small mixing bowl, combine eggs, soy flour, milk, ⅔ teaspoon olive oil, vanilla, cinnamon, and blueberries to form a thin batter. Heat ⅔ teaspoon oil in a nonstick sauté pan. Pour batter into pan to make small (2-inch) pancakes. Batter will make about 24 silver-dollar-sized pancakes. The pancakes will cook to a golden brown and will resemble buckwheat pancakes in color and flavor. As pancakes are cooked, place on two serving plates and keep warm. Repeat process until all batter is used.

*Available in some health food stores.

French Toast Sticks

Ingredients
  1 slice whole-grain bread
  4 large egg whites or ½ cup egg substitute
  vegetable spray
  confectioners' sugar
  1 cup strawberries, sliced
  1 tablespoon slivered almonds
  1 ounce extra-lean Canadian bacon or 3 slices turkey bacon

Instructions: Cut bread into sticks and soak in beaten eggs. (Scramble any egg mixture that remains.) Spray a nonstick pan with vegetable spray. Over medium-low heat, cook bread sticks, turning often until done. Roll cooked bread sticks in a little bit of confectioners' sugar. Top with sliced strawberries and slivered almonds. Cook bacon and serve on the side.

Huevos Rancheros

Ingredients
    1⅓ teaspoons olive oil
    1 whole egg
    2 egg whites
    chopped onion, green pepper, and tomato
    chili powder to taste
    1 corn tortilla
    2 ounces low-fat cheese
    1 tablespoon chopped cilantro

Side Dish
    1 cup honeydew melon, cubed

Instructions: Heat oil in skillet. Scramble egg, egg whites, chopped vegetables, and chili powder. Place scrambled eggs in tortilla and top with cheese and cilantro. Roll up tortilla.

Oatmeal

1 cup cooked oatmeal fortified with 2 tablespoons (1 ounce) protein powder (always add the protein powder after cooking the oatmeal).

Bagel and Lox

1 small plain bagel, 3 ounces lox or smoked salmon, and 3 tablespoons of light cream cheese.

LUNCHES

Turkey or Tuna Sandwich

4 ounces turkey breast or tuna with 1 teaspoon mayonnaise and 2 pieces of whole-rye bread.

Seafood Salad

Ingredients
4½ ounces seafood (shrimp, crab meat, lobster)
1 teaspoon light mayonnaise
1 mini-pita pocket or 1 piece rye bread*

For Dessert
½ orange

Instructions: Mix seafood and mayonnaise. Stuff in mini-pita pocket.

*You may eliminate the bread and place the seafood on top of a tossed salad. If you use the mayonnaise with the seafood, don't use salad dressing. Or substitute 1 tablespoon olive oil and vinegar dressing and hold the mayonnaise.

Tomato-Basil Salad

Ingredients
5 cups romaine lettuce, chopped
¼ cup chickpeas, rinsed and finely chopped
1 tablespoon fresh parsley, chopped
1⅓ teaspoons olive oil
1 tablespoon red wine vinegar
2 tablespoons fresh basil, chopped
1 teaspoon garlic, minced

¼ teaspoon chili powder

2 cups tomatoes, sliced

4 ounces skim-milk mozzarella cheese, shredded

For Dessert

1 apple or pear

½ cup strawberries

Instructions: Place lettuce on a serving plate. In a medium bowl, combine chickpeas, parsley, oil, vinegar, basil, garlic, and chili powder. Alternate slices of tomato and shredded mozzarella on the lettuce bed. Pour chickpea dressing over tomatoes and serve. Eat fruit for dessert.

BLT Sandwich

Ingredients

1 slice rye bread

2 ounces lean Canadian bacon

3 leaves lettuce

2 tomato slices

1 ounce low-fat cheese

1 teaspoon light mayonnaise

Side Dishes

½ orange

12 peanuts

Picnic-style Cold Tempeh Salad

Ingredients

4 ounces tempeh, cubed

1 tablespoon tamari sauce

1½ tablespoons mayonnaise

¼ cup plain yogurt

juice of ½ lemon
2 teaspoons prepared mustard
3 medium celery stalks
1 medium green pepper, diced
3 hard-boiled egg whites
1 slice red onion, diced
3 black olives, sliced
1 sprig fresh dill or parsley, minced

Instructions: Preheat oven to 350°. Toss tempeh with tamari sauce in baking dish and bake uncovered for 10 to 12 minutes. Set aside to cool. Mix mayonnaise, yogurt, lemon juice, and mustard. Add celery, green pepper, egg whites, and red onion. Fold in tempeh cubes and sprinkle with olives and herbs. Chill and serve on a bed of lettuce, if desired.

DINNERS

Grilled Sole with Leeks

Ingredients
1⅓ teaspoons olive oil
3 cups sliced leeks
6 ounces fillet of sole
4 ounces white wine (optional)
1 teaspoon minced garlic
1 shallot, minced
1 teaspoon dill salt to taste
pepper to taste
½ teaspoon lemon herb seasoning

Instructions: Preheat oven to 375°. Brush a medium baking dish with the olive oil. Layer bottom of dish with leeks. Place sole on top. In a medium bowl, combine wine, garlic, shallots, dill, salt, and pepper. Gently pour wine mixture into baking dish. Sprinkle with lemon herb seasoning. Tightly cover baking dish and place in oven. Bake for 25 to 30 minutes and serve.

Pork Medallions and Apples

Ingredients
3 ounces pork medallions or thinly sliced pork chops
½ apple
rosemary to taste
Dijon mustard to taste
1 to 2 tablespoons white wine (optional)
¼ cup water

Side Dishes
1 cup cooked broccoli
1 spinach salad with dressing (1 tablespoon olive oil and vine-
    gar to taste)

Instructions: Preheat oven to 450°. Place pork in a baking dish in a single layer. Top with apple slices, rosemary, and mustard. Pour wine and water around the pork. Bake for 15 minutes. Baste pork with pan juices. Reduce heat to 350° and continue cooking for 10 to 15 minutes, until pork is white, not pink, inside.

Chicken Fajitas

Ingredients
4 ounces boneless chicken breast
2 tablespoons salsa
2 tablespoons bottled lime juice
salt to taste
freshly ground black pepper to taste
¼ cup water or more
⅓ green pepper, cut into quarters, seeds and membrane
    removed
⅓ red pepper, cut into quarters, seeds and membrane removed
⅓ yellow onion, sliced into ¼-inch-wide rings, and microwaved
    on high for 2 minutes, stirring after 1 minute
1 fajita-size (8") tortilla

Condiments

½ cup chopped tomato

1⅓ tablespoons guacamole

For Dessert

½ cup strawberries

Instructions: Slice chicken breasts crosswise into ½-inch strips. Place in a glass dish with salsa, lime juice, salt, and pepper and enough water to cover. Cover with plastic wrap and refrigerate overnight. Into a large skillet, over high heat, pour in the liquid from the chicken and cook to reduce by half. Add the chicken strips and, using a wide wooden spatula, toss frequently. When chicken turns opaque but is not yet thoroughly cooked, add the peppers and onion. Continue cooking and tossing the mixture. Cook until the liquid has evaporated and it begins to sizzle. Give one more toss and remove from heat. Serve with tortilla and condiments.

Cioppino

Ingredients

1⅓ teaspoons olive oil

¾ cup chopped onion

1 cup chopped green pepper

1½ cups chopped canned tomatoes

4 cups chopped mushrooms

1 teaspoon minced garlic

1 tablespoon parsley, chopped

¼ teaspoon dried oregano

¼ teaspoon dried basil

⅛ teaspoon cayenne pepper

salt to taste

pepper to taste

½ cup lemon- and lime-flavored water

4 ounces dry red wine (optional)

1½ ounces cherrystone clams

1½ ounces sole
1½ ounces small shrimp, shelled and deveined
1½ ounces baby bay scallops

Instructions: In a medium saucepan, combine oil, vegetables, spices, water, and wine. Bring to a boil, reduce heat, and bring to a simmer. Add seafood, cover, and simmer for 5 to 7 minutes. Spoon into a bowl and serve.

Tofu-Vegetable Kebabs with Yogurt Olive Dip

Ingredients
¼ cup plain low-fat yogurt
3 black olives, sliced
2 teaspoons prepared mustard
1 teaspoon honey
½ teaspoon light miso
1 sprig fresh parsley, minced
2 medium zucchini, cubed
1 large onion, cut into small chunks
7 ounces extra-firm tofu, cubed
12 whole mushrooms
6 cherry tomatoes
1 teaspoon olive oil
salt to taste
pepper to taste

Instructions: Mix yogurt, olives, mustard, honey, miso, and parsley. Set aside. Blanch zucchini and onion in boiling water for two minutes, then drain. Onion may separate, which is to be expected. Alternate tofu, zucchini, onion, mushrooms, and cherry tomatoes on skewers, always ending with a mushroom. Brush with olive oil and salt and pepper lightly. Place under broiler or on outdoor grill. Turn after 5 minutes and grill another 5 minutes. Serve with yogurt-olive dip.

Snacks

- 2 hard-boiled egg whites, cut in half and stuffed with ¼ cup hummus
- 1 ounce low-fat string cheese
- ½ cup grapes
- 3 olives
- 1½ ounces deli-style turkey
- ½ apple
- 3 peanuts
- ¼ cup low-fat cottage cheese
- ½ cup pineapple
- 1 teaspoon slivered almonds
- 1 ounce cheese
- 4 ounces wine
- 1 cup 1% milk
- 3 macadamia nuts
- 1 Wasa cracker
- 1 ounce low-fat cheese
- 3 sliced olives (zap for 10 seconds in the microwave)
- 2 ounces firm tofu
- ⅓ teaspoon olive oil
- sprinkling of Lipton dry onion soup mix
- ⅛ cup chickpeas (blend until smooth)
- 1 sliced green pepper for dipping

Frozen Meals

The following frozen meals can fit into the Zone, but sometimes need a little tinkering. Therefore, read the food labels carefully.

Stouffer's Lean Cuisine
Beef Peppercorn
Grilled Chicken
Chicken and Vegetables

Healthy Choice
Grilled Chicken Sonoma (sprinkle a little Parmesan cheese on top)

Grilled Peppercorn Beef Patty
Garlic Chicken Milano (sprinkle a little Parmesan cheese on top)
Turkey Breast Medallions (add 2 teaspoons slivered almonds
   and have ¼ cup grapes for dessert)

Marie Callender
Grilled Turkey Breast Strips
Swedish Meatballs (a little high in fat)

Weight Watchers (these meals need quite a bit of work to get them into the Zone)
Fiesta Chicken (add 2 teaspoons slivered almonds and either 1
   ounce low-fat cheese or 1 additional ounce of chicken)
Creamy Rigatoni with Broccoli Chicken (add 2 ounces chicken
   and 9 sliced olives)

7

DINING OUT IN THE ZONE

Americans are eating out like never before. At least 50 percent of all meals are now eaten outside the home. Once you master preparing Zone meals at home, transferring that knowledge to the outside world is very easy.

What is the easiest (but the most expensive) way of dining out in the Zone? Go to a very expensive French restaurant. For around fifty dollars, you'll get a glass of great wine and a small amount of protein (no bigger and no thicker than the palm of your hand) surrounded by an artistically arranged outer ring of vegetables with a small side salad to cleanse the palate. And for dessert you'll have some fresh fruit. But the key to gourmet French cooking is the sauce, which is composed of fat. This is why most nutritionists hate the French: they eat too much fat, they smoke, they drink, and they don't exercise. But their biggest complaint about the French is that they seem to enjoy themselves. On the other hand, it's difficult to ignore the fact that the French have the lowest rate of heart disease in Europe, and they look good in designer clothing.

No one has ever accused the French of not eating well, but you now realize that a gourmet French meal is really a Zone meal. A gourmet French meal contains adequate (but not excessive) amounts of protein, lots of low-density vegetables, a little fruit for dessert, and a glass of wine (which the body treats like a carbohydrate) to balance off the protein. A little fat in the sauce not only adds to the taste, but also slows down the rate of entry of carbohydrates into the bloodstream.

Okay, eating at four-star French restaurants is a pretty expensive way to eat out in the Zone, since you could have had five meals at the all-you-can-eat pasta palace for the same price. But how do you stay in the Zone when you're going out to a typical restaurant, where a satisfied customer is one who has to unbuckle his belt after the meal? Here are some simple rules to follow at any restaurant, four-star or family-style.

Rule #1. Never eat the rolls. If you're going to eat carbohydrates, save it for dessert. Isn't that the reason you went to restaurant in the first place? More about this later.

Rule #2. Always choose your low-fat protein entree from the menu first, before you order anything else. This sets the stage for ordering the rest of your meal. Then ask the waiter to replace any starches or grains with extra vegetables.

Rule #3. While you're waiting for dinner, have a glass of red wine or a glass of bottled water while everyone else is munching on their rolls. Try conversation instead of eating to pass the time.

Rule #4. Once the dinner is served, look at the size of the low-fat protein entree you ordered. If it is significantly greater in size than the palm of your hand, plan to take the excess home (it sure beats eating cottage cheese the next day). Then look at your plate and determine whether the carbohydrates are favorable or unfavorable.

Rule #5. The volume of the low-fat protein you plan to eat determines the volume of the carbohydrate you are going to eat. If you're eating favorable carbohydrates, then plan to have double the volume of carbohydrates compared to the protein portion.

Rule #6. If you really came to the restaurant to eat dessert, then don't eat any carbohydrates at the meal. The waiter will still take your plate away. When he or she comes back with a dessert menu, order whatever you want, but plan to only eat half. The rest of the dessert? Offer it to your dinner companions. I'm sure they will be delighted to help out. Of course, if you want to eat a full dessert, have fresh fruit just like the French do.

Now that wasn't too difficult. This is very easy to do in the four-star French restaurant, where there isn't very much food to begin with, but much more difficult to undertake at the typical restaurant, where massive volumes of food are pushed in your direction. And this is what has happened to American restaurants in the last generation. Because we have the cheapest food on earth, people expect to get their money's worth by consuming massive amounts of calories. Everything is oversized. The only exceptions are the exclusive (and expensive) restaurants, where presentation and quality count far more than sheer bulk. And since mass is in, you make your money as a restaurant owner by making sure most of the food volume comes in the form of carbohydrates (which are cheap) as opposed to protein (which is relatively expensive).

THE FAST FOOD ZONE

It's just as easy to make hormonally correct meals in fast food restaurants, if you remember the Zone rules. Let's take McDonald's, for example. Here's a very quick meal. Buy the grilled McChicken sandwich and a salad. Throw away three-quarters of the bun, add the grilled chicken and one-quarter of the bun to the salad, and presto, you have a grilled chicken salad with a large crouton. It's quick, it's easy, and it's hormonally correct if you know the rules. Fast food restaurants can be a great help for those times when you don't have the time to cook or sit at a restaurant because they always have protein (unfortunately, much of it is high-fat hamburgers, so always try to choose the chicken entrees). The secret of fast food in the Zone is knowing when to stop adding carbohydrates. Some of the Zone meals that can be found in fast food restaurants are shown below.

Fast Food Zone Meals

Wendy's
  12 oz. of chili

McDonald's
  Grilled McChicken Sandwich (throw away ¼ of the bun)

Burger King
  BK Broiler without mayo (throw away ¼ of the bun)

Taco Bell

Chicken tacos

However, the best fast food meals can be found in your super-market at the salad bar. Simply grab a bunch of precut vegetables and fruits (especially the things you would never buy otherwise), and put them in the tin plate they provide, along with some olives (your monounsaturated fat). Then walk over to the deli and buy a quarter-pound of low-fat protein, such as turkey, chicken, or tuna. Add the low-fat protein to your precut vegetables, fruits, and olives, and you've got a great Zone meal. It may be a little expensive compared to a bagel and a cup of coffee, but isn't your health worth it?

ZONE MEALS FOR THE BUSINESS TRAVELER

How do you stay in the Zone if you are constantly on the road? Here are some easy tricks. If you are staying for a couple of days at a hotel that has a room refrigerator, then go out and buy some fruit and sliced low-fat deli meat or low-fat cottage cheese. For every piece of fruit, plan to eat 1 ounce of low-fat meat or 2 ounces of cottage cheese. These can be quick snacks before you go out to eat (thereby making it easier to stay in the Zone at the restaurant) for the times you can't prepare your own food. And before you go to bed, have a quick Zone snack as a hormonal "touch-up" so that you get a good night's sleep in a strange bed.

Keep in mind that Zone meals are your key to business success on the road, because they will determine your mental alertness throughout the day. Listed in the table below are some of the Zone winners that will give you an unfair advantage over your competitors. And, of course, never eat the rolls. Life is tough enough on the road without wandering out of the Zone.

Zone Meals for the Business Traveler

Breakfast

6-egg-white omelet plus oatmeal (don't eat the toast or the potatoes)

Breakfast buffet with scrambled eggs and fruit or scrambled
eggs and oatmeal (but choose only one)

Lunch

Grilled chicken Caesar salad with extra side of vegetables and
fresh fruit for dessert

Dinner

Fish with extra vegetables and no starches (that also means no
rolls) and fresh fruit for dessert

Holidays

During the Christmas season, the average American gains 5 to
10 pounds. Not so in the Zone. In fact, the typical holiday buffet
gives you an excellent opportunity to make great Zone meals. When
you are going through the buffet, always look for the low-fat protein first, and then just follow the eye and palm method outlined
earlier. Make sure that most of your carbohydrates come from vegetables and fruits, and try the best you can to ignore the grains,
breads, rolls, bagels, and pasta that usually characterize holiday
entertaining.

Holidays also usually mean alcohol consumption. Since the
body treats alcohol like a carbohydrate, always plan to have a protein chaser with every drink. An example might be a glass of wine
with a piece of soft cheese, or a bottle of beer with six cocktail
shrimp. Just make sure that you eat all the necessary protein before
your next drink. Again, it's a matter of balance.

In summary, eating out in the Zone is easy, if you know the
rules. "Just say no" to the overwhelming incoming tide of carbohydrates you're constantly exposed to when eating out. If you think
it's difficult, then think of carbohydrates as a drug. The more you
take of any drug, the more likely you are to suffer from a drug overdose. In this case, it's an excess production of insulin, which can
cause your premature death. That thought should make it easier to
pass on the rolls.

8

THE SOY ZONE

A very common confusion about the Zone is that you must eat animal protein to follow the program. Nothing could be further from the truth. To stay in the Zone only requires that you consume adequate protein. For vegans, the vegetarian version of the Zone uses vegetable sources of protein, primarily soy. Lacto-ovo vegetarians have an even greater protein variety because they can use low-fat egg products (such as egg whites) and low-fat dairy sources (cheeses, milk, and yogurt) in addition to soy products. However, as I describe in greater detail in my book *The Soy Zone*, the most powerful version of Zone that has the greatest potential health benefits uses primarily soy protein. Soy is an amazing food that everyone, whether a vegetarian or die-hard meat lover, should incorporate into their diet.

SOY: THE WONDER PROTEIN

Soybeans are unique because they are the only beans that contain slightly more protein than carbohydrate, and they contain certain phytochemicals known as isoflavones that have remarkable health benefits.

For a thousand years, the most widely available protein-rich source of soy protein was tofu. Many Americans are a bit wary of tofu, but it is actually an incredibly versatile food that easily absorbs flavor and can be used in a huge array of dishes. Now, with new technology, a great variety of soy meat substitutes that look and taste like meat products (hamburgers, sausages, and hot dogs) are also available. As a result, Americans are likely to begin making more soy-based meals.

The scientific data on the benefits of increased soy protein consumption is continually expanding. In fact, the FDA has recently allowed food manufacturers to make health claims about soy products and heart disease. Some of the benefits of increased soy consumption are listed below.

Health Benefits of Soy

Decreased cholesterol
Decreased heart disease
Decreased breast cancer
Decreased prostate cancer
Decreased osteoporosis
Decreased symptoms of menopause

Admittedly, many of these benefits come from epidemiological studies, which study large populations of people who eat soy, and then compare them to the similar populations that eat very little soy. But clinical studies do indicate one very unique distinguishing characteristic of soy protein: it lowers insulin and increases glucagon to a greater extent than does the same amount of animal protein. Since the goal of the Zone is to maintain insulin within a zone, the increased use of soy protein in your Zone meals, even if you're not a vegetarian, can be a very powerful tool for achieving that goal.

This unique hormonal property of improved insulin control, described in greater detail in *The Soy Zone*, accounts for many of the health benefits of soy protein. In addition, the isoflavones found in soy products also have the ability to alter the hormonal action of insulin. All in all, this makes soy protein one of the most beneficial foods you can eat in the Zone.

THE LONGEST-LIVED PEOPLE IN THE WORLD

I feel that one of the primary reasons for why a person changes eating patterns—whether that means entering the Zone or eating more soy protein—is to live a longer and better life. If that is the goal, then the best starting point for developing the ideal diet would be to study what the longest-lived people in the world actually eat.

It turns out the longest-lived people (with legitimate birth records to verify their ages) live on the Japanese island of Okinawa. Okinawans have a 40 percent lower mortality rate than the second longest-lived people, the mainland Japanese, and they have a greater percentage of centenarians (people living to 100) than any other country in the world. In fact, five times more Okinawans reach the age of 100 as mainland Japanese.

What accounts for the longevity of the Okinawans? First, they eat a huge amount of soy, nearly 100 grams per day. This is more than twice the amount of soy protein consumed by mainland Japanese and 25 times more soy than consumed by Americans. At the same time, they limit their calorie intake, consuming nearly 30 percent fewer calories than the Japanese. How do they decrease calorie intake while simultaneously increasing soy intake? By cutting down on rice while stocking up on vegetables, thus reducing the amount of carbohydrates consumed. Essentially, they are following an eating plan that is very similar to the Zone, particularly the Soy Zone.

As I explain in greater detail in Chapter 9, there are two main reasons why the Okinawan diet will improve longevity. First, soy protein decreases insulin levels, to an even greater degree than animal protein. Second, the restricted calorie intake lowers the levels of free radicals in your body, the damaging elements that can speed aging. Both of these anti-aging benefits can also be obtained by following a Zone diet rich in soy protein. You will learn all about the anti-aging process in Chapter 9, but for now just remember to add more soy to your diet, using protein powder, tofu, tempeh, soy hot dogs, soy sausages, or soy hamburgers.

This soy recommendation applies even if you are not a vegetarian, since many of the health and hormonal benefits of soy cannot be obtained as effectively from animal protein. Likewise, if you have already stopped eating meat, consuming more soy is particularly crucial because many vegetarian diets are too high in pasta, bread, and rice and too low in protein. You may have turned to a vegetarian diet to achieve better health, only to find that your health has begun to decline. Perhaps you have gained weight, or have been plagued by persistent colds and fatigue. These are all signs that you are out of the Zone, and have been eating too many high-density carbs and not enough protein. Soy protein can get you into the Zone, and keep you there forever. Not only will you gain all the advantages of the Zone, you'll also reap the health rewards that soy can provide.

Just to show how easy this is, I have listed some of the Vegetarian Zone meals from *The Soy Zone*.

Asparagus Frittata

1 Breakfast or Dinner Entrée

Ingredients

4 ounces firm tofu, cubed
1 whole egg
2 egg whites
¼ teaspoon dried basil
¼ teaspoon ground black pepper
¼ teaspoon sea salt
½ cup unsweetened tomato sauce
1 small onion, thinly sliced
1 bunch asparagus (about 8–10 stalks)
1 large red or yellow bell pepper, cut into ¼-inch strips
1⅓ teaspoons olive oil
pinch of salt

Instructions

1 Preheat oven to 400°.
2. In a medium bowl, mash tofu with a fork. Add egg, egg whites, basil, black pepper, and salt. Whisk mixture with fork and set aside.
3. Pour tomato sauce into small saucepan and gently warm over low heat.
4. Meanwhile, fill a large pot with lid with ½ inch water. Set steamer basket into pot and layer onions, asparagus, and bell pepper into steamer. Cover pot and bring to boil over high heat.

Reduce to medium heat and steam vegetables 5 to 6 minutes, or until just tender. If you don't have a steamer, boil the vegetables till tender, about 3 minutes. Transfer to plate.

5: In a medium oven-proof skillet, heat oil over medium-high flame until oil sizzles. Pour in egg/tofu mixture all at once and reduce heat to medium-low. Spread egg/tofu mixture evenly across pan to cook.

6: Before mixture has completely set, evenly distribute steamed vegetables over eggs. Transfer skillet to oven and cook for about 5 minutes, or until egg/tofu mixture completely sets and vegetables are hot. Add a pinch of salt and serve with tomato sauce.

Greek Salad With Garlic-Oregano Dressing

1 Lunch or Dinner Entrée

Ingredients

5 cups loosely packed romaine lettuce, washed, patted dry, and torn into small pieces

1 cup canned artichoke hearts, drained and cut into bite-size pieces

2 medium tomatoes, cut into wedges

1 small red onion, thinly sliced

¼ cup canned garbanzo beans, drained and rinsed

2 ounces feta cheese, crumbled

6 ounces extra-firm tofu, cut into ½-inch cubes

1⅓ teaspoons extra-virgin olive oil

1 tablespoon red wine vinegar

2 tablespoons vegetable stock or water

1 small garlic clove, minced

¼ teaspoon dried oregano, crumbled

¼ teaspoon freshly ground black pepper

Instructions

1: Arrange lettuce on large dinner plate. Top with artichoke hearts, tomatoes, onions, garbanzo beans, feta cheese, and tofu.

2: In a small bowl, mix together olive oil, red wine vinegar, vegetable stock or water, garlic, oregano, and black pepper. Pour over salad and toss to evenly distribute dressing. Serve.

Variation: If you have it on hand, try using cold baked or cold grilled tofu in this recipe. Many health food stores now carry pre-baked or pregrilled tofu in the refrigerator section.

Easy Barbecue Tempeh And Vegetables

1 Dinner Entrée

Ingredients

1⅓ teaspoons olive oil
½ small onion, diced
2 medium stalks celery, diced
1 clove garlic, pressed
1 red or green bell pepper, diced
4 ounces tempeh, cubed
⅓ cup textured vegetable protein (such as Morningstar Farms Burger Style Recipe Crumbles)
½ to ¾ cup vegetable broth
1 teaspoon prepared mustard
1 teaspoon apple cider vinegar
2 tablespoons prepared barbecue sauce

Instructions

1: Heat oil in large skillet and sauté onions and celery over medium-high heat until onions are translucent and slightly browned.
2: Add garlic, bell pepper, tempeh, and textured vegetable protein and sauté 3 to 5 minutes longer. If the mixture starts sticking to skillet, add 2 to 3 tablespoons vegetable broth.
3: Add vegetable broth, mustard, vinegar, and barbecue sauce. Simmer covered about 20 minutes, until tempeh is infused with flavor.

Very Berry Smoothie

4 Snack Portions or 1 Breakfast Entree

Ingredients

⅓ cup unsweetened pineapple juice

1⅓ ounces unflavored soy protein powder (portion containing 28 grams protein)

½ teaspoon pure vanilla extract

⅛ teaspoon ground nutmeg

1 cup frozen, unsweetened blueberries

1 heaping cup frozen, unsweetened strawberries

1⅓ teaspoons olive oil or almond oil

Instructions

1: Place juice and protein powder in blender container. Cover and blend until smooth.

2: Add vanilla, nutmeg, blueberries, strawberries, and oil. Blend until smooth, scraping down sides of blender if necessary.

Variation: For a thicker, icier smoothie, add 4 or 5 ice cubes.

9

THE ANTI-AGING ZONE: LIVING LONGER AND LIVING BETTER

Let's face it: We all want to stay young forever. We do everything in our power to reverse signs of aging, from buying fancy face creams that are "age-defying" to expensive cosmetic surgery like facelifts. We're all looking for that quick fix that can turn back the clock—no matter what the cost.

Now I'm going to give you a proposal. Let's say you can reverse the aging process simply by changing your lifestyle. You'll look younger, have the strength and stamina that you had 20 years earlier, and prevent those diseases that are telltale signs of age: heart disease, osteoporosis, cancer. Interested?

I thought you would be. In fact, I wrote an entire book called *The Anti-Aging Zone* that details how the Zone Diet works hand in hand with various lifestyle factors to reverse the aging process. The centerpiece of this plan is what I call the Anti-Aging Zone Lifestyle Pyramid. By employing the strategies outlined at each level of the pyramid, you'll be able to conquer what I call the four pillars of aging: excess insulin, excess free radicals, excess cortisol, and excess blood sugar. Each of these pillars acts in a different way to corrupt your hormonal communication system and accelerate aging.

My point is that the aging process can be reversed if you are willing to incorporate some basic lifestyle strategies into your daily activities that will fine-tune your hormonal systems. The key strategies include calorie restriction using the Zone Diet, moderate exercise, and stress reduction through meditation. Unfortunately, exercise and meditation are not equal to the Zone Diet in terms of their ability to reverse aging: following the Zone Diet is by far the most important step in your anti-aging efforts. I've ranked these strategies in order of importance and come up with the Lifestyle Pyramid that you see below.

Anti-Aging Zone Lifestyle Pyramid

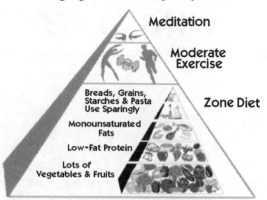

The base of the pyramid, which takes up the largest block of space, contains the most important component of the anti-aging lifestyle: a calorie-restricted diet, in particular the Zone Diet. Calorie restriction is the only scientifically proven method to reverse aging. The verdict is definitely in that it works. As I mentioned earlier, the Zone Diet naturally restricts your calories by limiting your intake of high-density carbohydrates. It provides far greater hormonal benefits than any other calorie-restricted diet and doesn't leave you feeling hungry and deprived, like diets based primarily on grains and other starches. Without following the Zone Diet, you simply won't be able to achieve the maximum benefits of age reversal.

The next step of the Zone Anti-Aging Lifestyle Pyramid is moderate exercise. Although the question of whether intensive exercise extends your lifespan remains unanswered, a lack of exercise, without a doubt, increases the aging process. With exercise, you need to strike the right balance. Intense levels of exercise put stress on the body by increasing the formation of free radicals and increasing levels of the stress hormone cortisol—both of which can speed aging. You want to aim for moderate but consistent exercise. You also need to keep in mind that even the best exercise program can be obliterated by the wrong diet.

At the top of the Lifestyle Pyramid, you'll find stress reduction, particularly through meditation. Meditation can help reverse the damage caused by stress by lowering levels of stress hormones, especially cortisol. Unfortunately, the jury is still out over whether meditation can actually increase your longevity. In theory, though, meditation should delay aging in the brain by protecting it against the ravages caused by excess production of cortisol. Just like exercise, meditation can't do the anti-aging job alone. You need to combine it with a hormonally correct diet like the Zone.

If you combine all three components of the Lifestyle Pyramid, you'll start disassociating your biological age (i.e., how your body functions and feels) from your chronological age (the number of candles on the cake). That means you may be 60, but look and perform like a 40-year-old, or be a 40-year-old and look and perform like a 20-year-old. The Zone Anti-Aging Lifestyle Pyramid can actually turn back your physiological age by 20 years! The key is to make these lifestyle changes permanent. Depending on how you choose to live your life, you are either speeding or reversing the aging process each day. At the end of each day (or even at the end of every meal), you should ask yourself: "Did I take steps to lengthen my life span or to shorten it?" Even if you're disappointed by your answer, remember that tomorrow you'll have another chance to reverse your physiological age.

How the Zone Reverses Aging

I believe that the Zone Diet is the single most important thing you can do to reverse aging for this reason: it reduces all four pillars of aging simultaneously. Following the Zone Diet, you'll restrict your calorie intake, which will reduce the formation of tissue-damaging free radicals. At the same time, you'll also reduce excess blood glucose because you are not consuming excess amounts of carbohydrates. By the same token, you'll reduce excess insulin, which is triggered by excess carbohydrate consumption. Last, you'll reduce the likelihood of excess cortisol production to maintain blood glucose levels, since at every meal you'll eat adequate levels of low-fat protein, which stimulates the secretion of glucagon (the hormone that restores blood glucose levels).

You don't need any special adaptations to the Zone Diet to maximize its age-reversing benefits. Simply follow the concepts that I outlined in the previous chapters, and you'll be taking the most important step you can take to reverse aging.

The next level of the Anti-Aging Zone Lifestyle Pyramid is moderate exercise. With the exercise component, you want to have a cross-training program that affects as many hormonal systems as possible. To reduce insulin, you should plan to do 30 minutes of aerobic exercise every day: brisk walking is one of your best exercise choices, but you can also play volleyball, run, swim, or take a step class. Try several types of exercise and find out what you really enjoy. In addition, you want to spend 5 to 10 minutes a day on a strength-training program.

Strength training is not thought of fondly by most people, but it is the only form of exercise that will build and maintain the muscle mass necessary for maximal functioning in the future. For upper-body strength, the best exercise is push-ups. The word *push-up* conveys dread in most individuals. Therefore, if you are not physically fit, start your daily strength exercise with push-aways from a wall. Stand two to three feet from a wall and extend your hands in a direct line from your shoulders until they reach the wall. Make sure the placement of the hands is low enough on the wall so that when you lower yourself your shoulders will be just above your hands. Lower your body toward the wall, and then push away to return to the original position. Do three sets of 10 to 15 repetitions with a one-minute rest in between sets.

If you can do this easily, then graduate to counter push-backs. Stand two to three feet from a countertop (again positioning your hands in a direct line from the shoulder) and extend your hands to reach the top of the counter. (When lowering yourself to the counter, your shoulders should be directly over your hands). Lower your body to the counter, and then push back to the original position. As you originally did with the push-aways from the wall, do three sets of countertop push-backs each with 10 to 15 repetitions.

Once these are mastered, then move to the knee push-up. Here you are on the floor with your knees bent and your arms extended to the floor (again in a direct line from your shoulder). Lower yourself until your chest (not your stomach) touches the floor, and then raise yourself back up to the original position. Once you have mastered this exercise for 10 to 15 repetitions in three sets, then you are ready to graduate to the dreaded push-up in which only your toes are touching the ground and your arms are totally extended (again so the hands and shoulders are in a direct line). Lower yourself to the floor until your chest reaches it, and then return to the original position. Once you can achieve 10 to 15 repetitions for three sets, then you have two additional options. One is to simply do more repetitions of push-ups in each set. The other is to raise your feet off the floor (like on a chair) and then do your push-ups. Of the two, the first (more repetitions) is easier and probably safer. Don't be disappointed if you have to start with the wall push-aways due to lack of current upper-body strength. It just means you have greater potential for improvement.

The best exercise for developing lower-body strength is the squat. In earlier days it was known as a deep knee bend. Just like the push-up, you start this exercise slowly, depending on your initial fitness level. As a start, just stand facing forward in front of a chair that has arms. Place your hands on the arms of the chair, and then slowly lower yourself to the seat of the chair. Still using the arms of the chair for support, raise yourself back up to a standing position. Do three sets of 10 to 15 repetitions with a one-minute rest between each set.

The next step is to do the same exercise, but without using the arms of the chair for support (however, the arms are always there to be used for support if needed, like a safety net). Again, your goal is to achieve 10 to 15 repetitions in three sets.

Graduating to the next level means using a chair with no arms. With your arms crossed over your chest, you do your squat. As you did with the push-ups, simply increase your repetitions until you reach 15 repetitions per set.

This strength-training program will take less than 10 minutes per day. Regardless of your fitness level, these exercises for upper- and lower-body strength should be done every day. Since they don't require any equipment, they can be done at home or on the road.

There is simply no excuse not to make them part of your Anti-Aging Zone Lifestyle.

These exercises (brisk walking and simple strength-training exercises) should be the core of your moderate exercise program. But this doesn't mean that more exercises can't be added. For more aerobic intensity, think about walking on hilly terrain as opposed to a flat landscape. When you travel, this might mean walking up and down the stairs of your hotel. Alternatively, you may want to invest in a home exercise machine like a rower, a stationary bicycle, or a treadmill to increase the intensity of the workout, or decrease the time spent exercising aerobically so that you get your 300 calories of daily energy expenditure. This will provide 2,000 calories per week of exercise, which provides maximum longevity benefits. For additional anaerobic training, you might want to get a set of adjustable dumbbells because they are easily stored and provide maximum flexibility in the number of weight-training exercises you can do. If you do any additional strength training, never do more than 45 minutes of strength training because beyond that point, cortisol levels begin to rise. Extended strength training beyond this time frame in a single session will start to accelerate the aging process.

Monitoring Your Progress

Since maintaining strength will be one of your most important components of functionality, you need to have some indication of how you are progressing on this component of your Anti-Aging Zone Lifestyle. Here's how you can measure your strength at home.

For determining your upper-body strength, males will do standard push-ups and females will do knee push-ups. Always make sure that your back is not sagging (just pull your abdominals in) and that you are touching the floor with your chest and not your chin. In other words, the number you can do is based on maintaining perfect form. Remember, no one is watching you, so you want to get a true test of your current upper-body strength.

Push-ups: Men

AGE:	20–29	30–39	40–49	50–59	60
EXCELLENT	55	45	40	35	30
GOOD	45–54	35–44	30–39	25–34	20–29
AVERAGE	35–44	25–34	20–29	15–24	10–19
FAIR	20–34	15–24	12–19	8–14	5–9
LOW	0–19	0–14	0–11	0–7	0–4

Knee Push-ups: Women

AGE:	20–29	30–39	40–49	50–59	60
EXCELLENT	49	40	35	30	20
GOOD	34–48	25–39	20–34	15–29	5–19
AVERAGE	17–33	12–24	8–19	6–14	3–4
FAIR	6–16	4–11	3–7	2–5	1–2
LOW	0–5	0–3	0–2	0–1	0

Don't be dismayed if you have a low score. Most Americans will. In fact, the average male teenager can't do 10 push-ups. But with consistent exercise, your upper-body strength will increase.

Lower-body strength is measured by the number of times you can do a squat with weights. Use a chair of standard height (approximately 18–20 inches) without arms. Males should hold 15-pound dumbbells in each hand (a total of 30 pounds), and females should hold 5-pound dumbbells in each hand (a total of 10 pounds). Keeping your legs open as wide as your hips, do a standard squat until you touch the seat of the chair and then return to your starting position. Do as many standard squats as you can while maintaining good form. Then check out how you rate in lower-body strength.

30-Pound Squats: Men

AGE:	20–29	30–39	40–49	50–59	60
EXCELLENT	55	45	40	35	30
GOOD	45–54	35–44	30–39	25–34	20–29
AVERAGE	35–44	25–34	20–29	15–24	10–19
FAIR	20–34	15–24	12–19	8–14	5–9
LOW	0–19	0–14	0–11	0–7	0–4

10-Pound Squats: Women

AGE:	20–29	30–39	40–49	50–59	60
EXCELLENT	49	40	35	30	20
GOOD	34–48	25–39	20–34	15–29	5–19
AVERAGE	17–33	12–24	8–19	6–14	3–4
FAIR	6–16	4–11	3–7	2–5	1–2
LOW	0–5	0–3	0–2	0–1	0

Finally, your cross-training program should include flexibility exercises. In addition to five minutes of stretching to warm up and cool down before and after more intensive exercises, you should plan to do at least 20 minutes every other day of continuous stretching. It doesn't matter if it's basic sports stretching or yoga; both are great.

So here is your basic Anti-Aging Zone exercise program:

1. 30 minutes of brisk walking every day.
2. 5 to 10 minutes of basic strength-building exercises (push-ups and squats) every day.

So far, not too hard. Try to do this every day, but if you do these basic exercises at least five days a week, you will be making progress in your anti-aging program. Then, if you want to add to this basic program, consider the following:

1. Replace your daily brisk walk with a slightly higher-intensity aerobic exercise (rowing, bicycling, or walking on a treadmill where you can increase the difficulty) until you have burned 300–400 calories. If the machine doesn't have a calorie counter, this would be about 30 minutes of exercise.
2. Do no more than 45 minutes of strength training with dumbbells (or free weights and exercise machines) three days per week.
3. Do 20 minutes of flexibility exercises on the days that you don't do any strength training.

The moderate exercise component of the Zone Anti-Aging Lifestyle Pyramid will reduce excess insulin and excess blood sugar, two of the four pillars of aging, without increasing cortisol or free radicals. Not quite as good as reducing all four pillars of aging as with the Zone Diet, but by increasing strength and aerobic fitness, you will increase your functionality in later life.

The final component of the Zone Anti-Aging Lifestyle Pyramid is meditation, because it can lower at least one pillar of aging: excess cortisol production, which is important for promoting brain longevity.

Meditation is not simply sitting back and thinking good thoughts or daydreaming. It is a very precise way to control cortisol. Meditation for the specific physiological purpose of cortisol reduction is key to your brain longevity program. This is not to say that the use of meditation to achieve spiritual goals is not a higher purpose, but that requires a far greater commitment. Here we are simply looking at meditation as another anti-aging tool. This is a very Western (i.e., goal-oriented) approach. In essence, it is practical meditation.

PRACTICAL MEDITATION

Practical meditation is not some purely mystical technique known only to a few gurus. Practical meditation is a series of defined actions. There appear to be common themes that run throughout recorded history on how to meditate. There is usually a constant chanting of a word or phrase or a focus on a physiological action (such as breathing), always returning to that focus on a word, phrase, or physiological function when your thoughts begin to wander (i.e., daydreaming). In essence, you are trying to clear the decks mentally.

Here is a thumbnail sketch of practical meditation: Find a quiet place with a comfortable chair. Close your eyes and repeat a word (the word *one* is a good choice) or phrase continually. At the same time, focus on your breathing. Try to always expand your stomach when you inhale. By focusing on the word or phrase and your breathing, you are trying to keep random thoughts from coming into your consciousness. If such random thoughts do appear, simply refocus your attention on the word and your breathing until they pass. Do this for 20 minutes a day, and there you have it, practical meditation.

Meditation (even practical meditation) takes practice (just like the Zone Diet and exercise), but with increasing skill, significant physiological changes related to reduction of cortisol levels can be achieved. These include the reduction of blood pressure and heart rate, and improvement in immune function.

Do practical meditation for 20 minutes a day, and you have a proven drug to reduce cortisol levels. It's a simple technique that helps alter hormonal response and in the process improves brain longevity.

The same three "drugs"—the Zone Diet, moderate exercise, and practical meditation—that can alter the pillars of aging for your body can also alter the hormonal environment in which the brain must function. Your ability to use these "drugs" correctly will determine how well you play the longevity game. Look around you, and see how you compare to your peers. Do you look younger? Are you in better shape? Do you have more energy? Are you more mentally alert? If so, you are younger than your years. If not, you're older. Aging is more than a state of mind; it requires constant application of the Anti-Aging Zone Lifestyle Pyramid. If you decide to throw in the towel and let your good lifestyle habits slide, you'll find yourself feeling older and weaker. If you choose to take charge and live a healthy life in the Zone, you'll stay strong and young for the rest of your life. The choice is up to you.

10

ZONE SUPPLEMENTS

So by following the Zone, engaging in moderate daily exercise, and practicing meditation, you have a great battle plan for a longer and better life. But what about all the vitamins and minerals that are supposed to reverse aging? Actually, it's macronutrients (protein, carbohydrate, and fat) that are your passport to the Zone, not micronutrient (vitamins and minerals) supplements. Are supplements important for the Zone? A few are, but never let the tail wag the dog. Supplements can enhance your experience in the Zone, but supplements will never get you into the Zone on their own.

What about vitamins and minerals? Isn't our food more deficient in these essential micronutrients than it was 50 years ago? The answer is yes. Why? Fifty years ago, most of the fruits and vegetables came from your backyard or just outside town at the nearby farm. Now they come from all over the world and can be stored for months after being harvested. Vitamins are incredibly sensitive to heat, light, and storage time. Minerals are more stable, but they are very sensitive to processing and cooking technologies. The first casualties in the war for cheap food will always be the vitamin and mineral content of that food. So should you spend a good chunk of your food bill down at the local health food store buying expensive vitamin and mineral supplements? No, but you can use certain supplements wisely to get the most out of the Zone Diet.

Not all vitamins and minerals are of equal importance. I list them below in terms of their importance.

ESSENTIAL SUPPLEMENTS

These are purified fish oils and Vitamin E. Here the research is overpowering, and their cost is relatively inexpensive in comparison to the enhanced health benefits they provide.

Fish Oil

Let's talk about fish oil first, since your grandmother probably used it in the form of cod liver oil. Cod liver oil is rich in Vitamin A and Vitamin D, and was used two generations ago to prevent a disease called rickets. Even though it was (and probably still is) one of the most disgusting foods known to man, its daily consumption was a given.

It turns out that the real reason that cod liver oil was so beneficial was not because of the vitamins it contained, but because of its high levels of the long-chain omega-3 fatty acids called eicospentaenoic acid (EPA) and docosahexaenoic acid (DHA). EPA turns out to be a key factor for controlling insulin levels, and DHA is needed to maintain and rebuild your brain. So even though your grandmother was forcing your parents to eat cod liver oil for the wrong biochemical reasons, she was doing an excellent job of controlling insulin and improving brain longevity. In fact, as I explain in *The Soy Zone*, DHA was the transformational factor that made modern man the master of the planet. Without adequate levels of DHA, your brain-power drops significantly. Equally important, many neurological conditions such as depression, multiple sclerosis, and attention deficit disorders are linked to low levels of DHA in the diet, and often supplementation with fish oils rich in DHA can show dramatic changes within a few weeks.

The need for these long-chain omega-3 fatty acids is only now being realized. Fifty percent of the weight of the brain is composed of fat. And one-third of the brain's mass is composed of long-chain omega-3 fats, like DHA. No other organ in the body has such a concentration of DHA. The greatest growth spurt for the brain occurs during the first two years of life, which is why human breast milk is so rich in DHA. Just how important are these omega-3 fats found in breast milk? One English study indicated that breast-fed children scored nearly 10 points higher on IQ tests compared to children who were formula-fed.

Just as DHA is important for the brain, EPA is also incredibly beneficial in reducing heart disease, cancer, arthritis, and other chronic disease conditions in humans. Why? Because of its effect on a group of hormones called eicosanoids. Why eicosanoids are so important is described in detail in *The Zone* and *The Anti-Aging Zone*, but simply stated, if you want to decrease the likelihood of developing most chronic diseases, then adequate intake of EPA from fish oils is key.

My prescription for fish oil: Even if you are eating two to three servings of fish per week, I still recommend taking a fish oil supplement of about 5 grams per day. That's about one teaspoon of fish oil. Fortunately, today's fish oils are nearly tasteless and can be taken in capsule form.

Vitamin E

The other essential vitamin supplement for the Zone Diet is Vitamin E. It is simply impossible to obtain adequate levels of Vitamin E through diet alone. As with fish oil, the data are compelling that increased supplementation with Vitamin E will have a dramatic clinical effect on diseases ranging from heart disease to Alzheimer's and immune system disorders. The primary benefit of Vitamin E is the destruction of fat-soluble free radicals.

My prescription for Vitamin E: I recommend taking a minimum of 100 I.U. per day, with 400 I.U. as a reasonable upper limit for adults and 50 to 100 I.U. a reasonable upper limit for children (because of their lower body weight).

IMPORTANT SUPPLEMENTS

If fish oils and Vitamin E are essential supplements for the Zone Diet (and any other diet for that matter), then there is a second tier of vitamins and minerals that I consider very important for anyone interested in their health. This tier of supplements includes Vitamin C and the mineral magnesium.

Vitamin C

Vitamin C is an anti-oxidant that reduces excess water-soluble free radicals (one of the pillars of aging). Vitamin C acts like a shuttle to get rid of all the nasty fat-soluble oxidation products that are constantly being formed in your body. And if you don't have enough Vitamin C, these oxidation products pile up and get stored in your fat cells, where they can cause trouble.

Fortunately, Vitamin C is plentiful, especially when following the Zone Diet. Unlike Vitamin E and purified fish oils, where supplementation is a must, fruits and vegetables tend to be rich in Vitamin C. The best sources of Vitamin C in fruits are kiwis, oranges, and strawberries. Vegetables such as red peppers, broccoli, spinach, and mustard greens are also rich in Vitamin C.

My prescription for Vitamin C: Although megadoses of Vitamin C are often touted, the best research indicates that a reasonable level for Vitamin C supplementation is in the range of 250 to 500 mg per day. Because Vitamin C is so inexpensive, supplementation of this vitamin is a good recommendation for everyone.

Magnesium

The one mineral supplement I highly recommend is magnesium. No mineral is as important as magnesium in the Zone. It's the critical mineral cofactor for the enzymes involved in the production of eicosanoids. In addition, it is a cofactor for more than 350 other enzymes. The latest research shows that adequate magnesium is critical for cardiovascular patients, which only makes it reasonable to assume that it is useful for the rest of us, especially since dietary surveys indicate that nearly 75 percent of Americans are deficient in this key mineral. Magnesium is found in every green vegetable, such as spinach and broccoli. However, the richest naturally occurring sources of magnesium are nuts. Other sources that are relatively rich in magnesium are leafy green vegetables, and seafoods like shrimp and crab. These foods are also among the primary foods used in the Zone Diet. Also not surprising is that the foods that are poor in magnesium are starches, breads, and pasta, the new staples of the American diet. No wonder Americans are magnesium-deficient.

My prescription for magnesium: Store-bought magnesium supplements are difficult to take because magnesium tastes terrible and
is poorly absorbed by the body. So go the natural route first. Eat lots
of nuts (especially those rich in monounsaturated fat, like almonds
and cashews), and the other foods rich in magnesium. If you insist
on taking store-bought supplements, the cheapest are capsules of
magnesium oxide. Capsules containing the chelated magnesium (for
better absorption) actually have less magnesium per capsule and are
more expensive. Regardless of the dosage form, try to take 300 to
400 mg of supplemental magnesium per day.

CHEAP INSURANCE POLICIES

I think of the third-tier supplements as cheap insurance policies.
Although their benefits to an individual on the Zone Diet are limited compared to the benefits of the supplements recommended
above, these supplements represent a very inexpensive way to create peace of mind.

Beta-carotene

The first of these third-tier supplements is beta-carotene. No
supplement in the world causes more confusion than beta-carotene.
Scientists always want to search for a magic bullet that can be put
into a capsule and sold as the essence of health. For many years
beta-carotene seemed to be such a magic bullet. After all, there
were many studies showing that higher blood levels of beta-
carotene were associated with lower risks of heart disease and cancer. The obvious conclusion was that beta-carotene was the key factor for preventing both diseases, but in this case the scientists were
looking at the tree instead of the forest.

No one thought for a minute that the reason there was a lot of
beta-carotene in the bloodstream of healthy people was that these
people were eating a lot of fruit! After all, if you are eating a lot of
fruit, it is unlikely that you are eating a lot of high-density carbohydrates, such as starches and pasta. It's now clear that beta-carotene
didn't have the mystical properties that researchers first thought; in
fact, it's just as possible that all the healthy fruit eaters had lower

rates of heart disease and cancer because they were keeping insulin levels low by not eating as many high-density carbohydrates.

Another important fact to remember about beta-carotene is that it must be taken with Vitamin C. Beta-carotene is a great anti-oxidant for fat-soluble free radicals (just like Vitamin E). This simply means it picks up free radicals and stabilizes them before they can do some real damage. But unless removed from the body, a stabilized free radical is still trouble looking to strike. To get these free radicals out of your system, you need adequate levels of water-soluble anti-oxidants (like Vitamin C) to take the free radicals from beta-carotene and transport them to the liver, where they can be excreted. And that was the problem with the beta-carotene studies: you have to add extra Vitamin C to transport the beta-carotene-stabilized free radicals to the liver for their final detoxification.

Does this mean that beta-carotene is somehow dangerous or a supplement you should avoid? Of course not, and in fact it has great utility as long as the other part of the equation (Vitamin C) is present at adequate levels. This is why Vitamin C is very important as a Zone supplement, and beta-carotene is less important.

My prescription for beta-carotene: I usually recommend 5,000 I.U. of beta-carotene as a supplement. But before you go out and buy extra beta-carotene supplements, try getting it from fruits and from vegetables like red peppers and spinach. And while carrots contain beta-carotene, unfortunately they enter the bloodstream very rapidly, thus raising insulin levels, which can be worse for your health than the benefit gained by the increase in beta-carotene.

Other supplements that I place into this third tier are Vitamins B3 (niacin) and B6 (pyridoxine), which are critical for the production of eicosanoids.

Niacin

Lack of niacin was discovered as the cause of pellagra. It became a widespread epidemic in this country at the turn of the century when poorer populations subsisted on white flour, white rice, and sugar, products all devoid of niacin. (Not surprisingly, these foods have become the staples of our country but now in the form of pasta, bagels, and rice cakes). Unlike most vitamins, niacin can be produced in the body through the conversion of the amino acid tryptophan into niacin. However, the process is not very efficient, but it does mean that if you are eating adequate levels of protein, you will probably avert an outright deficiency of niacin. The best source of niacin remains food, and particularly foods that are integral to the Zone Diet, including lean meat, poultry, fish, eggs, cheese, and milk. While whole grains are another good source, I don't recommend them because their higher carbohydrate densities will increase insulin levels, thus outweighing any benefit of increased niacin.

My prescription for niacin: If you are going to supplement with niacin, then 20 mg per day is a good dose.

Pyridoxine (Vitamin B6)

As with niacin, increased food processing has reduced the amount of Vitamin B6 in our food. This vitamin is a vital co-factor for making eicosanoids, so its presence is important.

My prescription for pyridoxine: I would recommend 5 to 10 mg per day. These amounts of B6 vitamin can also be found in any decent vitamin pill.

Folic Acid

Folic acid is another vitamin that has received research attention because of its ability to reduce both neural tube defects in children and levels of homocysteine, a risk factor for heart disease. The name folic acid comes from the Latin word for leaf because that is exactly where you find this vitamin—in leafy green vegetables.

My prescription for folic acid: Although the RDA for this vitamin is 200 micrograms per day, the most recent research (especially on heart disease) indicates that it makes sense to take at least 500 to 1,000 micrograms per day. It turns out that folic acid also works with Vitamins B3 and B6 to reduce the levels of homocysteine, another example of vitamin synergy (like Vitamin C and Vitamin E) in the body.

In this same tier of useful supplements are the minerals calcium, zinc, selenium, and chromium.

Calcium

You have been told that calcium is necessary for strong bones, since 99 percent of the calcium in your body is in your bones. But it's also needed to control muscle contraction and nerve conduction. Dairy products, including cheese, are without a doubt the best sources of calcium. Our national fat phobia has made most dairy products *persona non grata*, forcing many women to go out and get calcium supplements. But dairy products aren't the only sources of calcium because broccoli, cauliflower, green leafy vegetables, and calcium-precipitated tofu also provide this important mineral.

My prescription for calcium: I recommend 500 to 1,000 mg of calcium per day. Much of this can be obtained from low-fat dairy products.

Zinc

Another important mineral to consider is zinc. Zinc plays a critical role in the proper functioning of your immune system and, not surprisingly, in the production of eicosanoids. As you might expect, good sources of zinc are the building blocks of the Zone Diet, including chicken, beef, fish, oatmeal, and nuts.

My prescription for zinc: If you are going to supplement with zinc, then 15 mg per day should be sufficient. As with Vitamins B3 and B6, you will probably find this amount of zinc in a typical vitamin/mineral supplement.

Selenium

Another important mineral is selenium, which is an essential component of the enzyme known as glutathione peroxidase, which reduces excess free radicals. This is why selenium supplementation is useful in cancer treatment and prevention. Food sources higher on the food chain tend to be rich in selenium. These include seafood and beef. Nuts are also rich in selenium.

My prescription for selenium: The dose I advise for this supplement is 200 micrograms per day, and L-selenomethionine is your best store-bought choice for maximum selenium absorption.

Chromium

Chromium is part of a biochemical complex known as glucose tolerance factor. This complex makes insulin more effective in driving blood glucose into cells for utilization. Therefore, the more chromium you have, the less insulin you need to make. This is why chromium is called a potentiator of insulin action. Unfortunately, many supplement manufacturers have touted chromium as the only nutrient required to lose fat or gain muscle mass. Nothing can be further from the truth. Your diet will have a far greater effect on insulin than any supplement.

My prescription for chromium: If you choose to supplement your diet with chromium, I suggest taking approximately 200 micrograms per day.

EXOTIC AND NOT-SO-CHEAP SUPPLEMENTS

This last group of vitamins is interesting, but only if you have money to spare. It includes lycopene, leutin, CoQ10, and oligo-proanthocyanidins. All are exotic anti-oxidants. Two of the most interesting are the carotenoids lycopene and leutin.

Lycopene and Leutin

Lycopene has been associated with a decrease in prostate cancer and is found primarily in foods with red pigments, such as tomato and watermelon. Leutin is associated with a decrease in macular degeneration (which causes an ever-decreasing field of vision in the eye and leads to blindness). Where do you find luetin? In green leafy vegetables and red peppers.

My recommendations for lycopene and leutin: If you want to supplement your diet with these very expensive anti-oxidants, try 3 to 5 mg per day.

CoQ10

This is really not a vitamin, since the body can synthesize it, but the synthesis is usually very inefficient. CoQ10 functions like a souped-up Vitamin E and appears to be the last line of defense for preventing the oxidation of low-density lipoproteins (LDL), which appear to be a major factor in the development of atherosclerosis. There is also evidence of its benefit in the treatment of congestive heart failure.

My prescription for CoQ10: I recommend 30 mg per day.

Oligoproanthocyanidins (OPC)

These anti-oxidants are also known as polyphenolics. They are found in grapes and are part of the bioflavanoid family, which works together with Vitamin C. Since bioflavanoids have some solubility in both fats and water, they make a good shuttle system to help move stabilized free radicals from fat-soluble antioxidants, such as Vitamin E and beta-carotene, to water-soluble antioxidants, such as Vitamin C. The end result is that excess free radicals can be detoxified by the liver more rapidly.

My prescription for OPC: I would suggest 5 to 10 mg per day.

SUPPLEMENTS FOR VEGETARIANS

Although my recommendations are always the same for vegetarians, there are two special additions.

DHA from Algae

The only way that vegetarians can get adequate levels of the long-chain omega-3 fatty acid DHA, which is critical for brain function, is with supplementation. DHA can now be isolated from algae. The body will retroconvert some of this supplemented DHA into EPA. A far less efficient way is to consume large amounts of flaxseed oil. Even though flaxseed oil contains short-chain omega-3 fatty acids, their conversion into long-chain omega-3 fatty acids is very inefficient.

My prescription for algae-based DHA: 3 to 5 grams of algae oil (containing at least 1 gram of DHA total).

Vitamin B12

The one other supplement for vegetarians is Vitamin B12, since it is only found in animal protein sources.

My prescription for Vitamin B12: Because of the poor absorption of Vitamin B12, I would recommend taking 50 micrograms per day.

Summary of Recommendations

TYPE	DAILY AMOUNT
Essential	
Fish oil	5 grams
Vitamin E	100–400 I.U.
Important	
Vitamin C	250–500 mg
Magnesium	300–400 mg
Cheap Insurance	
Beta-carotene	5,000 I.U.
Vitamin B3 (niacin)	20 mg
Vitamin B6 (pyridoxine)	5–10 mg
Folic acid	500–1,000 ug
Calcium	500–1,000 mg
Zinc	15 mg
Selenium	200 ug
Chromium	200 ug
Exotic and Not-So-Cheap Insurance	
Lycopene	3–5 mg
Leutin	3–5 mg
CoQ10	30 mg
OPC	5–10 mg
Supplements for Vegetarians	
Algae oil containing DHA	3–5 grams
Vitamin B12	50 ug

11

FINE-TUNING THE ZONE

This will help you further master the Zone. If you are doing well using the eye-and-palm method, then you don't have to read this chapter carefully. However, the information contained in this chapter will enable you to fine-tune the Zone to your unique bio-chemistry.

The Zone is not a diet in the traditional sense. Diets can be thought of as short-term periods of deprivation and hunger to lose excess weight, only to return to your old eating habits, which originally caused the weight gain in the first place. The Zone Diet is a lifelong food management program based on balance and moderation for better insulin control. Think of the Zone as a hormonal checkbook. Like your regular checkbook, you don't have to balance it to the penny to make it work. You only want to assure yourself that there is enough money in the account so that the next check you write doesn't bounce. The Zone is similar. You want the best possible balance of protein, carbohydrate, and fat at each meal to achieve the right hormonal action, but you don't have to balance your meal to the exact gram each and every time.

YOUR HORMONAL CARBURETOR

The Zone Diet can be viewed as the constant balancing of protein to carbohydrate at every meal and snack to get the best hormonal output. This is similar in concept to balancing the gas and air in your car engine to get the best mileage. There is no one exact ratio for the optimal balance because of the genetic diversity of individuals. However, the balance of protein to carbohydrate can be described in terms of a bell curve, as shown below

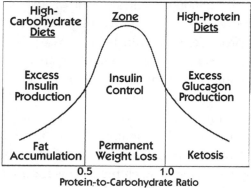

Entering the Zone Depends Upon the Protein-to-Carbohydrate Ratio

What this graph indicates is that if you are eating more than twice as many carbohydrates as protein (a protein-to-carbohydrate ratio of less than 0.5) at a meal, you are likely to make too much insulin, which can lead to increased fat accumulation. On the other hand, if you eating more protein than carbohydrate (a protein-to-carbohydrate ratio greater than 1.0) at a meal, you are likely to make too much of the hormone glucagon, which can lead to ketosis. Don't worry about these numbers, because if you use the eye and palm method described in Chapter 3, you should always be within these limits and therefore in the Zone.

The reason I show this graph is to indicate that there is a mathematical foundation for the Zone, and that you can fine-tune each of the meals you like to eat to always be in the Zone, just as you would adjust the carburetor in your car.

You may want even greater precision (especially for adjusting your hormonal carburetor), and there are two additional food accounting methods that I have found to be useful over the years.

THE ZONE "1–2–3" METHOD

Since many Americans are already accustomed to reading the nutritional labels on food, I have developed an easy-to-use system for building Zone meals. Rather than counting calories, however, you'll be counting grams of fat, protein, and carbohydrates. For packaged food, you can take a quick look at the food label to see how many grams of each macronutrient it contains. Some foods will contain proteins, carbohydrates, and fats in various combinations, but normally most will contain a bulk amount of just one of these three. And what about foods that aren't packaged or labeled, such as fresh meats, produce, and even bagels? You can quickly learn the carbohydrate, protein, and fat content of these types of foods by turning to Appendix B at the back of this book.

How do you actually use the 1–2–3 method? It's just as it sounds: for every *one* gram of fat you consume, you want to add *two* grams of low-fat protein and *three* grams of carbohydrate to every meal. Let's go back to the typical American female who needs about 3 ounces of low-fat protein at each meal. This is about 20 grams of protein. Therefore, her typical Zone meal would consist of 10 grams of fat, 20 grams of protein, and 30 grams of carbohydrates, or "1–2–3." The typical American male, who needs 4 ounces of low-fat protein at each meal, would eat about 30 grams of protein. Therefore, his typical Zone meal would contain about 15 grams of fat, 30 grams of protein, and 45 grams of carbohydrate, or again, "1–2–3."

Just to go through the math again, take the number of grams of protein you plan to consume (like 30) and divide it by 2 to give the number of fat grams.

30 grams of protein ÷ 2 = 15 grams of fat

Then take the number of fat grams (15) and add to the number of protein grams (30) to get the number of carbohydrate grams (45) for that meal as shown below:

30 grams of protein + 15 grams of fat = 45 grams of carbohydrate

This simple accounting system gives a protein-to-carbohydrate ratio of 0.7, about midway in the Zone as shown in the previous graph. These numbers are by no means set in concrete. They can be altered to your particular biochemistry. But by following this system, you can make adjustments to the Zone Diet with a high degree of precision. So let's see how the "1–2–3" system works in practice.

Protein

Here is a helpful hint for helping to better visualize what 20 to 30 grams of protein actually represents: Get an inexpensive kitchen scale, and then measure out 3 ounces of low-fat animal protein or 4½ ounces of fish. This would provide 20 grams of protein, suitable for most females. For males, measure out 4 ounces of low-fat animal protein or 6 ounces of fish. This would represent what 30 grams of protein looks like. Within a few days, you can eye these amounts at home, in restaurants, and at dinner parties. You'll soon realize that these amounts of protein are what you generally get at the most exclusive French restaurants.

Carbohydrates

Let's take a closer look at carbohydrates. When you read a food label, it lists the grams of total carbohydrate. However, that number also includes the grams of fiber, which has no effect on insulin. So to get an indication of the effect of a particular carbohydrate source on insulin stimulation, you have to subtract the fiber content. In the following table I show you the amount of insulin-stimulating carbohydrates in several typical food items.

Amounts of Insulin-Stimulating Carbohydrates in Various Foods

Food	Volume	Total Carbs (G)	Fiber (G)	Insulin-Stimulating Carbs (G)
Pasta	1 cup	40	2	38
Apple	1 medium	20	4	16
Broccoli	1 cup	7	4	3

You can quickly see that you would have to eat a tremendous volume of broccoli (approximately 12 cups) to consume the same amount of carbohydrates as eating a relatively small amount of cooked pasta. This is why starches, breads, and grains are considered high-density carbohydrates, whereas fruits are considered medium-density carbohydrates, and vegetables are considered low-density carbohydrates. The Zone Diet relies heavily on low-density carbohydrates, so large volumes of food must be consumed in order to have an appreciable impact on insulin. On the other hand, very small volumes of high-density carbohydrate stimulate excess insulin, which is why they are used in moderation in the Zone.

There is also a lot of confusion about simple and complex carbohydrates. In reality, all carbohydrates must be broken down into simple carbohydrates to be absorbed. The rate at which any carbohydrate enters the bloodstream as the simple sugar glucose is known as the *glycemic index.*

It turns out that some complex carbohydrates such as potatoes, rice, and carrots actually enter the bloodstream as glucose at a faster rate than does table sugar! As a result, the simple distinction of simple and complex carbohydrates is not of great use in helping you control insulin.

As I describe in greater detail in my upcoming book *The Soy Zone*, the key to understanding the effect of any carbohydrate source on insulin is not related to its glycemic index, but to its glycemic load. The concept of glycemic load takes into account both the density of carbohydrates in a given food volume and also their rate of entry into the bloodstream.

So now we can redefine a favorable carbohydrate as one that has a low glycemic load. The lower the glycemic load, the more favorable the carbohydrate choice is for the Zone, as shown below.

FAVORABLE AND UNFAVORABLE CARBOHYDRATES

Favorable (have a lower effect on insulin)
Most vegetables (except corn and carrots)
Most fruits (except bananas and raisins)
Selected grains (oatmeal and barley)

Unfavorable (have a greater effect on insulin)
Grains and starches (pasta, bread, bagels, cereals, potatoes, etc.)
Selected fruits (bananas, raisins, etc.)
Selected vegetables (corn and carrots)

If you are following the "1–2–3" program, the typical female would need to eat approximately 30 grams of carbohydrate at a meal, whereas the typical male would consume about 45 grams of carbohydrates at a meal. Listed below are the food amounts that supply 10 grams of carbohydrates.

Food Volumes That Supply 10 Grams of Carbohydrates

Food	Volume
Broccoli	3 cups
String beans	1 cup
Apple	½
Strawberries	1 cup
Pasta	¼ cup
Rice	⅕ cup
Bread	½ slice

So to supply 30 grams of carbohydrate for a Zone meal for a typical female, one could choose 1 cup of strawberries (10 grams), 1 cup of string beans (10 grams), and half a piece of bread (10 grams). This would supply 30 grams of carbohydrate, enough to balance 20 grams of protein. For a Zone meal for the typical male, he might have 1½ cups of broccoli (5 grams), 1 cup of strawberries (10 grams), an apple (20 grams), and ¼ cup of pasta (10 grams). This would provide 45 grams of carbohydrate, enough to balance 30 grams of protein. Mix and match your carbohydrates any way you want as long as they don't overwhelm the protein content of the meal.

As you can see from this example, it's not that you can never eat unfavorable carbohydrates; just treat them as condiments and use them in moderation.

Fats

The primary fat you will be adding to the Zone is monounsaturated fat. But keep in mind that the Zone is not a program of fat gluttony. Following the "1–2–3" method, the typical female would need about 10 grams of fat in a Zone meal, and the typical male would require about 15 grams. Listed below are some monounsaturated fat choices that when added to the protein content of a Zone meal will provide a total of 10 grams of fat.

Again, mix and match your fats to match your protein and carbohydrate amounts as long as you don't overconsume them.

Monounsaturated Fat Choices That Provide a Total of 10 Grams of Fat in a Typical Zone Meal

Food	Volume
Olive oil	1½ teaspoons
Guacamole	4 tablespoons
Slivered almonds	2 tablespoons
Almonds	12
Macadamia nuts	2

So our Zone meal for a typical female might have 1½ teaspoons of olive oil (in a vinegar and olive oil dressing), providing a total of 10 grams of monounsaturated fat. The typical male Zone meal might have 2 tablespoons of slivered almonds (10 grams) and 2 tablespoons of guacamole (5 grams), providing a total of 15 grams of monounsaturated fat. Even though you are adding fat to the Zone, it is still a low-fat program (in terms of fat grams), and more important, one that is very low in saturated fat.

So let's now look at the typical Zone meal for a female or male.

Typical Female Zone Meal   ## Typical Male Zone Meal

Protein

3 ounces chicken breast   4 ounces chicken breast

Carbohydrates

1 cup strawberries   1½ cups broccoli
1 cup string beans   1 cup strawberries
½ piece bread   1 apple
¼ cup pasta

Fat

1½ teaspoons olive oil   2 tablespoons slivered
                                    almonds
                              2 tablespoons guacamole

Each meal follows the "1–2–3" method, and you can see that no one is going to be deprived by either meal, even though the typical female Zone meal was less than 300 calories and the typical male Zone meal was slightly over 400 calories. Eat three similar-sized meals each day plus two Zone snacks, and your caloric intake is approximately 1,200 for a female and about 1,500 for a male. The Zone Diet is a lifetime program of reduced calories, but without deprivation (because of the large size of the meals) or hunger (because blood sugar levels are being maintained at a constant level).

ZONE FOOD BLOCKS

The other food accounting system that I developed is called Zone Food Blocks. Many people find this system easier to use than the "1–2–3" method, but it does take a little getting used to. Basically, it measures food in blocks rather than in grams.

Personally, I believe that Zone Food Blocks are ultimately easier because you don't have to remember as many numbers as with the "1–2–3" method. Zone Food Blocks are volumes or weights of various food sources that contain the same number of grams in pre-measured blocks of protein, carbohydrate, and fat. Now all you have to do is maintain those Zone Food Blocks in a 1:1:1 ratio to be squarely in the center of the Zone.

With the Zone Food Block method, one block of protein is equal to 7 grams, one block of carbohydrate is equal to 9 grams, and one block of fat is equal to 3 grams. This means that the typical American female will require 3 Zone Food Blocks each of protein, carbohydrate, and fat at each meal, whereas the typical American male would require 4 Zone Food Blocks of each at every meal.

Since people generally only eat 20 different food items, all you have to do is remember what the Zone Food Block sizes are for your favorite foods. Actually, remembering your telephone number is probably more difficult. Appendix C lists many of the most common foods, broken down into Zone Food Blocks. This is also the system described in my other books, including *The Zone* and *Zone-Perfect Meals in Minutes*.

ADJUSTING YOUR HORMONAL CARBURETOR

Is there one diet for everyone? The answer is both yes and no. There is one hormonally correct diet for everyone, and that is one that keeps insulin within the Zone. However, the balance of protein to carbohydrate to reach the Zone might be different from person to person, and we obviously don't all like to eat the same things. Whether you are using the eye and palm method, the "1–2–3" method, or the Zone Food Block method, the technique for adjusting your hormonal carburetor is essentially the same.

So how do you know if your last meal was hormonally correct? It's very simple. After you eat, look at your watch. Then, four hours later, ask yourself two questions:

Are you hungry?

Do you have good mental focus?

If the answer to both these questions is yes, then you know your last meal was hormonally correct, based on your biochemistry. You can always go back to that same exact meal in the exact same proportions to get the exact same hormonal output. Just like a drug. All you need is to create 10 hormonally winning meals (2 breakfasts, 3 lunches, and 5 dinners) that you can constantly rotate in your diet.

On the other hand, if the answer to either question is no, then you know your last meal was not hormonally correct. For example, if you are hungry and loopy (like after eating a big bowl of pasta), this means that you consumed too much carbohydrate relative to protein in your last meal, and pushed your insulin too high. Plan to have the same meal again, and keep the protein constant but reduce the carbohydrates by about 10 grams or one Zone Block of carbohydrate.

If you have a good mental focus but you are hungry, that's an indication that you had too much protein relative to carbohydrate. As a result, you pushed your insulin too low, so the brain is telling you to eat again, even though the brain is getting adequate blood sugar. If this is the case, next time you have that same meal, keep the protein constant, but increase the amount of carbohydrate by about 10 grams or one Zone Block of carbohydrate. By using either food accounting system, you are learning how to adjust your hormonal carburetor to your own unique biochemistry and using only the foods you like to eat.

CAN YOU EVER BE TOO THIN?

The Zone is designed to bring you to your ideal body weight and keep you there for a lifetime. However, you can become too lean. How do you know if you've reached this point? You'll be able to see your abdominal muscles. Usually this is only a problem for elite athletes, and may occur when one includes intensive exercise to the Zone. But if it does happen (God forbid, who would want to look like an Olympic athlete?), then what do you do? You don't want to add any protein to your diet because it is already protein-adequate. You don't want to add any more carbohydrate to your diet, since that would raise insulin levels. So there's only one nutrient left to add to your diet that has calories, but has no effect on insulin. It's our old friend fat, and in particular monounsaturated fat. Add more monounsaturated fat to your diet (such as olive oil, macadamia nuts, or guacamole) to give you enough calories to maintain your percentage of body fat at a level consistent with good health. Actually, many of the elite athletes I work with consume more than 50 percent of the calories as monounsaturated fat to maintain their percentage of body fat in the appropriate range for optimal sports performance. Should your body fat begin to increase too much, then cut back on the amount of extra monounsaturated fat added to your diet until your abdominal muscles begin to reappear.

THE ONCE-A-MONTH PORKY PIG MEAL

The Zone Diet is not restrictive, nor does it require perfect attention. In fact, you will get 75 percent of the benefits of the Zone by following it 75 percent of the time. As a result, there is no guilt on the Zone. If you have a bad meal, just make sure that your next meal is squarely in the Zone. No one is perfect, nor should anyone ever become obsessive regarding the preparation of Zone meals.

And even if you were perfect, I strongly recommend eating a

large carbohydrate meal (pasta, Mexican food, and so on) at least once a month, just so you can feel miserable the next day. You will be bloated, fatigued, mentally foggy—basically the feeling of being hit by a Mack truck. What you are suffering from is an insulin hangover. The reason why I recommend such torture once a month is to reinforce how powerful food can be, and that only one hormonally incorrect meal can send you directly to carbohydrate hell. It's okay, because your next meal will take you back to the Zone. Unfortunately, some of us need some powerful reinforcement from time to time to reaffirm how we want to spend the rest of our lives.

If you want to be even more precise (because, after all, the Zone is based on science), then I recommend that you read my books *Mastering the Zone* and *Zone-Perfect Meals in Minutes* for more detailed information on how to adjust your current diet to make it more hormonally correct.

12

SUCCESS STORIES FROM THE ZONE

Being in the Zone will help you think better, perform better, and look better. But the power of this dietary technology goes far beyond these benefits alone. It was developed to treat what I call "either/or" medical conditions, medical conditions that either have no treatment or those for which the treatments are less than desirable.

Hormonal control will be the key to twenty-first-century medicine, and much of this hormonal control comes from the food that you eat. You can take advantage of this fact when you enter the Zone. The end result is that some very remarkable changes are possible if you treat food with the same respect that you treat a prescription drug.

While I can tell you this over and over, perhaps you would like to hear what other people have to say about the Zone and how it has affected their lives. These are their stories. They may begin like yours, or like the story of someone you know. Their endings, however, come straight from the Zone.

Consider the story of Willard H., a prostate cancer survivor who wrote:

I just returned from the Mayo Clinic, where I go for my annual physical. All of my tests came out well. My PSA [a marker for prostate cancer] is undetectable. My cholesterol has continued to decrease from 210 to 150. Thanks and congratulations go to you and the Zone. I spoke with my physicians about the Zone. They were not experts on nutrition, but said they thought it was a good program.

Neither their encouragement nor discouragement would have made a difference with me. I'm on your program for life. I give a lot of credit to your program for keeping my PSA at the bottom end of the scale.

Now, five years later, Willard H. continues to write to me about his continuing good health and virtually zero PSA levels.

Reaching the Zone is all about improved quality of life. That's why I particularly like the letter that I got from Joan S., a multiple sclerosis patient, who wrote:

This "incurable" multiple sclerosis is reversing after sixteen years. It feels like I'm living a miracle. I'm glad I've kept daily notes, because it seems unbelievable. I keep pinching myself.

What is even more encouraging are letters from individuals who have been on medication for decades, like Audrey, who wrote me the following:

I have suffered from clinical depression for 37 years and spent thousands of dollars on therapy and medication. Plagued by weight gain and other side effects from the antidepressants, I became determined to go off the medications altogether. Working with my doctor, I have been medication free for 4 months, and my depression still has not returned. Before I heard about the Zone, I cut out sugar and alcohol. Last month, I heard about the Zone from a friend and decided to try it. I've found that I'm happier and able to think more clearly than I can ever remember. (I never thought that it was possible to feel this way.) What's more, the Zone has been able to reverse the lingering effects of the antidepressants. Before I went on the Zone, I was 140 pounds—25 pounds above what I used to weigh. Now I can happily report that I weigh 125 and can get into my favorite clothes! The Zone is helping me in so many areas of my life, especially physically and psychologically. When these two areas are stable, the rest of life just flows.

Another condition that responds rapidly to the Zone is high blood pressure, as Steve W. wrote:

I tried your program and am very satisfied. My blood pressure was 132/103. Even after cutting out desserts and having my weight drop to 172, my blood pressure had not changed. After 45 days on the Zone, my weight is in the low 160s and my blood pressure has dropped to 103/73. I guess you can say you probably saved my life. I am sorry I had to give up so many of my favorite things, such as bread, pizza, and rice. But I am developing new favorites, such as cherries, peaches, blueberries, turkey breast and more. I guess it's a small price to pay to live longer.

I also received a letter from Pat G., who wrote:

I weighed 205 pounds and was a Type 2 diabetic. My brain was always foggy from the use of my medications. After 4 months on the Zone, I have lost 41 pounds, and I feel great. My body is still changing. My muscles are building and becoming more toned while I am losing fat. I take no medications. My blood sugar levels continue to remain in the normal range. I have very little if any pain now from my back and my leg. My doctor can't believe it.

Pat's experience in the Zone and improved control of blood sugar is no different from that of lots of other people including Fedore L., who wrote,

During the month of September, I developed a strange taste of sawdust in my mouth and some needle-like pain in my liver, in addition to a small amount of foam in my urine. I decided to go to my doctor, and my blood tests of October 13 showed a fasting blood glucose level of 288, and inflammation of the liver. He prescribed a medication for diabetes, then asked me to come back in 6 weeks for another test. I seriously pondered whether to try the Zone and not the medication. I reported it to my doctor who, as expected, was not at all pleased. I bargained with him for four weeks of a trial. I confessed to him that I had abused my body for the last 40 years (I'm now 71), therefore wanted to give my body a chance for recovery. Scared to death, I followed the Zone to the letter. Four weeks later, my blood glucose test was 103, totally normal. Then, on purpose, I exited the

Zone a bit, and a week later my blood sugar had risen to 126. I am truly feeling that food must be perceived as a drug.

Relief from pain is crucial for one's quality of life. That's why I was happy to receive a letter from Belinda D. Belinda is a health care professional who was not only overweight, but also suffered from repetitive stress injuries that had required three separate surgeries. She was still taking 18 aspirin per day to ease the pain. Belinda wrote:

When I picked up your book in the bookstore, my first response was to put it back on the shelf and renew my promise not to try a diet program. What made me stop and buy the book was the section I read on chronic pain and arthritis. At that point, I was ready to try anything. Within a month of following the Zone, my pain levels were reduced to a point where I stopped taking all medication, and I was actually returning to basically pain-free living. The weight loss I have experienced has been an added bonus to the way I feel. For the record I have lost 40 pounds in the last five months. I have a way to go, but I feel no stress in getting to my ideal weight. My husband has been equally as successful in the Zone. He has returned to his ideal weight of 178 (from 220), and it is like having a new man around the house. The biggest improvement has come in his emotional well being. Thank you again for your work and for publishing the information in such a clear and concise manner.

There are many more stories like these, but I feel that the examples I have chosen are representative of my basic concept that food is a very powerful drug if used correctly.

But what about overweight individuals who exercise to lose weight? Consider Steve G., who three years ago weighed 313 pounds. Determined to change his life, Steve started biking and running 1½ hours per day and sticking to a 1,000-calorie diet rich in carbohydrates and low in fat. Within a year, he had reached 250. For the next year and a half, he did the same exercise and low-calorie, high-carbohydrate diet and nothing happened. His weight remained the same. As he wrote:

I noticed your book this past summer one day in a bookstore, and could not believe what perfect sense you made. I actually cut back on some of my exercise and added more fat to my diet. I applied your technology and the weight has been dropping off. I'm down to 205 now, and headed toward my ultimate goal of 174. On top of it all, I feel energized, whereas on every other diet, I always felt very drained. The Zone simply works.

Obviously, I am very gratified when I receive such letters, testimonials, and profound thanks from people whose lives have been dramatically improved by the Zone program. The real credit does not go to me, however, but to these readers. They took the initiative to change their own lives, and you can, too. I hope that some of these stories illustrate the potential of the Zone Diet to transform your health, and perhaps will inspire some changes of your own. Remember, the Zone Diet is not radical; it just requires you to look at food in a new way and take responsibility when you eat—a small price to pay for a longer and better life.

13

FREQUENTLY ASKED QUESTIONS

GENERAL

Why are both protein and carbohydrates required at every meal and snack?

Zone logic says that excess insulin will make you fat and keep you fat. Your goal is to maintain insulin in a Zone, not too high, not too low, throughout the day. The protein and carbohydrate content of a meal has a dramatic impact on insulin production and determines how well you keep insulin in that Zone for the next four to six hours.

Why is meal timing so important?

As with a medication, you want to control the body's utilization of protein and carbohydrate consistently throughout the day, and you should eat a minimum of three meals and two snacks. A Zone meal should provide you with four to six hours in the Zone, whereas a snack is good for approximately two to two and a half hours. Additionally, you must eat within one hour after waking, and don't forget your afternoon and late-night snacks. Eating every five hours, whether you're hungry or not, is necessary to stay in the Zone. In fact, lack of hunger without cravings for sugars and sweets coupled with good mental focus is a good indicator that you're in the Zone.

Like planning your daily activities, meal and snack times should be planned accordingly. Based on your wake-up time, determine those timepoints throughout the day when it's time to eat your next meal or snack.

If I follow the Zone Diet, does this mean I can never have rice, pasta, or bagels again?

No, but you should be using these carbohydrate sources in moderation, like condiments. Simply make sure that most of your daily intake of carbohydrates comes from vegetables and fruits and, whenever possible, cut down on your intake of grains and starches.

I thought complex carbohydrates (such as grains and starches) were good for you.

Grains and starches are high-density carbohydrates that are very easy to overconsume, which will elevate insulin. As an example, one cup of cooked pasta has the same amount of carbohydrates as 12 cups of broccoli. Low-density carbohydrates in the form of fruits and vegetables are virtually impossible to overeat, and their fiber content slows the entry rates of carbohydrates into the bloodstream and helps control insulin levels. In addition, don't forget that fruits and vegetables are loaded with vitamins and minerals, unlike grains and starches. Remember, it's not that you'll never consume grains and starches again, but when you do, they must be consumed in moderation, compared to fruits and vegetables.

Do I have to be obsessive about the Zone Diet to be successful?

No. Obviously, the greater the precision, the greater the results, but even if you only play by the general rules of the Zone and use the eye and palm method, you won't be too far away from the center of the Zone. Just remember to pay very close attention to your hunger and mental focus four to six hours after a meal. Using your eyes, you will be able to adjust your hormonal carburetor with increasing precision without having to obsess about portion size, grams, or calculations.

Isn't the Zone Diet a high-protein diet?

No, it's a protein-adequate diet. You should never eat excessive amounts of protein, nor should you consume any less than your body requires. At each meal, an adequate amount of protein is approximately 3 ounces for the typical female and 4 ounces for the typical male. Both snacks should contain one ounce of protein. These amounts of low-fat protein are hardly considered excessive.

I prefer to eat smaller, more frequent meals throughout the day. Is it possible to stay in the Zone?

Actually, the greater the number of small meals you eat, the better the insulin control. This is called *grazing*.

Should I be concerned about such a seemingly low daily caloric intake?

For most females the minimum total calories consumed is 1,100 to 1,200 calories per day, and for most males, the calories consumed is 1,400 to 1,500. While this might seem like a deprivation diet that leaves you constantly fatigued, the Zone Diet will actually eliminate hunger between meals, without the nagging cravings for sugars and sweets, while maintaining peak physical and mental energy throughout the day.

You aren't hungry, because the balance of protein to carbohydrate maintains stable blood sugar levels to the brain. Finally, on the Zone Diet, you are eating as if you are already at your ideal body weight because you are using a combination of your stored body fat and incoming calories to meet your daily caloric requirements. Therefore, once you achieve your ideal weight, you don't change your diet at all.

Doesn't any low-calorie diet cause fat loss? (A calorie is a calorie.)

Not necessarily. Research studies in the 1950s demonstrated this with several different diets consisting of 1,000 calories per day. All patients lost substantial weight on a high-protein (90% of calories) diet, high-fat (90% of calories) diet, and mixed (42% of calories as carbohydrate) diet, but most patients actually gained weight on a high-carbohydrate (90% of calories) diet. Cutting back on calories without lowering your insulin levels is a surefire prescription for feelings of deprivation, constant hunger, fatigue, and, finally, failure. Any time you reduce calories, you will lose some weight, but eventually you hit a hormonal plateau where the weight loss (and, more important, fat loss) stops, but feelings of hunger, deprivation, and fatigue continue. Unlike other reduced-calorie dietary programs, the Zone Diet is a hormonal control program that maintains adequate levels of blood sugar to the brain, which allows for significant calorie reduction without hunger, fatigue, or deprivation. This lifelong use of the Zone makes it the only "drug" that can successfully provide permanent fat loss.

How long will it be before I can expect to see results on the Zone Diet?

Within two to three days you should see a noticeable reduction in your carbohydrate cravings and an increased mental focus. Within five days you will notice a significant decrease in hunger throughout the day coupled with greater physical performance and less fatigue as the day wears on. Keep in mind that this is a fat loss program; don't expect rapid weight loss, which is often mostly water. The maximum fat loss you can expect, no matter how strictly you follow the program or how much you exercise, is one to one and a half pounds of fat per week. It is simply impossible to reduce excess body fat any faster on any dietary program. Within two weeks, you will notice that your clothes are fitting much better. Judge your success by the fit of your clothes and not by changes on your bathroom scale.

What is the minimum amount of daily protein intake?

I always recommend a minimum of 75 grams of protein throughout the day for adults. This is ideal for most women, whereas most men will require about 100 grams of low-fat protein each day.

Won't the Zone Diet cause osteoporosis and kidney failure?

The Zone is a protein-adequate diet in which small amounts of protein are portioned evenly throughout the day. No one should eat more protein than their body requires, but conversely, no one should eat less, because you will put yourself in a state of protein malnutrition. On the Zone Diet, you are not only eating adequate protein, but also spreading it over three meals and two snacks. It's almost as if you are receiving an intravenous drip of protein throughout the day. The newest research actually indicates that women who eat more protein have 70 percent fewer hip fractures than those who eat less than 75 grams per day. Furthermore, the additional research indicates that even for patients with kidney failure, earlier reports about protein restriction may have been overblown. And if you don't have kidney failure there is no evidence that eating the amounts of recommended protein in the Zone Diet has any negative effects.

Why don't the French have high rates of heart disease?

Nutritionists just hate the French. They smoke, they drink, they eat lots of fat, they don't exercise, they seem to have a very good time, and they have the lowest rates of heart disease in Europe. It's called the French Paradox. It's only a paradox if the results are contrary to your expectations. Obviously, there are a number of reasons for these surprising statistics, but I believe the major factor is that their meals are moderate in calories, rich in fruits and vegetables, always contain protein, and include fat. That's also a good definition of the Zone. Then there is the so-called Spanish Paradox. In the last 20 years, Spaniards have eaten more protein, more fat, and fewer grains, and their rates of cardiovascular disease are dropping.

The Chinese eat a lot of rice; don't they have low rates of heart disease?

No. According to the American Heart Association the rates of cardiovascular disease in urban Chinese males are nearly as great as in American males, and Chinese females, both rural and urban, actually have greater rates of cardiovascular disease than American females. In addition, the data from the American Heart Association indicate that the Chinese have greater overall adult mortality than is found in Americans. These data demonstrate the danger of using epidemiological data to make far-reaching dietary assumptions.

I'm concerned about pesticides on fruits and vegetables, and the hormones and antibiotics used in beef and chicken production. What should I do?

These are valid concerns. You should always try to eat organic fruits, vegetables, and range-fed beef and chicken. However, be prepared to pay a significantly higher price and to cope with their scarcity. Don't, however, make this an excuse for not eating the appropriate protein-to-carbohydrate balance at every meal.

I'm not overweight. Why would I need to follow the Zone Diet?

The Zone is not a diet. It's a lifelong hormonal control program. Loss of excess body fat is only a pleasant and very desirable side benefit. The important reason to follow the Zone Diet is that it is the only dietary program which has been demonstrated to reverse the aging process. Although the Zone Diet was originally developed for cardiovascular patients, it was extensively tested on world-class athletes. Between those two extremes lies everyone else. If you are at your ideal weight and want to think better, perform better, and live longer, then the Zone Diet is for you.

Can I continue taking my vitamins and minerals?

Vitamins and minerals are an excellent low-cost insurance policy to ensure adequate micronutrient (vitamins and minerals) intake. However, the Zone Diet—which is primarily composed of low-fat protein, fruits, and vegetables—provides an excellent source of vitamins and minerals, and requires much less supplementation. The only supplements that I strongly recommend are fish oils and extra Vitamin E.

What exactly do you mean by "use in moderation" when referring to unfavorable carbohydrates?

Try not to make unfavorable carbohydrates (grains, starches, breads, and pasta) more than 25 percent of the total carbohydrate grams in a meal. Use them as condiments, not as your primary carbohydrate source.

Should I be concerned about sodium?

Not if you are following the Zone Diet, because excess insulin activates another hormonal system that promotes sodium retention. However, it always makes sense not to use excessive amounts of sodium.

I'm a pure vegetarian. How can I make this diet work for me?

Simply add protein-rich vegetarian foods to your current diet to maintain the correct protein-to-carbohydrate ratio. Ideal choices would be firm and extra-firm tofu and isolated soybean protein powder. The new generation of soybean-based meat substitutes (hot dogs, hamburgers, sausages, and so on) is another excellent way of turning a carbohydrate-rich vegetarian diet into a vegetarian Zone diet. Traditional vegetarian protein sources, such as beans, have an exceptionally high amount of carbohydrate for the amount of protein they provide, which makes it impossible to achieve the desired protein-to-carbohydrate balance to enter the Zone.

Which protein powders are best?

Sources of isolated protein include egg and milk combinations and lactose-free whey powder. For vegetarians, isolated soy protein powders are excellent choices. Protein powders are available at most health food stores. Protein powders can be added to any carbohydrate-rich meal, like oatmeal, to make them more hormonally favorable. They can also be added to flours and mixes (like pancake, muffin, and cookie mixes) for cooking and baking to fortify the protein content.

What impact will various cooking methods have on the quality of macronutrients or micronutrients?

Cooking has little effect on macronutrients (except that excessive heat can damage and cross-link protein with carbohydrates). However, cooking can have a very negative effect on micronutrients (vitamins and minerals). Vitamins are extraordinarily sensitive to heat. In addition, minerals can be leached out of food when cooked with water. Therefore, steaming vegetables is an ideal way to retain micronutrients, yet make the vegetables more digestible. Fruits are usually eaten raw, retaining all of their micronutrients. The more carbohydrates are processed or cooked, the more rapid their entry rate into the bloodstream. This is why "instant" forms of carbohydrate like one-minute rice or instant potatoes should be avoided.

Should I eat my Zone meal or snack even if I'm not hungry?

Yes. This is the best time to eat in order to maintain insulin equilibrium from one meal to the next. If you're thinking hormonally, you want to maintain insulin in a Zone by eating every five hours. As with an IV drip, you want to control the entry rates of protein and carbohydrate evenly throughout the day. That's why everyone should consume three meals and two snacks each day.

Will this diet heal the damage done to my body over the years?

The body has a remarkable ability to repair itself, given the appropriate tools. The best of those tools is the diet, especially one that orchestrates the desired hormonal responses that accelerate the repair process.

Why don't I count all the protein, carbohydrate, and fat in everything I eat?

Because you would need a mini-computer to make all the calculations. This is why I recommend the eye and palm method to balance your plate. If you want more precision, then you can use either the "1–2–3" or Zone Food Block methods.

Will a liquid meal in the correct ratio get me to the Zone?

A liquid meal has a much greater surface area than solid food. Therefore, the digestion and entry rate of macronutrients into the bloodstream cannot be controlled that well, and there is a corresponding decrease in the desired hormonal control. Liquid meals are more convenient but hormonally not as desirable as solid food.

They can be used occasionally if you just don't have the time to cook, and are much more desirable than skipping a meal or snack.

Can children use the Zone?

The diet is ideal for children because they need to be in the Zone even more than adults do. The average preadolescent child (boy or girl) will need about 15 grams of protein per meal, with the appropriate amounts of fat and carbohydrate. After puberty, children should eat the same amounts as a typical adult. The one protein source that virtually every child will eat is string cheese. Although a little high in saturated fat, string cheese is a good way to introduce more protein into your child's diet. That leaves just the hard part for parents: getting your kids to eat fruits and vegetables instead of pasta and bread.

How do I know that two years from now the Zone Diet will not turn out to be like the other diets that initially produce great results?

First, the Zone is not a diet, but a lifelong hormonal control program that allows you to maximize your full genetic potential. Second, the Zone has been in the popular press for more than five years, and the newest research has confirmed everything I originally stated when *The Zone* was first published in 1995. Most important, the hormonal systems the Zone Diet is based upon have evolved over the last 40 million years and are unlikely to change soon. Many fad diets are based on gluttony and extremism. Either they let you eat all the carbohydrates you want (high-carbohydrate, low-fat diets) or all the protein and fat you want (high-protein diets), and neither type worries about the quantities consumed. The Zone Diet is based on balance (of protein and carbohydrate) and moderation (of calories), with limits on the amount of protein, carbohydrate, and fat consumed at every meal.

What if I make a mistake or go overboard?

Don't worry, you're only temporarily knocked out of the Zone. You can get back on track with your next meal or snack. Zone living is guilt-free.

I'm currently taking medications. How will this affect the Zone Diet?

Any change in diet (for better or worse) will affect the metabolism of the drug(s) you are taking. Always consult with a physician before starting the Zone Diet or any other dietary plan. In addition, many medications will actually raise insulin levels, making it difficult to enjoy the desired benefits no matter how strictly you follow the program. See if your physician could possibly switch you to a medication that does not negatively influence insulin levels. However, never change the dosage or stop taking your medication without first consulting your physician.

I haven't exercised in years. Should I?

Since you are not fatigued or listless on the Zone Diet, you may be inclined to start an exercise program for the first time in years. While not as important as your diet, exercise does play an important role in helping you control insulin levels. The best form of exercise is any routine you will perform on a regular basis. If you haven't exercised for a long time, building up to a brisk 30-minute walk is a great way to get started again. As your endurance builds, you may wish to increase the intensity and even add some form of weight training as part of your regular workout schedule. Never think that increased exercise can erase the problems associated with poor diet. I use the 80/20 rule: 80 percent of your ability to control insulin will come from the diet and 20 percent from exercise.

I exercise on a regular basis at high intensity. How can I optimize my workout schedule to get the maximum hormonal bang for the buck?

Whether you are training with weights or training aerobically, eat a Zone snack 30 minutes prior to exercise. This will set the hormonal stage to trigger the preferential burning of stored body fat as soon as your workout begins. Have another Zone snack within 30 minutes after the training session ends and a Zone meal no more than 2 hours later. Most important of all, don't forget your bedtime snack.

I get confused when it comes to the difference between proteins and carbohydrates. Are there any simple rules to help me when I shop?

Here is a simple rule for distinguishing between protein and carbohydrates: Protein moves around (or at least once did) and carbohydrates come from the ground, in the form of grains (pasta, breads, and cereals), vegetables, and fruits. When shopping, always try to stick to the periphery of the market. There you will find fresh fruits and vegetables, the deli case, the salad bar, and the meat department. Down the middle aisles, you'll find all the packaged carbohydrates, a surefire way to increase insulin levels and knock you out of the Zone.

What about alcohol?

The body treats alcohol as if it were a carbohydrate. For all intents and purposes, treat 4 ounces of wine, a bottle of beer, or 1½ ounces of distilled liquor as if it were 10 grams of carbohydrate or one Zone block of carbohydrate.

As long as my protein and carbohydrate balance at any meal or snack is based on Zone guidelines, couldn't I eat all I wanted and still keep insulin under control?

Any excess calories that can't be used immediately by the body will be stored as fat, even if the meal is perfectly balanced, and the extra calories will also increase overall insulin levels. The typical female should consume approximately 300 calories in a meal, and the typical male should consume approximately 400.

FAT FACTS

Why do I need extra fat? What does it do?

Paradoxically, it takes fat to burn fat, especially if the fat source is monounsaturated fat. Remember, the Zone Diet is not an excuse for fat gluttony, but there is a need to add back reasonable amounts of fat to each meal. First, monounsaturated fat doesn't affect insulin and thus acts as a control rod to slow carbohydrate entry into the bloodstream, thereby reducing the insulin response. Second, it releases a hormone (cholecystokinin, or CCK) from the stomach that tells the brain to stop eating. Third, it makes food taste better. Most of your fat intake should be in the form of monounsaturated fat, and the amount of fat you consume is dictated by the amount of protein you consume at each meal. If anything, be more liberal than restrictive with your monounsaturated fat intake.

Can I lose too much body fat?

Obviously, it's possible to lose too much body fat. Once you achieve a weight and look that you are happy with, and wish to stabilize your body weight, simply add more monounsaturated fat to your Zone Diet. Since you were always eating as if you were at your ideal weight, the protein and carbohydrate content of your diet remains the same. Therefore, to prevent any further weight loss, you must add more fat, preferably monounsaturated fat, as caloric ballast to prevent any further fat loss. This extra monounsaturated fat provides the extra calories to maintain your ideal body weight without affecting insulin levels. Many world-class athletes on the Zone Diet consume more than 50 percent of their daily calories in the form of fat.

What are the best sources for long-chain omega-3 fats?

The best sources are cold-water fatty fish, such as salmon, mackerel, and sardines. Other marine sources that have a lower omega-3 fat content are common fish such as tuna, swordfish, scallops, shrimp, and lobster. Try to consume about 10 grams of long-chain omega-3 fats per week. This would translate into two servings of salmon or four servings of tuna or similar fish per week. One teaspoon of refined fish oil contains about 1 gram of long-chain omega-3 fats. Remember that your grandmother used to give you a tablespoon of cod liver oil per day? That provided about 3 grams of long-chain omega-3 fats per day, or 20 grams per week.

I'm a vegetarian and can't use fish oil. What should I do?

There is a new generation of algae-based oils that are rich in long-chain omega-3 fats. This allows the vegetarian to get adequate levels of these critical fats.

FINE-TUNING

How do I adjust my hormonal carburetor?

Not everyone is genetically the same. Your hormonal carburetor is based on the protein-to-carbohydrate balance that generates the best hormonal response for you. That hormonal response is easily measured by asking yourself, "How do I feel?" four to six hours after a meal. If you maintain excellent mental clarity and have no hunger, then the protein-to-carbohydrate balance in your last meal was ideal for your biochemistry. Your goal is to make every meal with that same ratio in order to generate the same hormonal response. For the vast majority of people, this balance is 2 grams of low-fat protein for every 3 grams of carbohydrate. So the most efficient way to fine-tune your own carburetor is to start with this ratio and then experiment slightly on either side to determine your limits by using lack of hunger and mental clarity as the parameters you wish to optimize.

I thought fat was the enemy.

Fat has no direct effect on insulin. However, monounsaturated fats like olive oil play a critical role in controlling insulin by slowing the entry rate of carbohydrates into your bloodstream. How well you control the entry rate of carbohydrates into the body determines how well you control insulin, and consequently how your body performs for the next four to six hours.

I have developed some constipation. What should I do?

A Zone Diet will switch your body to a fat-burning metabolism instead of a carbohydrate-burning metabolism. The metabolism of fat requires greater amounts of water on a daily basis. Therefore, the first step is to increase your water intake by 50 percent. If this isn't sufficient to reduce the constipation, then you are probably releasing a particular type of stored fat known as *arachidonic acid* from your fat cells. For about 25 percent of the population, there will be a transitory release of arachidonic acid. The build-up of extra arachidonic acid is a result of your previous dietary patterns. This temporary increase in arachidonic acid in the bloodstream can give rise to constipation by reducing water flow into the colon. Adding extra long-chain omega-3 fats to your diet will minimize this transitory effect. The best source of long-chain omega-3 fats is fish, but another good source is fish oil capsules, as long as the fish oil has been extensively purified. For the first week on the Zone, I recommend taking an additional 6 grams of purified fish oil per day.

How should I alter this diet if I'm pregnant or nursing my child?

If you are pregnant or nursing, you should be using the Zone to ensure adequate protein intake. For pregnant women, increase your protein intake by 10 grams at every meal, with a corresponding increase of carbohydrate and fat. In essence, you are now consuming the meals that a typical male would eat. For nursing mothers, add an extra five grams of protein and the corresponding amount of carbohydrate and fat to each Zone meal.

Can I cut back on fat intake as long as I balance my protein and carbohydrate requirements?

You can, but ironically, you will not lose as much fat. The small amount of added fat acts as a control rod to reduce the entry rate of carbohydrates into the bloodstream, thereby reducing insulin secretion. By reducing insulin, you can access your stored body fat more effectively. Also, the fat causes the release of the hormone cholecystokinin (CCK), which promotes satiety between meals. Of course, any added fat to your diet should be primarily monounsaturated fat, such as olive oil, guacamole, almonds, or macadamia nuts.

I haven't lost any weight. What am I doing wrong?

Often your weight on the scale will not change even though you are losing body fat. This is because you are likely to be gaining new lean body mass. The result is that your weight is constant, but your body composition is changing. You can tell this from the better fit of your clothes.

14

WHY HIGH-PROTEIN DIETS FAIL

High-protein diets are once again sweeping the nation: rashers of bacon and sausage in the morning, cheeseburgers (without buns) for lunch, and big steaks for dinner. Eat as much protein as you want, just don't eat any carbohydrates. And as for saturated fat, eat all you want. Sound too good to be true? Well, it is. As we grow fatter as a nation, more and more Americans are turning in desperation to these highly unbalanced diets to lose weight quickly. Unfortunately, that hope of permanent fat loss will never be realized.

First, let me make it very clear again that the Zone is *not* a high-protein diet. Although it is commonly described that way by the popular press, you now know that the Zone doesn't come close to being a high-protein diet. A high-protein diet is exactly that: you're eating excessive amounts of protein, often rich in saturated fat, at every sitting. On the Zone Diet you are *never* eating more than 3 to 4 ounces of low-fat protein at any one meal. That is exactly what every nutritionist in America recommends.

Furthermore, on the Zone Diet, you are always eating more carbohydrates than protein. In fact, while the U.S. government recommends eating three to five servings of fruits and vegetables per day, the Zone Diet recommends eating ten to fifteen servings of fruits and vegetables daily. So if the Zone Diet is not a high-protein diet, then what exactly is a high-protein diet? And more important, why have high-protein diets failed to deliver the promise of safe and permanent weight loss?

High-protein diets have been around for more than 30 years. Millions of people have tried them and lost weight. The same millions have all gained the weight back, and usually more to boot. I am one of the harshest critics of high-protein diets because I think they are unhealthy and downright dangerous. Let me explain why.

These diets tell you to eat virtually unlimited amounts of protein and fat with virtually no carbohydrates. In the absence of a minimal amount of incoming carbohydrates, the body is quickly set into an abnormal metabolic condition known as *ketosis.* This condition occurs when there is not enough carbohydrate to metabolize fat completely, and waste products known as ketone bodies begin to accumulate in the blood. In addition, without an adequate amount of incoming carbohydrates, your brain can't function properly. For this reason alone, many people on high-protein diets often feel cranky and irritable—a sure sign that their brain is malnourished for carbohydrates.

In terms of weight loss, these high-protein diets look good at first glance. Almost everyone who tries them loses weight initially. But weight loss is different from fat loss. Weight loss is a combination of loss of water, muscle, and fat. Your goal is to make sure that virtually all your weight loss comes from excess body fat. The reason behind the quick weight loss seen with high-protein diets is that your body is working overtime to expel all the ketone bodies in your system. It does this by increased urination, which in turn causes water loss. This water loss will translate into weight loss, but at the same time will leach valuable electrolytes, like potassium, from the bloodstream. This can create a false sense of accomplishment and, more seriously, lead to potentially dangerous cardiac problems. Furthermore, it has been clinically proven that both weight loss and fat loss are no different after six weeks following a high-protein diet or the Zone. So why risk potential short-term cardiac problems if the fat loss is no different from that in the Zone?

After any extended period of time, high-protein diets don't have a great track record. As you continue to diet and force your body into ketosis, insidious changes are slowly taking place in your body. First, your fat cells begin adapting themselves and become "fat magnets" that now are 10 times more active in shuttling fat into fat cells than they were before you went on the high-protein diet. This means that when you go off the diet, you'll accumulate body fat at a frightening rate. Second, your brain didn't just fall off the turnip truck. It needs blood sugar for optimal performance, which it is no longer receiving from carbohydrates. Desperate, it instructs your body to start tearing down protein in existing muscle mass to convert into glucose for energy. This is why people who stay on high-protein diets for a long period of time have that very gaunt look in the face and start losing their hair. The body is actually stripping protein from these sites to make adequate glucose levels for the brain. Third, you are consuming far too much saturated fat. This not only makes you more prone to heart disease, but makes your cells less responsive to insulin. This in turn forces the body to start making more insulin, which is what made you fat in the first place. Finally, new evidence indicates that continued ketosis leads to increased oxidation of your lipids, an important factor in the development of heart disease. These are the biochemical reasons why high-protein diets ultimately fail, and why the millions who have lost weight on them have gained their weight back and more while risking their cardiovascular health. It has happened for the last 30 years, and it will continue to happen for the next 30 years and beyond.

To further illustrate the differences between the Zone Diet and a typical high-protein diet, we can look at what a typical day might consist of for the average American male.

COMPARISON OF A HIGH-PROTEIN DIET TO THE ZONE

High-Protein	Zone
	Breakfast
Eggs, scrambled or fried	8-egg white omelet with
Bacon	2 teaspoons olive oil
Ham	1 cup slow-cooked oatmeal
Sausage	1 cup strawberries
	Lunch
Bacon cheeseburger without bun	Chicken Caesar salad with 4 oz chicken and 1 tablespoon olive oil-and-vinegar dressing
Small tossed salad	2 cups steamed vegetables
	1 apple

Afternoon snack

None

1 oz turkey breast
1 kiwi
3 almonds

Dinner

Shrimp cocktail

6 oz grilled salmon covered
    with 2 tablespoons slivered
    almonds

Clear consommé
Tossed salad
Diet Jell-O

4 cups steamed vegetables
1 cup mixed berries

Late night snack

None

4 oz red wine
1 oz low-fat cheese

If you take the daily consumption of protein, carbohydrate, and fat for each of these two very different diets and put them into a bar graph, the differences become more apparent.

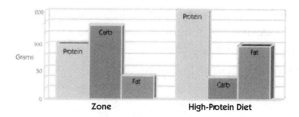

The Zone is *Not* a High-Protein Diet

You can quickly see that no rational person could ever mistake the Zone Diet for a high-protein diet. On a high-protein diet, you are eating far more protein than carbohydrate. On the Zone, you are eating more carbohydrate than protein. On a high-protein diet, you are eating large amounts of fat, and much of that is saturated fat. On the Zone, you are eating limited amounts of fat (even though you always add some extra fat to every meal), and much of this fat is heart-healthy monounsaturated fat.

This does not mean, however, that the Zone Diet is a high-carbohydrate diet. Most high-carb diets allow you to overindulge in unfavorable carbohydrates, whereas the Zone treats these as condiments. Now that you have a basic background in hormones, let me illustrate the differences between the Zone and high-protein and high-carbohydrate diets.

High-Carbohydrate Diets

Dietary mantra: "Eat all the carbohydrates you want, just don't eat any fat."

Hormonal effect: Increased insulin levels

Consequences: Increased fat accumulation; mood swings; loss of strength; carbohydrate cravings; constant hunger; decreased mental focus; increased likelihood of heart disease, Type 2 diabetes, and cancer; and acceleration of the aging process

High-protein Diets

Dietary mantra: "Eat all the protein you want, just don't eat any carbohydrates."

Hormonal effect: Increased glucagon levels

Consequences: Ketosis, low blood sugar, irritability, adaptation of fat cells to become "fat magnets," increased oxidation of lipids, loss of muscle mass, increased likelihood of heart disease if continued for any significant period of time, and acceleration of the aging process

The Zone

Dietary mantra: "Balance and moderation."

Hormonal effect: Keeps insulin within a zone by balancing insulin and glucagon

Consequences: Loss of excess body fat; improved control of blood sugar; increased mental and physical energy; stable moods; decreased likelihood of heart disease, Type 2 diabetes, and cancer; and slowing of the aging process

15

SCIENTIFIC VALIDATION OF
THE ZONE

The Zone Diet remains one of the most misunderstood concepts in nutrition, although the concept is simple. The Zone is based on keeping various hormones generated by the macronutrient (protein, carbohydrate, and fat) composition of each meal within specified zones: not too high, not too low.

In 1995 my first book, *The Zone*, outlined the biochemical basis of the Zone Diet. However, since the publication of my dietary program, it has been incorrectly labeled as a high-protein diet, and thus linked to those risky high-protein dietary programs that have absolutely no relationship to the Zone, as explained in Chapter 14. What the Zone Diet does represent is a protein-adequate, carbohydrate-moderate, low-fat diet to keep insulin within a zone: not too high, not too low. Furthermore, the Zone Diet is based on two principles: *balance* and *moderation*. You balance the protein, carbohydrate, and fat at each meal, and consume only a moderate amount of calories at each meal.

The Zone is simply a dietary program that recommends adequate amounts of low-fat protein and lots of vegetables and fruits, with a dash of monounsaturated fat. What could be controversial about that? Yet to hear the nutritional establishment, you might think the Zone is a fad diet that is medically unsafe and nutritionally unsound.

I believe that the controversy surrounding the Zone Diet is

based on two factors. First, it forces people to consider the hormonal consequences of a meal, and in particular, how to maintain insulin within a zone. This is a totally new concept to virtually all nutritionists. Second, the Zone Diet is based on the most recent advances in medical research, which many critics seem to be totally unaware of. Recently, a number of independent studies have been published that validate the power of the Zone to change health care in America. Here is some of the most relevant recently published research. For complete information on the studies, see the references at the end of the book.

1. **The number-one risk factor that predicts heart disease is elevated insulin.** Prospective studies conducted with individuals with no initial trace of heart disease have demonstrated that elevated insulin is a vastly more powerful predictor of heart disease than is cholesterol. In fact, elevated insulin increased the likelihood of having a heart attack by a factor of 5.5, compared to elevated "bad" cholesterol (LDL), which only increased the likelihood by 2.4 times. Another prospective study has also indicated that the only blood parameter associated with increased heart attacks is increased insulin levels. A third study, from the Harvard Medical School, has demonstrated that an elevated ratio of triglycerides-to-HDL cholesterol (an indirect marker of increased insulin levels) increases the likelihood of a heart attack by a factor of 16. Therefore, any dietary program, like the Zone, that lowers insulin will decrease the risk of heart disease.

2. **The more protein you eat, the less heart disease you have.** Recent long-term studies from Harvard Medical School indicate that when the ratio of protein-to-carbohydrate reaches the levels recommended for the Zone, there is a 26 percent decrease in heart disease risk. The group that had the lowest incidence of heart disease followed a diet that provided a protein-to-carbohydrate ratio of 0.7, squarely within the boundaries of the Zone.

3. **The more protein you eat, the fewer hip fractures you get.** In postmenopausal women, a new study has indicated that women who consumed more animal protein had a 70 percent reduction in the number of hip fractures.

4. **The most powerful drug to prevent heart attacks is neither aspirin nor any cholesterol-lowering drug, but diet.** The Lyon Diet Heart Study indicated that a 70 percent reduction in both fatal and non-fatal heart attacks could be achieved simply by consuming more omega-3 fats in the diet and more fruit. This decrease in both cardiovascular mortality and overall mortality on the Lyon Diet is far greater than what was achieved by taking aspirin or any other cholesterol-lowering drug. The Zone Diet is similar to the diet used in the Lyon Diet Heart Study, except that the Zone Diet emphasizes eating greater amounts of vegetables and fruit and increasing the consumption of omega-3 fatty acids even more than does the diet used in the Lyon Diet Heart Study.

5. **Increased dietary protein is associated with increased breast cancer survival and decreased blood pressure.** As long as you decrease the consumption of fatty red meat (which is rich in arachidonic acid), the higher your intake of protein will be, and the more likely you will be to survive breast cancer. Likewise, the higher the protein intake, the lower the blood pressure.

6. **You lose body fat faster on the Zone.** In fact, the fat loss was nearly twice as great following the Zone Diet than on a high-carbohydrate diet even though both diets contained the same number of calories and the same amount of fat. This study demonstrates conclusively that a calorie is not a calorie when it comes to fat loss.

7. **The Zone Diet can initiate significant hormonal changes in only one meal.** This research work was conducted at Harvard Medical School with overweight adolescents. The Zone meal generated a completely different hormonal profile than a standard meal even though both contained the same number of calories. Furthermore, after eating a Zone meal, the number of calories consumed at the next meal was significantly less, indicating that the Zone provides better hunger control than other macronutrient compositions containing the same number of calories.

8. **The Zone Diet can reduce excess insulin levels before any fat loss is achieved.** This answers the chicken-and-egg question: Which comes first, elevated insulin or increased body fat? It has been known for some time that insulin levels can be elevated before there is any accumulation of excess body fat. However, this study demonstrated that elevated insulin levels were lowered before any fat loss was achieved, indicating that it is excess insulin that causes the accumulation of body fat.

9. **The Zone Diet can alter your genetic code.** It has been known for more than 60 years that calorie-restricted diets improve longevity. Recently, it has been shown that calorie-restricted programs can also alter the expression of the genetic code. Because it is a calorie-restricted diet, the Zone Diet is guaranteed to reverse aging, but without hunger, deprivation, or fatigue, since blood sugar levels are properly maintained.

It remains amazing to me how the media continue to ignore the science behind the Zone Diet. Even more amazing is the fact that the Zone Diet (which promotes eating 10 to 15 servings of vegetables and fruits per day with small amounts of universally recommended servings of low-fat protein, no more than 3 to 4 ounces per meal, and using monounsaturated fat as its primary fat source) is not the most highly recommended diet in America. Whatever the reasons behind this misunderstanding of the Zone Diet, you have the power to make your own decision about what type of diet you want to follow for the rest of your life. I hope this book has convinced you that it should be the Zone Diet.

THE FUTURE OF YOUR HEALTH CARE IN AMERICA

As we enter the new millennium, America's health care system stands at a crossroads. No one can honestly believe that Americans are healthier than they were 20 years ago, because we have become the fattest people on earth. New research findings indicate beyond a shadow of a doubt that the fatter you are, the more likely you are to die a premature death.

The Zone Diet was developed to address this growing crisis. The Zone is not a diet; it represents an exceptionally powerful drug for preventing the primary chronic diseases that characterize the aging process and promote premature death. The Zone Diet is also the most important tool you have to achieve permanent fat loss.

And if you are concerned about the future, then you should also be terribly concerned about what is happening to today's children. Childhood obesity has doubled in the last 15 years, adult-onset (Type 2) diabetes is now appearing in teenagers as opposed to adults over the age of 40, the growth of childhood asthma is epidemic, and there has been exponential growth in the number of children with attention-deficit disorders. A very strong argument can be made that all of these disease outbreaks in our children are consequences of growing hormonal imbalances in their diets. Children can't cook, but their parents can. If you take the time and effort to control your child's insulin levels with the food that you prepare (or let them eat), you will be ensuring a better future for your children.

Everyone understands that a good diet is your best prescription for a healthy life, yet Americans are more confused than ever about what to eat. A good diet means balance and moderation. Neither high-protein nor high-carbohydrate diets meet that criteria. The

Zone does. Hopefully, this book has cleared up much of this confusion because ultimately any diet book must be based on common sense. Hippocrates told us some 2,500 years ago that we must treat food with the same respect with which we treat any drug. His words are still true today.

As the hope fades that managed care will save us from increasing medical expenses as our population grows older, what is the future for our health care system? It's pretty bleak, unless we make some significant changes in the way we eat. It is time for us all to start taking responsibility for our own health, rather than simply relying on doctors, drugs, and expensive medical procedure to improve and prolong our lives.

Only you can feed yourself (and your children), only you can exercise, and only you can practice stress reduction. These are the components of the Anti-Aging Zone Lifestyle Pyramid. The better you put into practice these lifestyle components, the sooner you will experience a longer and better life. And the most important component of the Anti-Aging Zone Lifestyle Pyramid is eating in the Zone.

The Zone Diet is based on balance and moderation, science, and common sense. It is a simple tool, but a powerful one that can help all of us enter the millennium with healthier bodies, improved performance, and an optimistic outlook toward the future. Enter the Zone, and today can be the first day of a longer, healthier, and happier life.

RESOURCES

After reading this book, you now realize that eating in the Zone may be your most powerful "drug" for increasing daily performance (both mental and physical), losing excess body fat, and living a longer and healthier life. Although I use the term *Zone Diet*, this is not a short-term program as much as a lifelong food management system for better health through enhanced hormonal control, using foods you like to eat.

This is the sixth book I have written about the Zone technology. My first book, *The Zone*, was written primarily for cardiovascular physicians to alert them to the power of food to alter hormone levels, specifically how the levels of the hormones insulin, glucagon, and eicosanoids vary with the macronutrient composition of each meal. However, *The Zone* is not the best introduction for a beginner to understand how simple the Zone technology is to follow. That's why I usually recommend reading *Zone-Perfect Meals in Minutes* as a great introduction to Zone basics, plus *Mastering the Zone* as a more detailed how-to book for using the Zone. Once you understand basic Zone logic, then refer back to *The Zone* to better understand the biochemistry behind it. And if you really want to learn how to reverse aging and extend your life, then I strongly recommend reading *The Anti-Aging Zone*. This is my manifesto for the entire Zone technology I've developed. Although *The Anti-Aging Zone* is more complex than *The Zone*, it provides the information and motivation to make the Zone your lifelong ally to increase and enhance your longevity by reversing the aging process.

Although each of my books represents the latest research on the complex relationship between diet and hormonal response, the field is constantly changing. Much of that information can be found on my Web site, www.drsears.com, which reviews the latest updates to this rapidly evolving field. The goal of my Web site is to serve as a clearinghouse of information not only about the Zone Diet but also about worldwide hormonal research, how diet can affect various hormones, and the impact of those hormones on your longevity. Since this information is rapidly changing, I urge you to visit drsears.com to let me help you sort this new information into a digestible form (no pun intended). In addition, I am constantly updating this site with new recipes (many of them vegetarian), new research information, and simple tips to make the Zone Diet incredibly easy to follow on a lifelong basis.

Please consider drsears.com as your personal cyberspace resource to understand and easily integrate the lifestyle steps necessary to enjoy a longer and better life. If you would like additional information to show you how simple and easy Zone living can be, you can also call toll-free at 1-800-404-8171 for a free information package.

ZONE FOOD CHOICES

THE 1–2–3 METHOD

Preparing Zone meals requires an understanding of the appropriate food choices you must make for the optimal hormonal benefits. There is nothing forbidden to eat in the Zone, just as long as you maintain the right balance of protein and carbohydrate from meal to meal. However, some choices will be far better than others for maximum insulin stabilization.

If you are using the "1–2–3" method to make Zone meals, then all you have to do is balance the number of grams of fat, protein, and carbohydrate at each meal. For the typical female, this means eating about 10 grams of fat, 20 grams of protein, and 30 grams of carbohydrate at each meal. For the typical male, this means consuming about 15 grams of fat, 30 grams of protein, and 45 grams of carbohydrate at each meal. **These numbers are not set in concrete.** You may have to do some adjusting for your personal biochemistry, but they will give you a good starting point.

START WITH PROTEIN

I can't emphasize enough that every meal and snack must have adequate protein, because that will determine the amount of carbohydrate you can have without causing an overproduction of insulin. Listed below are the amounts of various protein portions that contain 10 grams of protein. The average female will need two 10-gram portions (20 grams of protein) at every meal, and the average male will need three 10-gram portions (30 grams of protein) at every meal.

Low-Fat Protein Sources

Meat and Poultry

Beef (range-fed or game)	1½ oz
Canadian bacon, lean	1½ oz
Chicken breast, skinless	1½ oz
Chicken breast, deli	2 oz
Turkey breast, skinless	1½ oz
Turkey breast, deli	2 oz
Turkey, ground	2 oz
Turkey bacon	4 strips

Fish and Seafood

Bass (freshwater)	1½ oz
Bass (sea)	2 oz
Calamari	2 oz
Catfish	2 oz
Cod	2 oz
Clams	2 oz
Crabmeat	2 oz
Haddock	2 oz
Lobster	2 oz
Mackerel	2 oz
Salmon	2 oz
Sardines	1½ oz
Scallops	2 oz
Snapper	2 oz
Trout	2 oz
Tuna (steak)	1½ oz
Tuna, canned in water	1½ oz

Eggs and Dairy

Egg whites	3 eggs
Eggs	1 egg
Egg substitutes	⅓ cup
Cottage cheese, low-fat	⅓ cup
Low-fat cheese	1½ oz
Nonfat cheese	1½ oz

Vegetarian

Protein powder	10 grams
Soybean hamburger crumbles	½ cup
Soybean Canadian bacon	5 slices
Soybean frozen sausage	1½ links
Soybean hamburger	⅔ patty
Soybean hot dog	1½ links
Tofu, extra-firm	3 oz
Tofu, firm	4 oz
Tofu, soft	6 oz

CARBOHYDRATES

Once your protein portion is set for a meal, you must balance it with carbohydrate. Each portion size listed below contains 10 grams of carbohydrate. Bear in mind that there are both favorable and unfavorable carbohydrates. The favorable carbohydrates will have the least impact on insulin secretion, whereas unfavorable carbohydrates will have a significantly higher impact even though they contain the same number of carbohydrate grams. Therefore, keep your use of unfavorable carbohydrates to a minimum.

The typical female will need three 10-gram portions of carbo-hydrate at each meal, whereas the typical male will need about four 10-gram portions of carbohydrate at each meal. Mix and match the carbohydrates if you wish, as long as you consume the appropriate number of 10-gram portions.

Favorable Carbohydrates (Use Primarily)

Cooked vegetables

Artichoke	4 large
Artichoke hearts	1 cup
Asparagus	12 spears
Beans, green or wax	1½ cups
Beans, black	¼ cup
Bok choy	3 cups
Broccoli	3 cups
Brussels sprouts	1½ cups

Cabbage (red or green)	3 cups
Cauliflower	4 cups
Chickpeas	¼ cup
Collard greens, chopped	2 cups
Eggplant	1½ cups
Kale	2 cups
Kidney beans	¼ cup
Leeks	1 cup
Lentils	¼ cup
Mushrooms, whole, boiled	2 cups
Onions (all types), chopped, boiled	½ cup
Okra, sliced	1 cup
Sauerkraut	1 cup
Squash, yellow, sliced, boiled	2 cups
Spinach	3½ cups
Swiss chard	2½ cups
Tomato, canned, chopped	1 cup
Tomato, pureed	½ cup
Tomato sauce	½ cup
Turnip, mashed	1½ cups
Turnip greens, chopped, boiled	4 cups
Zucchini	2 cups

Raw vegetables

Alfalfa sprouts	10 cups
Bamboo shoots	4 cups
Bean sprouts	3 cups
Beans, green	2 cups
Bell peppers (green or red)	2
Broccoli	4 cups
Brussels sprouts	1½ cups
Cabbage, shredded	4 cups
Cauliflower	4 cups
Celery, sliced	2 cups
Chickpeas	¼ cup
Cucumber (medium)	1½
Endive, chopped	10 cups
Escarole, chopped	10 cups

Jalapeño peppers	2 cups
Lettuce, iceberg	2 heads
Lettuce, romaine, shredded	10 cups
Mushrooms, chopped	4 cups
Onions, chopped	1½ cups
Radishes, sliced	4 cups
Scallions	3 cups
Shallots, diced	1½ cups
Snow peas	1½ cups
Spinach, chopped	20 cups
Tomato	2
Tomato, cherry	2 cups
Tomato, chopped	1½ cups
Water chestnuts	⅓ cup
Watercress	10 cups

Fruits (fresh, frozen, or canned light)

Apple	½
Applesauce (unsweetened)	½ cup
Apricots	3
Blackberries	¾ cup
Blueberries	½ cup
Boysenberries	½ cup
Cherries	8
Fruit cocktail, canned in water	⅓ cup
Grapes	½ cup
Grapefruit	½
Kiwi	1
Nectarine	½
Orange	½
Orange, mandarin, canned in water	⅓ cup
Peach	1
Peaches, canned in water	½ cup
Pear	½
Pineapple, cubed	½ cup
Plum	1
Raspberries	1 cup
Strawberries, diced fine	1 cup

Grains

Barley, dry	½ tablespoon
Oatmeal, slow-cooking (dry)	½ oz
Oatmeal, slow-cooking (cooked)	⅓ cup

Unfavorable Carbohydrates (Use in Moderation)

Cooked vegetables

Acorn squash	½ cup
Beans, baked	¼ cup
Beans, refried	¼ cup
Beets, sliced	½ cup
Butternut squash	½ cup
Carrots, sliced	1 cup
Corn	¼ cup
French fries	5 pieces
Lima beans	¼ cup
Parsnips	⅓ cup
Peas	½ cup
Pinto beans	¼ cup
Potato, baked	¼
Potato, boiled	⅓ cup
Potato, mashed	¼ cup
Sweet potato, baked	⅓ cup

Fruits

Banana	⅓
Cantaloupe	¼ melon
Cranberries	¾ cup
Cranberry sauce	3 teaspoons
Dates	2 pieces
Guava	½ cup
Honeydew melon, cubed	⅔ cup
Kumquat	3 pieces
Mango, sliced	⅓ cup
Papaya, cubed	¾ cup
Pineapple, diced	½ cup

Prunes, dried	2
Raisins	1 tablespoon
Watermelon, diced	¾ cup

Fruit juices

Apple juice	⅓ cup
Apple cider	⅓ cup
Cranberry juice	¼ cup
Fruit punch	¼ cup
Grape juice	¼ cup
Grapefruit juice	⅓ cup
Lemon juice	⅓ cup
Lemonade, unsweetened	⅓ cup
Lime juice	⅓ cup
Orange juice	⅓ cup
Pineapple juice	¼ cup
Tomato juice	1 cup
Vegetable juice	¾ cup

Grains and breads

Bagel (small)	¼
Biscuit	½
Bread crumbs	½ oz
Bread, whole-grain	½ slice
Bread, white	½ slice
Breadstick, hard	1 small
Breadstick, soft	½ piece
Buckwheat, dry	½ oz
Bulgar wheat, dry	½ oz
Cereal, breakfast	½ oz
Corn bread	1 square inch piece
Cornstarch	4 teaspoons
Couscous, dry	½ oz
Cracker, graham	1½
Cracker, saltine	4
Cracker, Triscuit	3
Croissant, plain	¼
Crouton	½ oz

Donut, plain	⅓
English muffin	¼
Granola	½ oz
Grits, cooked	⅓ cup
Melba toast	½ oz
Millet, dry	½ oz
Muffin, blueberry (mini)	½
Noodles, egg (cooked)	¼ cup
Pancake (4")	1
Pasta, cooked	¼ cup
Pita bread	¼ pocket
Pita bread (mini)	½ pocket
Popcorn, popped	2 cups
Rice, brown (cooked)	⅕ cup
Rice, long-grain (cooked)	⅓ cup
Rice, white (cooked)	⅕ cup
Rice cake	1
Roll, bulky	¼
Roll, dinner (small)	½
Roll, hamburger	½
Taco shell	1
Tortilla corn (6")	1
Tortilla, flour (8")	½
Waffle	½

Others

Sugar, brown	2 teaspoons
Sugar, granulated	2 teaspoons
Sugar, confectionery	1 tablespoon
Syrup, maple	2 teaspoons
Syrup, pancake	2 teaspoons
Teriyaki sauce	1 tablespoon
Tortilla chips	½ oz

Alcohol

Beer, light	6 oz
Beer, regular	4 oz

Distilled spirits	1 oz
Wine (red or white)	4 oz

Add Some Fat

Now that you have balanced your protein and carbohydrate, you must add some fat. Each of the portions listed below contains 5 grams of fat. The typical female will need to add two 5-gram portions of fat to each meal, while the typical male will need to add approximately three 5-gram portions to each meal.

Best Fats (Rich in Monounsaturated Fats)

Almonds	6
Almond oil	⅔ teaspoon
Avocado	2 tablespoons
Canola oil	⅔ teaspoon
Cashews	6
Guacamole	2 tablespoons
Macadamia nuts	2
Olives, black (medium)	12
Olive oil	⅔ teaspoon
Peanuts	12
Peanut oil	⅔ teaspoon
Peanut butter, natural	1 teaspoon
Pistachios	6
Sesame oil	⅔ teaspoon
Tahini	1 tablespoon

Preparing a Zone meal is now like going to a Chinese restaurant. You choose the appropriate number of protein grams from column A (protein), balance with the appropriate number of carbohydrate portions from column B (carbohydrate), and add the appropriate number of fat grams from column C (fat). If you make your meals like this for a couple of days, you will realize that the eye-and-palm method of balancing your plate provides virtually the same results.

APPENDIX C

ZONE FOOD CHOICES

THE ZONE FOOD BLOCK METHOD

Just as with the "1–2–3" approach to making Zone meals, you can use the Zone Food Block method. Now all you have to do is add up the number of Zone blocks (instead of grams) of fat, protein, and carbohydrate at meals and then stop. For the typical female, this means eating about three Zone blocks of protein, three Zone blocks of carbohydrate, and three Zone blocks of fat at every meal. For the typical male this means consuming about four Zone blocks each of protein, carbohydrate, and fat at each meal. Again, let me emphasize that these numbers are not set in concrete. You may have to do some adjusting for your personal biochemistry, but they will give you a good starting point.

START WITH PROTEIN

I can't emphasize enough that every meal and snack has to have adequate protein, because this will determine the amount of carbohydrate Zone blocks you can have without causing an overproduction of insulin. Listed below are the sizes of various types of protein that contain one Zone block of protein, which is equivalent to 7 grams of protein. Notice this is a slightly different amount than used in the "1–2–3" method.

Low-fat Protein Sources

Meat and Poultry

Beef (range-fed or game)	1 oz
Canadian bacon, lean	1 oz
Chicken breast, skinless	1 oz

Chicken breast, deli	1½ oz
Turkey breast, skinless	1 oz
Turkey breast, deli	1½ oz
Turkey, ground	1½ oz
Turkey bacon	3 strips

Fish and Seafood

Bass (freshwater)	1 oz
Bass (sea)	1½ oz
Calamari	1½ oz
Catfish	1½ oz
Cod	1½ oz
Clams	1½ oz
Crabmeat	1½ oz
Haddock	1½ oz
Lobster	1½ oz
Mackerel	1½ oz
Salmon	1½ oz
Sardines	1 oz
Scallops	1½ oz
Snapper	1½ oz
Trout	1½ oz
Tuna (steak)	1 oz
Tuna, canned in water	1 oz

Eggs and Dairy

Egg whites	2 eggs
Eggs	1 egg
Egg substitutes	¼ cup
Cottage cheese, low-fat	1¼ cup
Low-fat cheese	1 oz
Nonfat cheese	1 oz

Vegetarian

Protein powder	7 grams
Soybean hamburger crumbles	⅓ cup
Soybean Canadian bacon	3 slices
Soybean frozen sausage	1 link

Soybean hamburger	½ patty
Soybean hot dog	1 link
Tofu, extra-firm	2 oz
Tofu, firm	3 oz
Tofu, soft	4 oz

CARBOHYDRATES

Once you have determined the number of Zone blocks of protein you plan to consume for a meal, you have to balance it with carbohydrate. Each Zone block of carbohydrate contains 9 grams of carbohydrate. Notice this is slightly different than the "1–2–3" method. Bear in mind that there are both favorable and unfavorable carbohydrates. The favorable carbohydrates will have the least impact on insulin secretion, whereas unfavorable carbohydrates will have a significantly higher impact even though they contain the same number of grams of carbohydrate. Thus, keep your use of unfavorable carbohydrates to a minimum.

The typical female will need three Zone blocks of carbohydrate at each meal, whereas the typical male will need four Zone blocks of carbohydrate at each meal. The following portion sizes represent one Zone block of carbohydrate.

FAVORABLE CARBOHYDRATES
(USE PRIMARILY)

Cooked Vegetables

Artichoke	4 large
Artichoke hearts	1 cup
Asparagus	12 spears
Beans, green or wax	1½ cups
Beans, black	1/4 cup
Bok choy	3 cups
Broccoli	3 cups
Brussels sprouts	1½ cups
Cabbage (red or green)	3 cups
Cauliflower	4 cups
Chickpeas	¼ cup

Collard greens, chopped	2 cups
Eggplant	1½ cups
Kale	2 cups
Kidney beans	¼ cup
Leeks	1 cup
Lentils	¼ cup
Mushrooms, whole, boiled	2 cups
Onions (all types), chopped, boiled	½ cup
Okra, sliced	1 cup
Sauerkraut	1 cup
Squash, yellow, sliced, boiled	2 cups
Spinach	3½ cups
Swiss chard	2½ cups
Tomato, canned, chopped	1 cup
Tomato, pureed	1½ cup
Tomato sauce	½ cup
Turnip, mashed	1½ cups
Turnip greens, chopped, boiled	4 cups
Zucchini	2 cups

Raw Vegetables

Alfalfa sprouts	10 cups
Bamboo shoots	4 cups
Bean sprouts	3 cups
Beans, green	2 cups
Bell peppers (green or red)	2
Broccoli	4 cups
Brussels sprouts	1½ cups
Cabbage, shredded	4 cups
Cauliflower	4 cups
Celery, sliced	2 cups
Chickpeas	¼ cup
Cucumber (medium)	1½
Endive, chopped	10 cups
Escarole, chopped	10 cups
Jalapeño peppers	2 cups
Lettuce, iceberg	2 heads
Lettuce, romaine, shredded	10 cups

Mushrooms, chopped	4 cups
Onions, chopped	1½ cups
Radishes, sliced	4 cups
Scallions	3 cups
Shallots, diced	1½ cups
Snow peas	1½ cups
Spinach, chopped	20 cups
Tomato	2
Tomato, cherry	2 cups
Tomato, chopped	1½ cups
Water chestnuts	⅓ cup
Watercress	10 cups

Fruits (fresh, frozen, or canned light)

Apple	½
Applesauce (unsweetened)	⅓ cup
Apricots	3
Blackberries	¾ cup
Blueberries	½ cup
Boysenberries	½ cup
Cherries	8
Fruit cocktail, canned in water	⅓ cup
Grapes	½ cup
Grapefruit	½
Kiwi	1
Nectarine	½
Orange	½
Orange, mandarin, canned in water	⅓ cup
Peach	1
Peaches, canned in water	½ cup
Pear	½
Pineapple, cubed	½ cup
Plum	1
Raspberries	1 cup
Strawberries, diced fine	1 cup

Grains

Barley, dry	½ tablespoon

Oatmeal, slow-cooking (dry)	½ oz
Oatmeal, slow-cooking (cooked)	⅓ cup

UNFAVORABLE CARBOHYDRATES (USE IN MODERATION)

Cooked Vegetables

Acorn squash	1½ cup
Beans, baked	¼ cup
Beans, refried	¼ cup
Beets, sliced	½ cup
Butternut squash	½ cup
Carrots, sliced	1 cup
Corn	¼ cup
French fries	5 pieces
Lima beans	¼ cup
Parsnips	⅓ cup
Peas	½ cup
Pinto beans	¼ cup
Potato, baked	¼
Potato, boiled	⅓ cup
Potato, mashed	¼ cup
Sweet potato, baked	⅓ cup

Fruits

Banana	⅓
Cantaloupe	¼ melon
Cranberries	¾ cup
Cranberry sauce	3 teaspoons
Dates	2 pieces
Guava	½ cup
Honeydew melon, cubed	⅔ cup
Kumquat	3 pieces
Mango, sliced	⅓ cup
Papaya, cubed	¾ cup
Pineapple, diced	½ cup
Prunes, dried	2

Raisins	1 tablespoon
Watermelon, diced	¾ cup

Fruit Juices

Apple juice	⅓ cup
Apple cider	⅓ cup
Cranberry juice	¼ cup
Fruit punch	¼ cup
Grape juice	¼ cup
Grapefruit juice	⅓ cup
Lemon juice	⅓ cup
Lemonade, unsweetened	⅓ cup
Lime juice	⅓ cup
Orange juice	⅓ cup
Pineapple juice	¼ cup
Tomato juice	1 cup
Vegetable juice	¾ cup

Grains and Breads

Bagel (small)	¼ cup
Biscuit	½ cup
Bread crumbs	½ oz
Bread, whole-grain	½ slice
Bread, white	½ slice
Bread stick, hard	1 small
Bread stick, soft	½ piece
Buckwheat, dry	½ oz
Bulgar wheat, dry	½ oz
Cereal, breakfast	½ oz
Corn Bread	1 square inch piece
Cornstarch	4 teaspoons
Couscous, dry	½ oz
Cracker, graham	1½
Cracker, saltine	4
Cracker, Triscuit	3
Croissant, plain	¼
Crouton	½ oz
Donut, plain	⅓

English muffin	¼
Granola	½ oz
Grits, cooked	⅓ cup
Melba toast	½ oz
Millet, dry	½ oz
Muffin, blueberry (mini)	½
Noodles, egg (cooked)	¼ cup
Pancake (4")	1
Pasta, cooked	¼ cup
Pita bread	¼ pocket
Pita bread, mini	½ pocket
Popcorn, popped	2 cups
Rice, brown (cooked)	⅕ cup
Rice, long-grain (cooked)	⅓ cup
Rice, white (cooked)	⅕ cup
Rice cake	1
Roll, bulky	¼
Roll, dinner (small)	½
Roll, hamburger	½
Taco shell	1
Tortilla, corn (6")	1
Tortilla, flour (8")	½
Waffle	½

Others

Barbecue sauce	2 tablespoons
Cake (small slice)	⅓
Candy bar (regular)	¼
Catsup	2 tablespoons
Cocktail sauce	2 tablespoons
Cookie (small)	1
Honey	½ tablespoon
Ice cream, regular	¼ cup
Ice cream, premium	⅕ cup
Jam or jelly	2 tablespoons
Plum sauce	1½ tablespoons
Molasses, light	½ tablespoon
Potato chips	1½ oz

Pretzels	½ oz
Relish, pickle	4 teaspoons
Salsa	½ cup
Sugar, brown	2 teaspoons
Sugar, granulated	2 teaspoons
Sugar, confectionery	1 tablespoon
Syrup, maple	2 teaspoons
Syrup, pancake	2 teaspoons
Teriyaki sauce	1 tablespoon
Tortilla chips	½ oz

Alcohol

Beer, light	6 oz
Beer, regular	4 oz
Distilled spirits	1 oz
Wine (red or white)	4 oz

Add Some Fat

Now that you have balanced your protein and carbohydrate Zone blocks, you have to add some fat. Each of these portion sizes of fat contains 3 grams of fat, which is again different from the "1–2–3" method. The typical female will need to add three Zone blocks of fat to each meal, whereas the typical male will need to add approximately four Zone blocks of fat to each meal.

Best Fats (Rich in Monounsaturated Fats)

Almonds	3
Almond oil	⅓ teaspoon
Avocado	1 tablespoon
Canola oil	⅓ teaspoon
Cashews	3
Guacamole	1 tablespoon
Macadamia nuts	1
Olives, black (medium)	4
Olive oil	⅓ teaspoon
Peanuts	6
Peanut oil	⅓ teaspoon

Peanut butter, natural	½ tablespoon
Pistachios	3
Sesame oil	⅓ teaspoon
Tahini	½ tablespoon

Preparing a Zone meal is once again like going to a Chinese restaurant. You choose the appropriate number of Zone blocks from column A (protein), balance with the appropriate number of Zone blocks from column B (carbohydrate), and add the appropriate number of Zone blocks from column C (fat). As with the "1–2–3" method, if you make your meals like this for a couple of days, you will realize that the eye-and-palm method of balancing your plate provides virtually the same results.

BIBLIOGRAPHY

Chapter 1: What Is the Zone?

"Guidelines call more Americans overweight." *Harvard Health Letter* 10:7 (1998).

"New guidelines mean more Americans are overweight." *Mayo Clinic Health Letter* 9:4 (1998).

Sears, B. *The Zone.* New York: ReganBooks, 1995.

Chapter 2: Food and Hormones

Bruning, P.F., J.M.G. Bonfrer, P.A.H. van Noord, A.A.M. Hart, M. de Jong-Bakker, and W.J. Nooijen. "Insulin resistance and breast cancer." *International Journal of Cancer* 52:511–516 (1992).

Depres, J.-P., B. Lamarche, P. Mauriege, B. Cantin, G.R. Dagenais, K.S. Moorjani, and P.J. Lupien. "Hyperinsulinemia as an independent risk factor for ischemic heart disease." *New England Journal of Medicine* 334:952–957 (1996).

Gaziano, J.M., C.H. Hennekens, C.H. O'Donnell, J.L. Breslow, and J.E. Buring. "Fasting triglycerides, high-density lipoproteins, and risk of myocardial infarction." *Circulation* 96:2520–2525 (1997).

Heini, A.F. and R.L. Weinsier. "Divergent trends in obesity and fat intake patterns: An American paradox." *American Journal of Medicine* 102:259–264 (1997).

Hollenbeck, C. and G.M. Reaven. "Variations in insulin stimulated glucose uptake in healthy individuals with normal glucose tolerance." *Journal of Clinical Endocrinology and Metabolism* 64:1169–1173 (1987).

Holmes, M.D., M.J. Stampfer, G.A. Colditz, B. Rosner, D.J. Hunter, and W.C. Willett. "Dietary factors and the survival of women with breast cancer." *Cancer* 86:751–753 (1999).

Lamarch, B., A. Tchernot, P. Mauriege, B. Cantin, P.-J. Lupien, and J.-P. Depres. "Fasting insulin and apolipoprotein B levels and low density particle size as risk factors for ischemic heart disease." *Journal of the American Medical Association* 279: 1955–1961 (1998).

Markovic, T.P., A.B. Jenkins, L.V. Campbell, S.M. Furler, E.W. Kragen, and D.J. Chisholm. "The determinants of glycemic responses to diet restriction and weight loss in obesity and NIDDM." *Diabetes Care* 21:687–694 (1998).

Munger, R.G., J.R. Cerhan, and B.C.-H. Chiu. "Prospective study of dietary protein intake and risk of hip fracture in postmenopausal women." *American Journal of Clinical Nutrition* 69:147–152 (1999).

Pelikonova, T., M. Kohout, J. Base, Z. Stefka, J. Kovar, L. Kerdova, and J. Valek. "Effect of acute hyperinsulinemia on fatty acid composition of serum lipids in non-insulin dependent diabetics and healthy men." *Clinica Chimica Acta* 203:329–337 (1991).

Schapira, D.V., N.B. Kumar, G.H. Lyman, and C.E. Cox. "Abdominal obesity and breast cancer risk." *Annals of Internal Medicine* 112:182–186 (1990).

Sears, B. *The Zone.* New York: ReganBooks, 1995.

Sears, B. *Mastering the Zone.* New York: ReganBooks, 1997.

Sears, B. *Zone-Perfect Meals in Minutes.* New York: ReganBooks, 1997.

Sears, B. *The Anti-Aging Zone.* New York: ReganBooks, 1999.

Stoll, B.A. "Western nutrition and the insulin resistance syndrome: a link to breast cancer." *European Journal of Clinical Nutrition* 53:83–87 (1999).

Stoll, B.A. "Essential fatty acids, insulin resistance, and breast cancer risk." *Nutr Cancer* 31:72–77 (1998).

Chapter 3: Getting Started in the Zone

Ascherio, A., C.H. Hennekens, J.E. Buring, C. Master, M.J. Stampfer, and W.C. Willett. "Trans-fatty acids intake and risk of myocardial infarction." *Circulation* 89:94–101 (1994).

Ascherio, A. and W.C. Willett. "Health effects of trans-fatty acids." *American Journal of Clinical Nutrition* 66:1006S–1010S (1997).

Ascherio, A., M.B. Katan, P.L. Zock, M.J. Stampfer, and W.C. Willett. "Trans-fatty acids and coronary heart disease." *New England Journal of Medicine* 340:1994–1998 (1999).

Sears, B. *The Zone*. New York: ReganBooks, 1995.

Sears, B. *Mastering the Zone*. New York: ReganBooks, 1997.

Sears, B. *Zone-Perfect Meals in Minutes*. New York: ReganBooks, 1997.

Sears, B. *The Anti-Aging Zone*. New York: ReganBooks, 1999.

Sears, B. *The Soy Zone*. New York: ReganBooks, 2000.

Silver, M.J., W. Hoch, J.J. Koesis, C.M. Ingerman, and J.B. Smith. "Arachidonic acid causes sudden death in rabbits." *Science* 183:1035–1037 (1974).

Chapter 4: A Zone Makeover for Your Kitchen

Sears, B. *Zone-Perfect Meals in Minutes*. New York: ReganBooks, 1997.

Chapter 8: The Soy Zone

Kagawa, Y. "Impact of Westernization on the nutrition of Japanese: Changes in physique, cancer, longevity, and centenarians." *Preventive Medicine* 7:205–217 (1978).

Mimura, G., K. Murakami, and M. Gushiken. "Nutritional factors for longevity in Okinawa—present and future." *Nutritional Health* 8:159–163 (1992).

Sears, B. *The Soy Zone*. New York: ReganBooks, 2000.

Weindruch, R. and R.L. Walford. *The Retardation of Aging and Disease by Dietary Restriction*. Springfield, IL: Charles C. Thomas, 1988.

Weindruch, R. "Caloric restriction and aging." *Scientific American* 274: 46–52 (1996).

Chapter 9: The Anti-Aging Zone

Sears, B. *The Anti-Aging Zone*. New York: ReganBooks, 1999.

Chapter 10: Zone Supplements

Sears, B. *Zone-Perfect Meals in Minutes*. New York: ReganBooks, 1997.

Chapter 11: Fine-Tuning the Zone

Sears, B. *Mastering the Zone*. New York: ReganBooks, 1997.

Chapter 13: Frequently Asked Questions

American Heart Association. *Heart and Stroke Facts*. 1997 Statistical Supplement. American Heart Association, Dallas, TX (1998).

Kekwick, A. and G.L.S. Pawan. "Calorie intake in relation to body-weight changes in the obese." *Lancet* ii:155–161 (1956).

Holt, S., J. Brand, C. Soveny, and J. Hansky. "Relationship of satiety to postprandial glycemic, insulin, and cholecystokinin responses." *Appetite* 18:129–141 (1992).

Hunt, J.R., S.K. Gallagher, L.K. Johnson, and G.I. Lykken. "High- versus low-meat diets: effects on zinc absorption, iron status, and calcium, copper, iron, magnesium, manganese, nitrogen, phosphorous, and zinc balance in postmenopausal women." *American Journal of Clinical Nutrition* 62:621–632 (1995).

Mallick, N.P. "Dietary protein and progression of chronic renal disease: Large randomized controlled trial suggest no benefit from restriction." *British Medical Journal* 309:1101–1102 (1994).

Munger, R.G., J.R. Cerhan, and B. Chiu. "Prospective study of dietary protein and risk of hip fracture in postmenopausal women." *American Journal of Clinical Nutrition* 69:147–152 (1999).

Phinney, S.D., P.G. Davis, S.B. Johnson, and R.T. Holman. "Obesity and weight loss alter polyunsaturated metabolism in humans." *American Journal of Clinical Nutrition* 52:831–838 (1991).

Renauld, S. and M. de Lorgeril. "Wine, alcohol, platelets and the French paradox for coronary heart disease." *Lancet* 339:1523–1528 (1992).

Sears, B. *The Zone*. New York: ReganBooks, 1995.

Serra-Majem, L., L. Ribas, R. Tresserras, and L. Salleras. "How could changes in diet explain changes in coronary heart disease mortality in Spain? The Spanish paradox." *American Journal of Clinical Nutrition* 61: 1351S–1359S (1995).

Spencer, H., L. Kramer, M. DeBartolo, C. Morris, and D. Osis. "Further studies on the effect of a high protein diet as meat on calcium metabolism." *American Journal of Clinical Nutrition* 37:924–929 (1983).

Spencer, H., L. Kramer, and D. Osis. "Do protein and phosphorus cause calcium loss?" *Journal of Nutrition* 118:657–660 (1988).

Chapter 14: Why High-Protein Diets Fail

Folsom, A.R., J. Ma, P.G. McGovern, and H. Eckfeldt. "Relation between plasma phospholipid saturated fatty acids and hyperinsulinemia." *Metabolism* 45:223–228 (1996).

Jain, S.K., K. Kannan, and G. Lim. "Ketosis (acetoacetate) can generate oxygen radicals and cause increased lipid peroxidation and growth inhibition in human endothelial cells." *Free Radical Biology and Medicine* 25:1083–1088 (1998).

Jain, S.K., R. McVie, R. Jackson, S.N. Levine, and G. Lim. "Effect of hyperketonemia on plasma lipid peroxidation levels in diabetic patients." *Diabetes Care* 22:1171–1175 (1999).

Jain, S.K. and R. McVie. "Hyperketonemia can increase lipid peroxidation and lower glutathione levels in human erythrocytes in vitro and in Type 1 diabetic patients." *Diabetes* 48:1850–1855 (1999).

Kern, P.A., J.M. Ong, B. Soffan, and J. Carty. "The effects of weight loss on the activity and expression of adipose-tissue lipoprotein lipase in very obese individuals." *New England Journal of Medicine* 322:1053–1059 (1990).

Storlien, L.H., A.B. Jenkins, D.J. Chisholm, W.S. Pascoe, S. Khouri, and E.W. Kraegen. "Influence of dietary fat composition on development of insulin resistance in rats. Relationship to muscle triglyceride and omega-3 fatty acids in muscle phospholipid." *Diabetes* 40:280–289 (1991).

Storlien, L.H., D.A. Pan, A.D. Kriketos, J. O'Connor, I.D. Caterson, G.J. Cooney, A.B. Jenkins, and L.A. Baur. "Skeletal muscle membrane lipids and insulin resistance." *Lipids* 31:S261–265 (1996).

Chapter 15: Scientific Validation of the Zone

Boyko E.J., D.L. Leonetti, R.W. Bergestrom, L. Newell-Morris, and W.Y. Fujimoto. "Low insulin secretion and high-fasting insulin and c-peptide predict increased visceral adiposity." *Diabetes* 45:1010–1015 (1996).

De Lorgeril, M., P. Salen, J.-L. Martin, I. Monjaud, J. Delaye, and N. Mamelle. "Mediterranean diet, traditional risk factors, and rate of cardiovascular complications after myocardial infarction. Final report of the Lyon Diet Heart Study." *Circulation* 99:779–785 (1999).

Depres, J.-P., B. Lamarche, P. Mauriege, B. Cantin, G.R. Dagenais, S. Moorjani, and P.-J. Pupien. "Hyperinsulinemia as an independent risk factor for ischemic heart disease." *New England Journal of Medicine* 334:952–957 (1996).

Gaziano, J.M., C.H. Hennekens, C.H. O'Donnell, J.L. Breslow, and J.E. Buring. "Fasting triglycerides, high-density lipoproteins, and risk of myocardial infarction." *Circulation* 96:2520–2525 (1997).

Haffner, S.M., R.A. Valdez, H.P. Hazuda, B.D. Mitchell, P.A. Morales, and M.P. Stern. "Prospective analysis of the insulin-resistance syndrome (syndrome X)." *Diabetes* 41:715–722 (1992).

Holmes, M.D., M.J. Stampfer, G.A. Colditz, B. Rosner, D.J. Hunter, and W.C. Willett. "Dietary factors and the survival of women with breast cancer." *Cancer* 86:751–753 (1999).

Hu, F.B., M.J. Stampfer, J.E. Manson, E. Rimm, G.A. Colditz, F.E. Speizer, C.H. Hennekens, and W.C. Willett. "Dietary protein and the risk of ischemic heart disease in women." *American Journal of Clinical Nutrition* 70:221–227 (1999).

Lamarch, B., A. Tchernot, P. Mauriege, B. Cantin, P.-J. Lupien, and J.-P. Depres. "Fasting insulin and apolipoprotein B levels and low density particle size as risk factors for ischemic heart disease." *Journal of the American Medical Association* 279: 1955–1961 (1998).

Lee, C.-K., R.G. Klopp, R. Weindruch, and T.A. Prolla. "Gene expression profile of aging and its retardation by caloric restriction." *Science* 285:1390–1393 (1999).

Ludwig, D.S., J.A. Majzoub, A. Al-Zahrani, G.E. Dallal, I. Blanco, and S.B. Roberts. "High glycemic index foods, overeating, and obesity." *Pediatrics* 103:E26 (1999).

Markovic, T.P., A.B. Jenkins, L.V. Campbell, S.M. Furler, E.W. Kraegen, and D.J. Chisholm. "The determinants of glycemic response to diet restriction and weight loss in obesity and NIDDM." *Diabetes Care* 21:687–694 (1998).

Munger, R.G., J.R. Cerhan, and B.C.-H. Chiu. "Prospective study of dietary protein intake and risk of hip fracture in postmenopausal women." *American Journal of Clinical Nutrition* 69:147–152 (1999).

Odeleye O.D., M. de Courten, D.J. Pettit, and E. Ravassin. "Fasting hyperinsulinemia is a predictor of increased body weight gain and obesity in Pima Indian children." *Diabetes* 46:1341–1345 (1997).

Scandinavian Simvastatin Survival Study Group. "Randomized trial of cholesterol lowering in 4,444 patients with coronary heart disease: The Scandinavian simvastatin survival study (4S)." *Lancet* 344:1383–1389 (1994).

Skov, A.R., S. Toubro, B. Ronn, L. Holm, and A. Astrup. "Randomized trial on protein vs carbohydrate in ad libitum fat reduced diet for the treatment of obesity." *International Journal of Obesity* 23:528–536 (1999).

Stamler, J., P. Elliott, H. Kesteloot, R. Nichols, G. Claeys, A.R. Dyer, and M.A. Stamler. "Inverse relation of dietary protein markers with blood pressure." *Circulation* 94:1629–1634 (1996).

Steering Committee of the Physician Health Study Research Group. "Preliminary report findings from the aspirin component of the ongoing physician health study." *New England Journal of Medicine* 320:262–264 (1988).

Zavaroni, I., E. Bonora, M. Pagliara, E. Dall'aglio, L. Luchetti, G. Buonanno, P.A. Bonati, M. Bergonzani, L. Gnudi, M. Passeri, and G. Reaven. "Risk factors for coronary artery disease in healthy persons with hyperinsulinemia and normal glucose tolerance." *New England Journal of Medicine* 320:702–706 (1989).

MASTERING
THE
ZONE

Also by Barry Sears, Ph.D.

THE ZONE

MASTERING
THE
ZONE

THE NEXT STEP IN
ACHIEVING SUPERHEALTH AND
PERMANENT FAT LOSS

Barry Sears, Ph.D.

ReganBooks
An Imprint of HarperCollinsPublishers

HarperCollins books may be purchased for educational, business, or sales promotional use. For information please write: Special Markets Department, HarperCollins Publishers, Inc., 10 East 53rd Street, New York, NY 10022.

FIRST EDITION

Designed by Nancy Singer

Library of Congress Cataloging-in-Publication Data

Sears, Barry, 1947–
    Mastering the zone : the next step in achieving superhealth and permanent
fat loss / Barry Sears.
      p. cm.
    Includes bibliographical references and index.
    ISBN 0-06-039190-1
    1. Weight loss. 2. Nutrition. 3. Health. I. Title.
RM222.2.S389 1997
613.2'5--dc21   96-39111

97 98 99 00 01 ❖/RRD 10 9 8 7 6 5 4 3 2 1

CONTENTS

ACKNOWLEDGMENTS

No book is ever written alone, and this book is no exception. First and foremost I want to thank the thousands of individuals who have been using the principles of the Zone over the last several years. Their feedback has been instrumental in refining the program by identifying pitfalls and offering shortcuts to help make getting into the Zone easier than ever before. Just as important is the patience and support of my family, especially my wife, Lynn Sears, who was instrumental in editing much of this book. Likewise my brother, Doug, who has been my partner and close collaborator over the past fourteen years, as the dietary technology that is the core of the Zone has emerged. Without his support, the concept of the Zone might never have seen the light of day. Special thanks also goes to my first employee, my mother, who finally retired after twenty years of service. She and my brother helped make many of my early concepts take shape into reality. I would also like to thank Sherry Sontag and Jill Sullivan for their valuable editorial comments.

The Zone recipes are the work of Scott C. Lane, who is the Executive Chef and Quality Assurance Manager of one of the major food manufacturing companies in the United States. As a graduate of the Culinary Institute of America and a college instructor in the culinary arts, Scott brings a unique perspective in making great-tasting meals with advanced food technology.

I would be remiss in not thanking Michael and Mary Dan Eades for their fruitful and insightful discussions over the past years about the concept of hyperinsulinemia, and how this medical problem can be addressed at the clinical level. These discussions have significantly helped to refine my dietary concepts on eicosanoid control. More important, we have become extremely close friends during our years together.

My thanks go out as well to Todd Silverstein for his invaluable editorial advice and support and to the rest of the ReganBooks/ HarperCollins team for their hard work on this project.

Finally, I wish to thank Judith Regan, my publisher, for her belief in the Zone, and her continued support in bringing the concept to the public.

PREFACE

I hoped that by writing *The Zone,* I would be taking the first step in unearthing the Rosetta Stone of nutrition on how food affects hormonal response. Furthermore, I hoped to provide a readable summary of my work to other medical researchers, as well as to the lay public, who knew very little about those seemingly mystical and almost magical hormones known as eicosanoids that ultimately control our lives. Frankly, I never expected *The Zone* would sell so well. I am gratified, but still overwhelmed by the response. Yet I realize that many readers of *The Zone* still find it difficult to apply the concepts of the Zone to their daily lives. I hope that *Mastering the Zone* will remove many of those barriers, because in reality, the Zone Diet is incredibly easy to follow on a lifetime basis. *Mastering the Zone* is a compilation of the advice I have given over the years on how to easily integrate the principles of the Zone into your own life, whether you're a cardiovascular patient or a world-class athlete, or somewhere between these extremes.

Obviously, I had a strong personal reason for this quest to understand the Zone: my own health. With a family history of early death from heart disease, I knew I couldn't change my genes, but I could possibly control their expression by manipulation of levels of eicosanoids in my body. Frankly, I was willing to bet my life on the Zone.

Now that I'm forty-nine, the obvious question is, how am I doing? Every cardiovascular indicator says that I have the heart of a twenty-five-year-old. More important, I feel I have uncovered a fundamental pathway to achieving SuperHealth that is easy for everyone to follow. What is SuperHealth? In essence, it is doing everything in your power to squeeze as much quality out of life as possible, and in the process begin to dissociate biological age from chronological age.

Writing both books has been like keeping a personal diary of my own scientific journey toward understanding how food controls hormonal response. I never anticipated the twists and turns of that journey, nor the fact it would take me nearly fourteen years to decipher this Rosetta Stone of nutrition. The Zone is not intuitively obvious, but it is based on a combination of cutting-edge biotechnology and common sense.

I hope that after you read this book, you can say the magic phrase, "I can do this," because if you can, you have taken a major step forward to enhance the quality of your life by achieving SuperHealth. And in my opinion, the only way to achieve SuperHealth is by reaching the Zone and staying there on a lifelong basis.

This book is not intended to replace medical advice or be a substitute for a physician. If you are sick or suspect you are sick, you should see a physician. If you are taking a prescription medication, you should never change diet (for better or worse) without consulting your physician, because any dietary change will affect the metabolism of that prescription drug.

Prevention will always be the best medicine. However, prevention can only be undertaken by the individual, and that includes eating correctly. This is the foundation of a healthy lifestyle. You have to eat, so you might as well eat wisely.

Although this book is about food, the author and publisher expressly disclaim responsibility for any adverse effects arising from the use of nutritional supplements to your diet without appropriate medical supervision.

1

YOUR GRANDMOTHER COULD DO IT. WHY CAN'T YOU?

Mastering the Zone. Sounds very New Age, like Yoda teaching Luke Skywalker about the Force. But it's not. Instead it's very similar to the advice your grandmother gave you about eating. Eat everything in moderation, eat lots of fruits and vegetables, and have some protein at every meal. Your grandmother didn't know it, but she was teaching you the basic principles for developing a life-long strategy of hormonal balance. If you can achieve this hormonal balance, you are well on your way to the Zone.

What is the Zone? It is the balance of hormonal responses that occurs every time you eat. A perfect equilibrium: not too high, not too low. Why should you want to get there? Simply said, if you can keep yourself in the Zone, then you will:

A. think better, because in the Zone you are maintaining stable blood sugar levels,
B. perform better, because being in the Zone allows you to increase oxygen transfer to your muscle cells,
C. look better, because in the Zone you are shedding excess body fat at the fastest possible rate, and
D. never be hungry between meals, because staying in the Zone means your brain is being constantly supplied with its primary fuel: blood sugar.

All these benefits of being in the Zone will emerge within a one- to two-week period if you follow the instructions in this book.

But the best reason to want to stay in the Zone on a lifelong basis is to achieve SuperHealth.

For most people, health is defined as the absence of disease. SuperHealth goes beyond that. In a state of SuperHealth you will reduce the likelihood of developing chronic disease, the types of illnesses that represent the bulk of our health care costs. If you have read *The Zone,* you know that SuperHealth is exactly what you are aiming for. And the only way to obtain SuperHealth is to take control of your diet, and use it to keep yourself in the Zone on a continual basis. The more time you spend in the Zone, the more control you have over the ultimate quality of your life.

When I wrote *The Zone* in 1995, I tried to show that the age-old inherent common sense about dietary balance is really cutting-edge twenty-first-century hormonal control technology that can be mathematically defined with a precision your grandmother never dreamed of. While your grandmother's diet was prepared intuitively, you can do it scientifically.

This book marks the next step on that quest. It will show you how to make a wide range of food choices, from gourmet meals to fast-food drive-thru fare and everything in between, while still staying in the Zone. Although thinking of food hormonally may be revolutionary, eating in the Zone is not. In fact, eating in the Zone is a lot like eating your grandmother's cooking (except for the fast food).

For those of you already in the Zone, this book offers new information on making the Zone part of your lifelong routine, from tips on eating out and shopping, to information about adjusting the Zone Diet to your own body chemistry, to more than a hundred and fifty new Zone meals that will make it easier for you to stay there. For those of you still struggling to reach the Zone, this volume will make your journey much faster and easier.

Once you use these tips, getting into the Zone and staying there becomes second nature because you will be eating the foods you already like to eat and adapting the recipes you currently use every day into great Zone meals.

Let me help you visualize the Zone on a plate: a moderate serving of low-fat protein (such as fish or chicken) with a significant amount of vegetables covered with slivered almonds, and fruit for dessert. Every time you eat, make sure that your carbohydrates come with a protein chaser and a dash of fat. To be a little more precise, for every cup of vegetables, or half a piece of fruit or ¼ cup of pasta that you plan to eat (these serving sizes will be explained later on), add an ounce of low-fat protein like chicken or fish. Then add a bit of monounsaturated fat, like a little olive oil or a few slivered almonds. Do this at every meal and snack, and, presto, you're pretty close to being in the Zone for the next four to six hours. And during that four- to six-hour period, you will be thinking better, performing better, and losing stored body fat—all without hunger. This book will teach you how.

Once you understand what the Zone is and how it works, you will also understand that virtually every dietary recommendation made by the U.S. government and leading nutritional experts is hormonally dead wrong. What is their recommendation? Eat a high-carbohydrate diet. Unfortunately, these authorities seem to have forgotten that the best way to fatten cattle is to feed them excessive amounts of low-fat grain. The best way to fatten humans is also to feed them excessive amounts of low-fat grain, in the form of pasta and bagels. Another popular dietary slogan these days says, "If no fat touches my lips, then no fat reaches my hips." But that is simply not true. Our war on dietary fat really began in earnest fifteen years ago as fat phobia became the norm. And the results are now clear: Americans have become more obese than anyone on the face of the earth.

Obviously, fat was not the enemy. If fat isn't the enemy, then what is? The answer is insulin. It's excess insulin that makes you fat and keeps you fat. And your body produces excessive amounts of insulin when you eat either (1) too many fat-free carbohydrates, or (2) too many calories at a meal. Therefore, when I talk about the Zone, it is really a zone of insulin. Not too high, not too low: a zone of insulin controlled by your diet.

To eat in the Zone is to treat food with the same respect you would give a prescription drug. However, this doesn't mean food must taste like a drug. On the contrary, Zone cooking allows for great-tasting food packed with maximum nutrition. Mastering the Zone is a recipe for lifelong hormonal control, a recipe that pretty much lets you forget about counting calories or grams of fat.

Throughout this book, I will refer to my program as the Zone Diet. Most people think of a diet as a limited time they live in a state of deprivation that allows them to return to old eating habits. The Zone Diet is neither deprivation nor short-term. It is not deprivation because while you're in the Zone, you maintain peak mental and physical performance while consuming the foods you like to eat. And being in the Zone is a lifetime habit, not a short-term fad. The hormonal responses generated by food that allow you to reach the Zone haven't changed for the past 100,000 years, and they are not going to change in your lifetime.

Like any lifestyle change, getting into the Zone takes patience and practice. But within two weeks, if not sooner, you will begin to see a dramatic change in your life. Carbohydrate cravings will be gone, mental focus will be increased, physical performance will be enhanced, and you will lose excess body fat at the fastest possible rate. And you will be well on your way to achieving SuperHealth. That's the kind of lifestyle change anyone should be happy to swallow.

This book is divided into three basic parts. The first describes how to determine your unique protein and carbohydrate requirements and how they work together to form your hormonal carburetor. The second part deals with the construction of balanced Zone meals and contains more than one hundred and fifty new Zone recipes. The final part provides helpful hints that will allow you to stay in the Zone for a lifetime.

If SuperHealth is what you want to achieve, then reaching the Zone and staying there is the way to make it happen. Your grandmother knew this intuitively. Treat this book as a personal user's guide and achieve a precision never imagined by your grandmother. And once you're in the Zone, why would you ever want to leave?

2

YOUR PROTEIN PRESCRIPTION: THE FIRST STEP TO THE ZONE

You're nearly ready to travel toward the Zone, but just as with any trip, some preparation is necessary before you begin the journey. As I said in the first chapter, reaching the Zone is all about insulin control. If you have read *The Zone,* you know that the most important step needed to control insulin is fulfilling your body's unique protein requirements.

Why is protein so important? First, your body requires incoming protein on a continual basis to repair and maintain its critical systems. Your muscles, your immune system, and every enzyme in your body are composed of protein. Every day your body loses protein constantly. Without adequate incoming dietary protein, these critical body functions begin to run down.

But more important, protein is so vital because it stimulates the hormone glucagon. Glucagon has the opposite physiological action to insulin. In fact, glucagon acts as the major governor of excessive insulin production. It is excess insulin that makes you fat, makes you hungry, makes you mentally foggy, decreases your physical performance, and increases the likelihood of chronic disease.

If your goal is to enter the Zone and stay there, then you have to control insulin production, and to do that, protein is the key.

So how much protein should you eat at a meal? Here is the simple answer and handy rule of thumb: **Never consume more low-fat protein in one sitting than you can fit on the palm of your hand.** This means the maximum amount of protein you should eat at a meal is approximately 5 ounces of skinless chicken breast or its equivalent.

Of course, your protein requirement is unique to you and no one else. One size does not fit all. So can you be even more precise about exactly how much protein you need?

The answer is yes, and to make it very easy for you to actually apply, use, and remember just how much protein you need, I have created a nutritional measurement that I call a block. I don't care if you have a Ph.D. in nuclear physics, you probably don't want to have to calculate how many grams of protein you need each day, let alone each meal. But you can apply the block method to any source of protein, be it tofu, tuna, or a steak filet. Your stomach breaks all of them down into simple amino acids for absorption.

My blocks all contain 7 grams of protein. There, I've done the gram counting for you. Now any source of protein is on the same level in terms of amino acid content. Differences in protein density are eliminated. All you have to do is refer to a few simple measurements. One block of protein could be 1 ounce of meat, such as sliced turkey, chicken, or beef. One block of protein could be 1½ ounces of fish, or two egg whites, or ¼ cup of cottage cheese, or 3 ounces of extra-firm tofu. It's all equal to your body. One practical reason I like using blocks is so you can measure the amount of protein you need at each meal on the fingers of one hand.

In Appendix B you will find most of the protein sources (including vegetarian sources) you normally eat, in their appropriate block sizes. With a little practice you'll find that your eyeball becomes a very good judge of protein block size.

Using blocks, you now have a more precise way to determine how much protein is in the food you eat. You can also use blocks to tell you how much protein you need at each meal. **If you are a typical American female, you will need between two and three blocks of protein at every meal, and if you are the typical American male, you will need between three and four blocks of protein at every meal.** This amount of protein is adequate to maintain your muscles and your immune system, but won't exceed your daily requirements.

What if you want even greater precision? First, you have to determine your percent body fat by using the worksheet in

Appendix C. From that you can determine your lean body mass. And from your lean body mass you can begin to figure out exactly how much protein you need every day.

What is lean body mass? You can view your body as consisting of two components. The first is your total fat mass. The other component of your total weight is everything else. This "everything else" component is known as lean body mass. Lean body mass consists of water, muscle, bones, tendons, etc. Your body requires adequate levels of protein to maintain this amount of lean body mass. Obviously, your fat mass doesn't require any incoming dietary protein to maintain it.

Determining your total fat mass can be a downright scary proposition, but you have to do it to establish your starting point. Simply multiply your total weight by your percent body fat. For example, if you weigh 160 pounds and have 25 percent body fat, then your total fat mass will be

$$160 \times 0.25 = 40 \text{ pounds}$$

This means that 40 pounds of pure fat is sitting on your body. Since fat contains 3,500 calories per pound, this means you have approximately 140,000 calories of stored useable fat energy, and this stored energy is the equivalent of the calories in more than 2,000 pancakes!

So to continue the example, if you have 40 pounds of total fat, then what is your lean body mass? Simply subtract your total fat mass (40 pounds) from your total weight (160 pounds). As I said, your fat mass doesn't require any protein to maintain it, only your lean body mass does. So if you weigh 160 pounds and subtract 40 pounds of fat, what is left behind is 120 pounds of lean body mass. This measure gives you half of your Protein Prescription.

The other half of your Protein Prescription is determined by how active you are. Do you primarily watch TV all day (and that includes looking at computer screens all day at work), or are you a world-class athlete working out twice a day? Obviously, the more active you are, the more protein you will need. So we run a continuum from purely sedentary individuals (who only need 0.5 grams of protein per pound of lean body mass per day) to elite athletes (who require double that amount, or 1.0 grams of protein per pound of lean body mass per day). Between those extremes will be your activity level.

To calculate your protein requirements, multiply your lean body mass by your physical activity factor (see below). Now we're finally ready to determine your Protein Prescription: the actual amount of protein that you will require to maintain your lean body mass. Just multiply your lean body mass by your activity factor.

Protein Prescription = Lean Body Mass x Activity Factor

Continuing our example, if you had 120 pounds of lean body mass and were sedentary, you would require 60 grams of protein per day (120 pounds of lean body mass x 0.5 grams of protein/pounds of lean body mass). Now divide that 60 grams of protein by 7 grams of protein per block, and you see that you would require about nine protein blocks per day. On the other hand, if you were an elite athlete with 120 pounds of lean body mass, you would require 120 grams of protein per day (120 pounds of lean body mass x 1.0 grams of protein per pound of lean body mass). Divide that 120 grams of protein by 7 grams of protein per block, and you see that you would require about seventeen protein blocks per day. Note that the number of protein blocks required each day to maintain your lean body mass doesn't depend on your gender, only on your lean body mass and physical activity factor.

Listed below are levels of activity in terms of total weekly exercise so you can determine your own protein requirements.

PHYSICAL ACTIVITY FACTOR	GRAMS OF PROTEIN PER POUND OF LEAN BODY MASS
Sedentary	0.5
Light activity (e.g., walking)	0.6
Moderate activity (1.5 hours per week)	0.7
Active (1.5 to 2.5 hours per week)	0.8
Very active (greater than 2.5 hours per week)	0.9
Elite athlete (or weight training five times per week)	1.0

Keep in mind that people tend to overestimate their physical activity, just as they underestimate how much they actually eat. So here are some guidelines. If you walk 30 minutes a day seven times a week, then consider this light activity. If you work out three days a week for about 30 minutes a day, this would constitute moderate activity (this is about 1.5 hours per week of formal exercise). If you are working out five times a week for about 30 minutes (or about 2.5 hours per week), consider yourself active. If you do weight training at least three times a week in addition to working out for more than 2.5 hours per week, you are in the very active category. And finally, if you work out intensely twice a day, consider yourself an elite athlete.

Here is another key Zone rule: **Never consume any more protein than your body needs to maintain your lean body mass, but never eat less. Eating too little is to subject yourself to protein malnutrition.** In other words, stay in balance.

Now that you have your Protein Prescription, treat it like a prescription for a drug. First, you're going to have to take fairly equal doses throughout the day. If you were taking a hypertensive drug, you wouldn't take 5 mg in the morning, 500 mg at noon, and 250 mg at the evening. At least I hope not. More likely you would take three equal doses to maintain blood levels throughout the day and to maintain a therapeutic zone for the drug. Your Protein Prescription is the same. You're going to spread it throughout the day into three meals and two snacks, just like a prescription drug. In Chapter 6, I will show you how to do just that.

Remember, I am not talking about consuming a lot of protein at any one time. The human body can handle only relatively small amounts of protein at a meal. That amount of protein is a maximum of only about 35 grams (about 5 ounces) of low-fat protein per meal. That amount is about the amount you can fit onto the palm of your hand (remember the first quick Zone rule on protein). Or, now that you know about blocks, you can say that it's five blocks of protein. On the Zone Diet, that amount of protein (even for Olympic athletes) should never be exceeded at any meal. By eating small amounts of protein throughout the day, you are spreading your protein requirement evenly into your body, as if you are using an intravenous drip.

This is not to say you have to eat animal protein to be on the

Zone Diet. On the contrary, there are several great vegetarian sources of protein that you can use on this program. One of the best is firm or extra-firm tofu. Most of the carbohydrate has been fermented out of this type of tofu, making it very protein-rich. (Soft tofu, on the other hand, has not been fermented as much and is much richer in carbohydrate.) In many ways, firm and extra-firm tofu are the vegetarian equivalent of cottage cheese.

Unfortunately, tofu is not very protein-dense, so you have to use a lot (about 3 ounces) to get a block of protein. However, some of the inherent limitations of tofu have been overcome by a new generation of soybean-based imitation meat products that actually taste pretty good. Soybean hamburgers, hot dogs, sausages, etc., are all interesting sources of protein that can provide appropriate levels of protein in a vegetarian diet. Taking this one step further, there is also a new generation of soybean protein powders called soybean protein isolates that are not only very protein-dense but also contain a complete spectrum of amino acids (long one of the criticisms of soybean as a protein source). Adding protein powder to a meal (like stirring it into oatmeal in the morning) can be another great way to improve the hormonal balance of a purely vegetarian menu.

What about other traditional vegetarian sources of protein? Unfortunately, they carry either massive amounts of carbohydrate with them (like beans), or they are not very protein-dense (like broccoli). Furthermore, the high fiber content in such vegetarian sources prevents a significant amount of the protein from being digested. Rather than having to make all these correction factors, just make life easier for yourself and treat beans, broccoli, and other vegetable sources as excellent forms of carbohydrates and forget their protein content.

Knowing how much protein you need is only the first step toward the Zone. A Zone Diet is not a high-protein diet, it is a protein-adequate diet. But to have the Zone Diet work correctly you actually have to consume slightly *more* carbohydrate than protein. And like protein, there are limits on carbohydrate consumption: not too much nor too little. Just *how* much is a question that begs to be answered.

3

CARBOHYDRATES: MANNA FROM HEAVEN?

We are led to believe that carbohydrates are the closest thing to manna from heaven. After all, carbohydrates are fat-free. Just as Americans have become obsessive about fat-free foods, they have simultaneously embraced the idea that eating carbohydrates is next to godliness.

You're told that if you are an athlete, eating them will make you run faster. If you are a cardiovascular patient, they will make you well. If you are fat, eating them will make you thin. Sound familiar? It should, because virtually every nutritional publication in this country espouses the moral superiority of carbohydrates to any food that contains fat, and that includes protein.

Yet many of those millions of Americans who have worshipped at the altar of carbohydrates for the past fifteen years show an amazing degree of ignorance about what carbohydrates actually are. Ask most people, and they will tell you that carbohydrates are pasta, bagels, or sweets. If you look them in the eye and ask them what a fruit or vegetable is, they'll usually respond by telling you it's a fruit or it's a vegetable as if those foods are some unique species just recently discovered in the Amazon rain forest. In fact, fruits and vegetables are also carbohydrates.

As I stated in *The Zone*, people are genetically designed to eat primarily fruits and vegetables as their major source of carbohydrates. Grains as a reliable source of food simply did not exist 10,000 years ago. Consequently, the great majority of individuals have still not genetically adapted to eating high-density forms of carbohydrates, such as grains, starches, bread, and pasta.

Carbohydrates act as powerful drugs, a fact that most people just don't realize. As with any drug, excessive intake will cause side effects. In this case, excessive carbohydrate consumption causes your body to overproduce insulin. And too much insulin can make you fat and sluggish, and it can be dangerous.

Excess insulin acts like a loose cannon on the deck of a ship. Elevated insulin induces foggy thinking by reducing blood sugar levels to the brain (think of how hard it is to concentrate three hours after having eaten a big pasta lunch). Elevated insulin will decrease your overall physical performance. Most important, the biochemical effects from elevated insulin will profoundly affect your health. In fact, elevated insulin is the primary predictor of whether you will have a heart attack.

All that said, I want to make it clear that I am not anti-carbohydrate, but I am pro-balance and pro-moderation with respect to carbohydrates and their effect on insulin. Everyone needs to be keenly aware of the effect of carbohydrates on insulin.

If this sounds like carbohydrate-bashing, then let's go back into history and ask just how good carbohydrates were for ancient civilizations. Before the beginning of agriculture 10,000 years ago, people survived very well by eating low-fat protein and fruits and vegetables. This was the diet of most hunter-gatherer societies. It was only with the beginning of agriculture that people made the corresponding switch to a grain-based diet.

Not surprisingly, many diseases of "modern civilization" appeared during this switch to a grain-based diet. How do we know? The mummies tell us. Ancient Egyptian religion placed a great emphasis on preserving the body of the deceased for the afterlife through mummification. Furthermore, mummification was common in all social classes. What was religion then provides a powerful scientific tool now as mummies give us an excellent physical sampling of ancient Egyptian society.

Ancient Egyptians were the first society to follow a diet similar to the one recommended by the guidelines in the new U.S. food pyramid. They ate lots of bread, some vegetables and fruits, and small amounts of meat in the form of fish and waterfowl, and their only fat came from olives. If there was ever an ideal society to study the effects of a high-carbohydrate, low-fat diet, it would be the ancient Egyptians.

What do the mummies have to tell us? A lot of bad news is found under those wraps. First, many of the diseases that we assume appeared only with the advent of modern civilization were in full bloom in the ancient Egyptian society. Tooth decay is one. Although the Egyptians ate no refined sugar, they suffered from terrible tooth decay. This isn't all that surprising when you realize that chewing bread long enough will release a massive amount of sugar into the mouth.

If you want to do a simple experiment, purchase some diagnostic strips that diabetics use to test sugar in their urine. When these sticks turn blue, a significant amount of sugar is present. Now take a piece of bread and chew it for a few minutes in your mouth. Then place the diabetic sugar strip in your mouth and, presto, the strip turns blue. The enzymes in your mouth are turning the bread into pure sugar. It's not so surprising that the Egyptians had such a high degree of tooth decay. This simple experiment also gives you a good idea of how much sugar rushes into your system after you have eaten a piece of bread or a big pasta meal.

Tooth decay is one thing. What about heart disease? The ancient Egyptian diet is similar to the diet recommended by doctors in the United States today to prevent heart disease. You would think that there should be no trace of heart disease in mummies. Wrong.

Analysis of dissected arteries from mummies indicates extensive signs of advanced heart disease. In fact there are estimates that the extent of heart disease in ancient Egypt wasn't all that different from that in present-day America. Furthermore, the medical texts of ancient Egypt, written nearly 3,500 years ago, leave a clear impression that heart disease was widespread. In those texts are descriptions of the symptoms of a heart attack that could have been written yesterday by the American Heart Association. And if that isn't enough, remember the average age of death in ancient Egypt was far younger than it is today, which means heart disease appeared to be rampant in a much younger population.

Finally, what about obesity? Following the ancient Egyptian diet, it would be virtually impossible for anyone to be fat, right? Wrong again. The excess skin flaps in the midsections of mummies indicate extensive obesity in the ancient Egyptians. Of course, no one has ever seen a fat Egyptian in hieroglyphics. Why? Probably for the same reason that anthropologists 2,000 years from now will never see a fat American female in an unearthed copy of *Cosmopolitan* or *Vogue*. Excess body fat simply didn't play well in ancient Egypt, just as it doesn't play well in present-day America.

As philosopher George Santayana said, "Those who don't learn from history are condemned to repeat it." The Egyptian mummies are history, and it appears that the American public is repeating their fate.

You don't have to rely on the study of ancient Egyptians to come to the same conclusion about excess consumption of grains or starches. For example, a study published in 1996 in *Lancet* demonstrated that Italians who consumed the highest levels of pasta had the highest levels of breast cancer. But nowhere did anyone see a headline in any leading newspaper stating that pasta increases the risk of breast cancer. Obviously, pasta-bashing is politically incorrect.

Furthermore, two other studies from the same research group in Italy indicate that excessive pasta consumption is also linked to increases in colon cancer and stomach cancer. On the other hand, every major study has indicated that people who increased their consumption of fruits and vegetables had reduced rates of cancer and heart disease.

All this leads to the quick Zone rule on carbohydrates: Let most of your carbohydrates come from fruits and vegetables, and use grains, starches, pasta, and bread in moderation. In Table 3–1, carbohydrates are divided into two classes: favorable and unfavorable.

Table 3-1
Carbohydrate Quick List

FAVORABLE	UNFAVORABLE
Fruits	Starches (potatoes, rice, etc.)
Vegetables	Grains (cereals, pasta, bread, etc.)

Now eating more fruits and vegetables and fewer grains, starches, and pasta is a good way to begin heading toward the Zone. But can you become even more precise in controlling insulin? The answer is definitely yes. To start, you'll need a consistent measurement of the amount of carbohydrate in the foods you eat to determine their ability to stimulate insulin secretion. This could be done by measuring calories or grams, but there is a much easier way. Simply apply the block method to carbohydrates. When you redefine carbohydrates into blocks, it becomes very easy to get precisely into the Zone.

Some carbohydrates, such as fruits and vegetables, are not very carbohydrate-dense. In other words you have to eat a lot of them to get the same amount of carbohydrate found in very carbohydrate-dense sources, such as grains, starches, and pasta. By using carbohydrate blocks, you have a simple way to measure the amount of carbohydrate you need to eat, despite different densities of carbohydrates from various sources.

That is true even with the complicating factor of the fiber content of carbohydrates. The amount of insulin your body will produce is based on only the amount of carbohydrate that actually enters into the bloodstream as the simple sugar glucose. Fiber doesn't count. Therefore, when calculating carbohydrate blocks, you subtract the fiber to end up with the actual amount of carbohydrate that actually enters the bloodstream.

And it is only the carbohydrate that actually enters the bloodstream, the *insulin-promoting* carbohydrate, that I count to construct my easy-to-use carbohydrate blocks. For example, 1½ cups of broccoli has the same amount of insulin-promoting carbohydrate as ¼ cup of cooked pasta. Anyone can eat 1 cup of cooked pasta, but eating 6 cups of cooked broccoli is pretty hard work! Yet they both contain the same amount of insulin-promoting carbohydrate. Since the Zone Diet recommends eating primarily fruits and vegetables for its carbohydrate sources, it is a diet that is exceptionally rich in fiber, yet moderate in the amount of insulin-promoting carbohydrates consumed.

Ultimately, all carbohydrate blocks contain 9 grams of insulin-promoting carbohydrate. Why 9 grams? Because 9 grams of insulin-promoting carbohydrate is the exact amount you need to eat to hormonally balance the 7 grams of protein in my definition of a protein block. Now all you have to do is keep the amount of protein blocks equal to the number of carbohydrate blocks at any meal. And you will have an exceptionally easy way to construct Zone meals, as I will show in later chapters.

You can also appreciate that eating most of your carbohydrates from fruits and vegetables will supply not only large amounts of fiber, but also very significant levels of vitamins and minerals for a given amount of insulin-promoting carbohydrate. On the other hand, high-density carbohydrates such as grains, starches, and pasta supply relatively little fiber, vitamins, and minerals for the same given amount of insulin-promoting carbohydrate. I have illustrated this in Table 3-2, which compares the fiber, vitamin, and mineral content of different types of carbohydrate containing the same amount of insulin-promoting carbohydrate.

Table 3-2
Comparison of Fiber, Vitamin, and Mineral Content of Different Carbohydrates Containing One Block of Insulin-Promoting Carbohydrate

CARBOHYDRATE TYPE	FIBER	VITAMIN C	MAGNESIUM	CALCIUM
Favorable				
Broccoli (1½ cups)	3.6 g	55 mg	27 mg	104 mg
Red Pepper (3 peppers)	3.6 g	423 mg	21 mg	21 mg
Strawberries (1 cup)	1.9 g	91 mg	34 mg	45 mg
Orange (½)	1.6 g	40 mg	7 mg	25 mg
Unfavorable				
Pasta (2 ounces dry)	0.3 g	0.5 mg	6 mg	2.5 mg
White Rice (½ ounce dry)	0.1 g	0.0 mg	4 mg	1 mg

It doesn't take a rocket scientist to figure out that you will obtain a lot more fiber, vitamins, and minerals eating favorable carbohydrates (fruits and vegetables) than by eating unfavorable carbohydrates (grains, starches, and pasta). In fact, it's hard to understand why any nutritionist would recommend large amounts of pasta or rice as the base of any healthy diet.

One added complicating factor for carbohydrates is the glycemic index. The higher the glycemic index of a carbohydrate, the faster it enters the bloodstream as sugar. You may have been told in health class that all carbohydrates are either simple or complex. Well, they are in the mouth, but not in your stomach. All carbohydrates, whether simple or complex, have to be broken down into simple sugars before being absorbed by the body and entering the bloodstream. But it was only in 1980 that anyone bothered to ask the seemingly obvious question: "How fast does any carbohydrate actually get into the bloodstream?" The answer is exceedingly important if you're a Type II diabetic. (Indeed, 95 percent of all diabetics are Type II diabetics. They actually make too much insulin, and that's why virtually all of them are overweight.) The answer is also important if you are overweight, as high levels of insulin prevent the use of your stored body fat.

The only simple sugar that can actually enter the bloodstream is glucose, and the faster glucose appears in the bloodstream, the more insulin you make. Therefore, carbohydrates with a high glycemic index will have a greater effect on insulin secretion compared to carbohydrates with a lower glycemic index. The more insulin you make, the worse your diabetic condition becomes if you're a Type II diabetic (or the fatter you become if you happen to be overweight).

You might think that simple carbohydrates would enter the bloodstream faster than complex carbohydrates. When the first experiments were done at the University of Toronto, this often wasn't the case.

Some simple carbohydrates, such as table sugar, enter the bloodstream more slowly than more seemingly dietetically correct breakfast cereals, such as cornflakes. In other cases, it was found that the sugar in ice cream was entering the bloodstream far more slowly than complex carbohydrates found in a bagel. What was going on? It turns out that a lot of things were.

First, let's look at table sugar. Table sugar is composed of half glucose and half fructose, which is quickly broken down into both simple sugars. The glucose half is rapidly absorbed and enters the bloodstream quickly because it is already in the form your body can use. Fructose, although rapidly absorbed, has to be converted into glucose in the liver before it enters the bloodstream in the useable form of glucose. And this is a very slow process. The end result is that the overall rise of blood glucose is retarded. Since fruits primarily contain fructose, they have a very low glycemic index and stimulate insulin production far less than other carbohydrates, such as grains or starches.

For instance, the long-considered dietetically correct breakfast cereal is essentially pure glucose linked by chemical bonds. These bonds are very easily broken in the stomach, allowing glucose to rush into the bloodstream at a faster rate than the carbohydrate from table sugar. Therefore, it is time to rethink what is simple and what is complex.

Then consider ice cream, which also has a low glycemic index. The fat in the ice cream acts like a control rod, slowing the entry of any carbohydrates into the bloodstream. That's why the sugar in ice cream enters the bloodstream at a much slower rate than the glucose in a bagel.

Fiber can also play a role in determining the glycemic index, but not all fiber. There are two types of fiber, soluble and insoluble. Insoluble fiber includes such things as cellulose and bran, whereas soluble fiber includes such things as pectin, which is found in apples. (Remember what your grandmother said about an apple a day.) Soluble fiber represents another type of control rod that slows the rate of entry of any carbohydrate into the bloodstream. The type of fiber you find in a breakfast cereal is insoluble fiber, which has virtually no effect on carbohydrate entry.

Finally, how you cook a carbohydrate will also have a large effect on its glycemic index. The more you cook or process a carbohydrate, the more you break down its cell structure, allowing faster digestion. This is why refried beans have a much higher glycemic index than slightly cooked kidney beans. And when you go to convenience carbohydrates such as instant potatoes and instant rice, the glycemic index is dramatically increased. Obviously you pay a hormonal price for convenience.

And the food with perhaps the highest glycemic index on record? It's those puffed rice cakes, which have become the staple of every dieter on a high-carbohydrate, low-fat program.

Finally, let me say a word about alcohol. For all intents and purposes, the body treats alcohol as if it were a carbohydrate. As a result, any alcohol consumption has to be treated as if you were consuming carbohydrates, and each type of alcohol (wine, beer, or distilled spirits) represents a different carbohydrate block amount (found in Appendix B).

Here's another Zone rule on carbohydrates: Primarily use carbohydrates that are both low-density (thereby providing maximum fiber, vitamins, and minerals) and low-glycemic (so carbohydrates enter the blood at a slow and controlled rate). Conversely, unfavorable carbohydrates are high-density and high-glycemic carbohydrates. This is not to say you can never eat unfavorable carbohydrates, but they should be used with greater moderation, probably no more than a quarter of your total carbohydrate blocks, especially if you are genetically prone to being insulin-sensitive to carbohydrates.

How can you tell your degree of insulin sensitivity to carbohydrates without complicated medical testing? Simply eat a big pasta meal at lunch. If you begin falling asleep by three o'clock in the afternoon, then you are definitely insulin sensitive to carbohydrates.

Bear in mind that being insulin sensitive is very different from having constantly elevated levels of insulin (this is called hyperinsulinemia). When you are hyperinsulinemic, you are fast-tracking yourself to a heart attack. If you have an existing heart condition, you are also probably hyperinsulinemic, and it is likely that you come from that genetic pool of individuals who are genetically prone to producing high levels of insulin in response to any carbohydrate.

Now, of course, your body does need a constant intake of carbohydrate for optimal brain function. Too little carbohydrate in the bloodstream, and your brain will not function efficiently. Too much carbohydrate in the bloodstream, and your body responds by increasing the secretion of insulin to drive down blood sugar to a level too low to allow your brain to function effectively.

What your body needs is a zone of incoming carbohydrate. Not too much, not too little, just like protein. This maintains a zone of insulin. As I have said before, elevated insulin is the reason you get fat and stay fat.

But just how does excess carbohydrate consumption and corresponding insulin secretion increase your body fat? As I said in *The Zone,* insulin is your body's storage and locking hormone. The elevated insulin levels generated from a large carbohydrate meal prevent your body from using any of its stored fat for energy. In other words, it prevents you from burning the fat you already have.

Not only that, but humans can store unlimited amounts of excess calories as fat, and insulin is the key trigger. A unique evolutionary mechanism has evolved to limit our immediate use of incoming dietary fat for energy when excess carbohydrates are available in the bloodstream. Since incoming dietary fat is not used immediately for energy, the elevated presence of insulin (due to higher carbohydrate intake) ensures that the incoming dietary fat is driven into the adipose tissue for future storage: a clever but insidious process in the land where carbohydrate is king. This same evolutionary process is the reason that the combination of fat and excess carbohydrates (like a potato with butter) in a meal can be such an accelerator for fat accumulation.

Fear not. By now you have the beginnings of some very powerful dietary tools (protein, fat, and fiber) to work to decrease insulin secretion caused by carbohydrates. Protein stimulates glucagon, which reduces insulin secretion, and fat and fiber slow down the rate of entry of any carbohydrate to further reduce insulin secretion. Use these tools wisely.

Here is a summary of some simple Zone rules on carbohydrate.

1. Eat primarily low-density carbohydrates, like fruits and most fiber-rich vegetables.
2. Make sure that you consume primarily carbohydrates that have a low glycemic index.
3. Keep track of the total number of carbohydrate blocks that you are consuming in a given meal. By eating low-density carbohydrates, it is very easy to avoid overconsumption of carbohydrate blocks.

And the amount of carbohydrate you need to consume to maintain insulin in a tight zone? That is determined by the amount of protein you require at the same meal. This is the essence of the Zone Diet, the balance of protein and carbohydrates at every meal.

However, you need one last critical ingredient. The most dreaded three-letter word in America: FAT.

4

IT TAKES FAT TO BURN FAT

You're not dreaming. As ironic as it sounds, it does take fat to burn fat. But for this seemingly paradoxical statement to have meaning, you have to be thinking hormonally, not calorically.

How can fat be such an ally in burning your own stored body fat? I'll give you the reasons. First, incoming dietary fat has no effect on insulin. Carbohydrate is the major stimulator of insulin, and even protein can have a slight stimulatory effect on insulin, but fat is a big zero when it comes to insulin stimulation. So eating fat will not cause your body to store more fat.

Second, fat slows down the entry of carbohydrates into the bloodstream. In essence, fat acts like a control rod in a nuclear reactor to prevent an overproduction of insulin. The slower the rate that carbohydrates enter the bloodstream, the lower the insulin production. And the lower the insulin levels, the more likely you are to release stored body fat for energy. So in fact, fat is really your ally in chipping away stored body fat.

Third, fat causes the release of the hormone cholecystokinin (CCK) from the stomach. CCK goes directly to the brain to say, "Stop eating." So in essence, fat is your primary hormonal off-switch for eating.

Therefore, when you take much of the fat out of your diet and replace it with carbohydrate, you not only rob food of its taste, but you distort the hormonal signals that stop you from overconsuming calories, and *increase* your likelihood of storing fat by increasing insulin levels.

I'm not advocating fat gluttony, just recommending that you add enough additional fat to your diet to help your body reduce insulin secretion.

For although fat has no direct effect on insulin, you do want to keep your intake of saturated fat low (but again probably not for the reasons that you might expect). All the membranes in your body operate best in a zone of fluidity. If membranes are too fluid, they don't provide the rigidity required for proper function. They begin to look like a Salvador Dali watch. The body recognizes this fact and will make enough saturated fat to increase the viscosity of the membrane to maintain the necessary fluidity zone even if you are eating no saturated fat at all. On the other hand, if you are eating a lot of saturated fat, the cell membranes become too rigid, and resemble molasses in winter. Since the body has no mechanism to make polyunsaturated fat, it is unable to improve the fluidity of the membrane. In this rigid membrane environment, your body's receptors (especially the insulin receptor) don't function very well, and the body has to pump out more insulin to bring down blood sugar levels. This leads to insulin resistance and eventually hyperinsulinemia. Therefore, it simply makes good sense to keep your saturated fat intake to a minimum.

While reducing saturated fat is strongly recommended, it doesn't mean throwing the baby out with the bathwater. You do need a constant intake of *polyunsaturated* fats, which are the building blocks of eicosanoids.

What are eicosanoids? Simply stated, they are the most powerful hormones in your body. They control every cell, every organ, every system. Only a handful of physicians know about them, let alone the general public. This is because these hormones are extremely short-lived, never travel through the bloodstream, and are all but invisible to scientific study. Yet in a sense they are the molecular glue that holds your body together, and that's why the 1982 Nobel Prize in medicine was awarded for research, which underscores just how important these hormones are.

Eicosanoids are the hormones that will dictate whether you suffer a heart attack, how well you can rally your immune system, whether you have pain or inflammation, plus a myriad of other controlling functions. Yet as with all hormonal systems, their function is a matter of balance. If you have read *The Zone,* you know there are both "good" and "bad" eicosanoids, and you require a balance of both types to maintain SuperHealth. In essence, you want to maintain an eicosanoid zone.

And what can destroy that delicate balance of eicosanoids? An overproduction of insulin. This is why maintaining relatively constant levels of insulin is so important to the Zone Diet. Excessive levels of insulin cause a corresponding overproduction of one particular polyunsaturated fatty acid called arachidonic acid.

Your body needs some arachidonic acid because you will always need some amount of bad eicosanoids to maintain that hormonal balance. However, excessive levels of this fatty acid may be one of the most dangerous events you will ever encounter. Many chronic disease conditions (heart disease, cancer, diabetes, arthritis, etc.) are a consequence of elevated levels of bad eicosanoids derived from arachidonic acid. If you inject a rabbit with high amounts of arachidonic acid, it will be dead within minutes.

And where do you find excessive levels of arachidonic acid? In fatty red meats, egg yolks, and organ meats. Just as you should avoid saturated fats, you should also keep these dietary sources of fat that are rich in arachidonic acid to a minimum.

But simply avoiding dietary sources rich in arachidonic acid is not enough. You should also avoid consuming too much of another kind of polyunsaturated fat, known as omega–6 essential fatty acids. With excessive intake of this type of polyunsaturated fat, you run another risk, as you can potentially begin to overload your system and force it into making too many "bad" eicosanoids and create a hormonal cascade that can hugely undermine your efforts to achieve SuperHealth (see Chapters 4 and 12 on eicosanoids in *The Zone*). This is because excessive levels of omega–6 fatty acids (especially if coupled with high levels of insulin) can eventually increase the levels of arachidonic acid.

What are common sources rich in omega–6 fatty acids? Primarily oils like sunflower, safflower, and soybean. Since you will get all the omega–6 essential fatty acids you need by eating adequate levels of low-fat protein, you want to limit any added dietary fat sources rich in omega–6 fatty acids.

What your body really needs are adequate amounts of another kind of polyunsaturated fats, called omega–3 fatty acids, particularly the most important fatty acid in this family, eicosapentaenoic acid (EPA). EPA helps your body avoid the same negative hormonal cascade that excess intakes of omega–6 fatty acids can trigger. If you are keeping your intake of omega–6 fatty acids low, then you won't need that much EPA (probably only 200–400 mg per day). The best source of EPA is fish (with salmon the richest). Eating adequate amounts of EPA should be a primary dietary goal. If you don't like fish you can always get some EPA in your diet the same way your grandmother did: by taking cod liver oil.

If you are restricting the amounts of saturated fat and arachidonic acid, moderating the amounts of omega–6 polyunsaturated fats, and taking in relatively limited amounts of omega–3 essential fatty acids like EPA, then what type of fat should you eat to help yourself burn fat? The answer is monounsaturated fat. It's a hormonally neutral fat. It has no adverse effect on membrane fluidity. It has no effect on eicosanoids, it's easy to find, and it tastes great. Excellent sources of monounsaturated fat are olives, avocado (especially in the form of guacamole), and certain nuts such as macadamia, pistachio, cashew, and almond. Of course, you may always use olive oil. Besides, who could find fault in the concept of eating macadamia nuts, almonds, olives, and guacamole to burn excess body fat?

As with protein and carbohydrate blocks, there are also fat blocks. A fat block is only 1.5 grams of fat, which translates into one macadamia nut or ⅓ teaspoon of olive oil. As you can see, this is not a program of fat gluttony, but a method of using controlled amounts of fat to get the maximum tuning of what I call your hormonal carburetor.

And it is learning how to use your hormonal carburetor that is the true key to mastering the Zone.

5

YOUR HORMONAL CARBURETOR

To reach the Zone you must keep insulin in a tight range. Not too high, not too low. It's a lot like the carburetor in your car, which balances the gas and air going to your car's engine. Have you ever tried to run a car all on gas or all on air? You can't do it. You need a combination of both to make the engine run. The better you control that ratio of gas to air, the less wear and tear to the engine and thus the greater the mileage you get from your car.

In principle, your body behaves no differently. You can't run the body on all carbohydrate or all protein. You need a combination of both. You need a hormonal carburetor. Unfortunately, your body doesn't come fully installed. That's where the Zone Diet comes in. It keeps insulin in a tight range and things running smoothly, so that you can extend your own mileage.

Since no two people are alike, the range of effective protein-to-carbohydrate ratios for this human hormonal carburetor will vary, but for everyone it has boundaries. These boundaries are based on the ratio of insulin-promoting carbohydrates to absorbable protein consumed at every meal.

For the vast majority of individuals this carburetor works best at a 1:1 ratio of protein to carbohydrate blocks (this is how the block sizes for protein and carbohydrate were chosen). Nobody's hormonal carburetor ranges very far from that. And in Chapter 7, I will show you how to make any slight adjustments you may need.

But first you have to learn how to maintain this carburetor. As with all science, the more precise you are, the better the results. Still, your eye can provide you with a pretty good indicator of how you are doing in terms of hitting this ratio. Not surprisingly, I call this technique the eyeball method. Not as precise as the block method (described below), the eyeball method is easier to follow, especially when dining out. Just use this simple rule: Whatever the amount of low-fat protein you plan to eat, let that size (and really the volume) determine the amount of carbohydrates you're going to eat at the same time. If the carbohydrates you plan to eat are *unfavorable* carbohydrates (grains, starches, pasta, bagels, etc.), then make their volume equal to the volume of the low-fat protein portion you are going to eat. If you plan to eat *favorable* carbohydrates (fruits and vegetables), then you can double the volume of the low-fat protein portion. This method won't give quite the same precision of hormonal control as the block method, but at least your hormonal carburetor will never be too far out of tune.

Now, let's begin learning about the block method. A 1:1 ratio of protein-to-carbohydrate blocks is the equivalent of 7 grams of protein for every 9 grams of insulin-promoting carbohydrates (a protein-to-carbohydrate ratio of about 0.75). Don't let the math scare you. If you follow the techniques given in this book, hitting these ratios to maintain an ideal hormonal balance will become second nature (as will making the needed adjustments). And one of the most important adjustments is to add fat.

For every protein block and carbohydrate block you consume, you should add one fat block. This is not adding a lot of fat, since one fat block is defined as only 1.5 grams of fat, but this extra fat (especially monounsaturated fat) will be key to maintaining the ideal functioning of your hormonal carburetor. It's like going to a Chinese restaurant. Choose one item from column A (protein blocks), one item from column B (carbohydrate blocks), and one item from column C (fat blocks).

When you finish constructing your meal, the number of protein blocks, carbohydrate blocks, and fat blocks on your plate will be the same. So here is the block rule for constructing Zone meals: Always have equal numbers of protein, carbohydrate, and fat blocks at every meal.

Since a carbohydrate block (9 grams) is larger than a protein block (7 grams), you always consume more carbohydrate than protein at every meal on a Zone Diet. Therefore a Zone Diet can't be called a low-carbohydrate diet. Likewise since people are not con-suming excessive amounts of carbohydrates on a Zone Diet, it can't be called a high-carbohydrate diet. I guess the only way to describe a Zone Diet is a carbohydrate-moderate diet. Also, since fat blocks are very low in total fat, the Zone Diet can't be called a high-fat diet. In fact the total amount of fat in a Zone Diet is very low in absolute grams.

Overall moderation is the real key to understanding the Zone. Not too much, not too little. Not too much protein, but not too lit-tle. Not too much fat, but not too little. Not too much carbohydrate, but not too little.

Most diets are actually almost formulated to let you be a glut-ton. High-protein diet advocates say eat all the protein and fat you want, but drastically restrict carbohydrates. High-carbohydrate diet advocates say eat all the carbohydrate you want, but drastically restrict fat. Between both extremes lies the Zone.

Controlling insulin is key to reaching the Zone, but you don't have to give up carbohydrates to achieve this goal as long as you are willing to pay close attention to the ratio of protein and carbo-hydrate blocks at each meal. In fact, in a recent clinical study done at the University of Geneva in 1996, fat loss in patients following what was essentially a Zone Diet was exactly the same as for the patients following a much more restrictive carbohydrate diet, even though insulin levels were much lower in the highly restrictive car-bohydrate diet. This is why the Zone Diet is based more on bal-ance than on elimination. When insulin levels drop too low, many of the negative side effects (fatigue due to electrolyte loss, irritabil-ity, constipation, loss of muscle mass, etc.) associated with the high-protein diets of the 1970s become readily apparent. And this is why the constant balance of protein to carbohydrate at every meal is so important in the Zone Diet.

In many ways, I would liken current extreme diets to the early days of birth control pills, when it was thought that massive amounts of hormones were needed to prevent ovulation. Now we know that far smaller amounts do an excellent job. Likewise, the drastic restriction of carbohydrates will decrease insulin, but you don't have to restrict them nearly as much to lose excess body fat if you pay closer attention to your hormonal carburetor, which you now know is controlled by the protein-to-carbohydrate ratio of the meals you eat.

Finally, what about calories? Don't they count? Well, they do and they don't. Let me explain. Caloric thinking says, "A calorie is a calorie," and since a gram of fat has more than twice the calories of a gram of carbohydrate, the fastest way to reduce calorie intake is to drastically reduce dietary fat. But hormonal thinking says, "A calorie of fat has a different hormonal effect than a calorie of protein, which has a still different hormonal effect than a calorie of carbohydrate." So on the Zone Diet, it's not the number of calories on which you should focus. It's their hormonal effects.

This was demonstrated in a classic study by Kekwick and Pawan at the Middlesex Hospital in London nearly forty years ago. Under hospital-ward conditions, various 1,000-calorie-per-day diets were compared to see their effect on weight loss. If weight loss was simply a matter of calories, then regardless of the makeup of the calories, all patients would have experienced the same weight loss. Yet a 1,000-calorie-per-day diet consisting of 90 percent carbohydrates actually caused the patients to gain weight, while they lost weight on all the other 1,000-calorie-per-day diets that had a much lower carbohydrate content.

The hormonal carburetor also takes care of controlling calorie intake for you. Evolution has equipped us with unique hormonal control mechanisms that tell us to stop eating too many calories. The key player in that hormonal stop is called cholecystokinin, or CCK, and fat is the primary stimulator of CCK. As I said in Chapter 4, by reducing the fat in a meal, you are in essence short-circuiting your "stop eating" hormone.

Sound familiar? It probably does if you are on a high-carbohydrate, low-fat, and low-protein diet. Hungry all the time? Don't think you have enough willpower to stop eating so much? You don't need willpower to stop eating calories, you need science. That's what the Zone Diet is all about.

But also bear in mind that this is not an invitation to caloric gluttony. Excessive consumption of too many calories, no matter how well balanced hormonally, will lead to accumulation of excess body fat. But if you stick to your Protein Prescription (outlined in Chapter 2), it will be virtually impossible to consume too many calories on the Zone Diet because of all the hormonal control systems you are putting in play to stop overconsuming total calories.

In fact, the Zone Diet is a low-calorie diet ranging from 1,000 to 1,600 calories a day for most individuals. Should you be concerned about achieving this seemingly low number of calories on a Zone Diet? No, because, paradoxically, the biggest complaint about the Zone Diet is that people can't eat all their food, particularly if they are consuming most of their carbohydrate blocks in the form of favorable carbohydrates (fruits and vegetables with their low carbohydrate densities). To explain this seeming paradox, I have to go into a little more detail.

As I described in *The Zone*, the average American male or female carries at least 100,000 calories of stored body fat at any one time. Put in perspective, this is equivalent to eating 1,700 pancakes. That's a pretty big meal.

The calories you need are already sitting in your body. You just need a hormonal ATM card to release them. That's what your hormonal carburetor can be viewed as, your internal hormonal ATM card that will help you release some of those "fat pancakes" on your body. If you have the right hormonal ATM card, you won't have to eat as many calories to provide your daily caloric requirements. That is because the rest of the calories you need to fulfill your energy needs will come from those "fat pancakes" (having the right ATM card does assume you are in the Zone). On the other hand, if you don't have the correct hormonal ATM card (because you are eating a high-carbohydrate diet), you'll need to take in more incoming calories. And those 1,700 or more "fat pancakes" already on your body will stay there.

That same hormonal ATM card also lets you maintain relatively constant blood sugar levels by releasing stored carbohydrate from the liver. The end result is that you maintain high levels of mental acuity and focus along with a lack of hunger because the brain is now getting all the blood sugar it needs to function optimally. So once you tune up your hormonal carburetor, you will continually access stored body fat, maintain peak mental alertness, and not be hungry for four to six hours after a meal. Does it sound like it's worthwhile to control that carburetor at every meal? I would like to think so, unless you want to be continually mentally sluggish, perform poorly throughout the day, and risk being constantly over-weight.

Obviously, you want to tap into your caloric bank account only until you reach your ideal weight. A good rule of thumb is that your weight as an adult should be what it was at age eighteen. An even better estimation of an ideal body weight comes from the old (i.e., 1959) Metropolitan Life Tables relating size to weight. As Americans have gotten fatter, the recommended weights on such tables have been moved higher, so the older tables actually give better recommendations.

In reality there is no ideal weight, only an ideal percent body fat. That will be 15 percent for males and 22 percent for females. If you have any question about your body fat, simply stand stark naked in front of a mirror. If you're a male and don't have any "love handles," then you're probably close to 15 percent body fat. If you're a female and you have no "cellulite," then you're probably at about 22 percent body fat. Appendix C provides simple tables to determine your percent body fat.

The Zone Diet is designed as if you were already at your ideal percent body fat because at that point you're maintaining your lean body mass while you have used up your extra "fat pancakes." Once you get to your ideal percent body fat, you don't change your diet, because you've been eating as if you were already there from day one. Since the Zone Diet is controlled by your protein require-ments, the only time you ever change your protein intake is when you change your physical activity level or see a significant change in your lean body mass.

Can you achieve even a lower percent body fat? Of course you can, and should. But it's going to take more effort, and that usually means exercise. And is there a lower limit when your body fat can become too low? Certainly. For most males it's about 7 percent and for females about 13 percent. But now we're talking about world-class athletes. Below these levels of body fat, performance suffers. Individuals in this lower range of body fat will need more incoming calories to prevent their percent body fat from falling below a level at which performance will be compromised.

How do these people increase their calories? Will they add more protein to their diet? No, because their protein consumption is already adequate to maintain their lean body mass. Will they add more carbohydrate to their diet? No, because extra carbohydrate will increase insulin and destroy the delicate hormonal carburetor that they are trying to maintain.

What's left? The answer is that they have to add more fat to their diet. That's right, extra fat. This extra fat acts like a caloric ballast to add more calories to their diet and let them maintain a percent body fat in which their performance is optimal. In fact, some of the elite athletes I work with need nearly 60 percent of their calories as fat to maintain peak performance. But for most elite athletes, their fat content on the Zone Diet will be approximately 40–45 percent of total calories. This extra fat should be primarily monounsaturated fat, and should their body fat begin to increase beyond a determined level, they can simply decrease the amount of extra dietary fat they have begun to eat so that their percent body fat remains at the level at which they perform best.

Before you start buying extra jars of macadamia nuts or bottles of olive oil, remember that we are talking about very lean, highly athletic individuals. Here's a good rule of thumb to determine the level of leanness for males. As mentioned earlier, if you don't have any "love handles," then you are about 15 percent body fat. When you can raise your arm and see your ribs, then you have about 13 percent body fat. At about 10 percent body fat you can clearly see your abdominal muscles. If you're a female, simply add another 7 percentage points to the male numbers at each level of leanness, and the same criteria apply. When you can see your abs (for both males and females), then it's time to start adding more fat to your diet.

And this is the only difference between diets designed for Olympic athletes and Type II diabetics. The Olympic athletes will need more protein (because of their greater lean body mass and higher levels of physical activity) and more fat (to maintain their percent body fat in an ideal range). Other than that their meal plans are virtually the same. In Chapter 8, entitled "A Week in the Zone," you will see these diets laid out in more detail.

So how do you construct meals with the ideal block ratio of protein, carbohydrate, and fat to keep insulin in a tight zone like a drug? The next chapter shows you how. Let's spend a day in the Zone.

6

PUTTING IT ALL TOGETHER: A DAY IN THE ZONE

Constructing Zone meals starts with your individual Protein Prescription. Simply take the blocks of protein you require in the course of a day, and spread these blocks throughout the day like a prescription drug. Your daily meal plan is going to consist of three meals per day and two snacks (each snack containing one block).

Another key to the Zone is timing: Never let more than five hours go by without a Zone meal or snack. The body requires food intake on a relatively precise time schedule, just like taking a drug. This timing will maintain the appropriate hormonal levels throughout the day. For example, if you eat breakfast at 7 A.M., then plan to have lunch no later than noon. Since most people eat dinner at 7 P.M., you will have to have a one-block snack at 5 P.M. as a hormonal "touch-up." Finally, you want to have another hormonal touch-up before you go to bed because you are entering an eight-hour cycle of sleep.

I can't emphasize enough how important this late-night snack is because it sets the stage for the correct hormonal environment to facilitate all the repair processes that take place during sleep. In addition, it prevents any nocturnal hypoglycemia, as your brain still requires a supply of energy throughout the night. In fact, the best time to eat is when you're not hungry, which means your blood sugar levels are being maintained. This is just like determining the best time to take hypertensive medications, which is when your blood pressure is still under control.

Once you know your protein block requirements, the only thing you have to remember is the size of the blocks of the protein sources you like to eat. Just memorize these from Appendix B and use your fingers to keep track at each meal. And since your carbohydrate block requirements are exactly the same number as your protein blocks, you can keep track of those on your other hand. Just make sure those blocks are always in balance.

So let's say you are eating four protein blocks at each meal and one block of protein at each snack (a typical amount for an American male). Your meal schedule would look like this:

	BREAKFAST	LUNCH	AFTERNOON SNACK	DINNER	LATE-NIGHT SNACK
Protein Blocks	4	4	1	4	1

Now for every protein block in a meal or snack, plan to add one carbohydrate block. This will make your meal schedule look like this:

	BREAKFAST	LUNCH	AFTERNOON SNACK	DINNER	LATE-NIGHT SNACK
Protein Blocks	4	4	1	4	1
Carbohydrate Blocks	4	4	1	4	1

So far, it seems pretty easy. Now here is the hardest part for most people to grasp. You have to add fat, especially if you want to lose excess body fat. As paradoxical as that sounds, it's true if you understand hormonal thinking. If you really want to control insulin, you always have to add some extra fat to your meals.

But remember you are eating just enough added fat to tune up your hormonal carburetor. Now your meal schedule is finally complete:

	BREAKFAST	LUNCH	AFTERNOON SNACK	DINNER	LATE-NIGHT SNACK
Protein Blocks	4	4	1	4	1
Carbohydrate Blocks	4	4	1	4	1
Fat Blocks	4	4	1	4	1

By reducing everything you eat to precalculated food blocks, you now have a mathematically precise way of adjusting your hormonal carburetor based on the food you like to eat and therefore *will* eat. This is not based on the food someone else hopes you will eat, but the food you actually like to eat today. Everything is now based on your Protein Prescription. And as you can see, constructing Zone meals is actually pretty simple.

To show you how simple it is, let's look at some examples of four blocks of protein, carbohydrate, and fat. Figure 6–1 shows examples of four blocks of most low-fat protein (I threw the bacon in just to give an example of high-fat protein).

Obviously fourteen strips of bacon is not your best possible protein choice, because (1) it's not very dense in protein, and (2) it car-

Figure 6-1. Summary of Protein Blocks

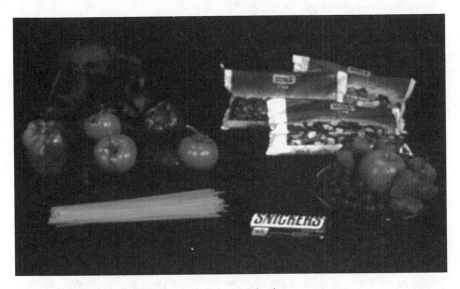

Figure 6-2. Summary of Carbohydrate Blocks

ries a lot of saturated fat, but that is the amount you would require if bacon were your protein choice. The other choices, such as 4 ounces of skinless chicken breast, or 6 ounces of flounder, or 1 cup of egg substitutes, or even 12 ounces of firm tofu, are all better selections. Every one of these choices contains four blocks of protein.

Now that you've chosen your protein for a meal, it's time to choose a carbohydrate that contains four blocks. Possible selections are shown in Figure 6–2.

Obviously, like the bacon, the Snickers bar would not be your best choice, but it does contain four blocks of carbohydrate. If a Snickers bar is not your idea of a great source of carbohydrate, then what about 2 ounces of uncooked pasta? If pasta is your choice, your four blocks doesn't give you much to eat, because 2 ounces would wipe out your carbohydrate allotment for that meal. Could you have made better carbohydrate choices than a Snickers bar or 2 ounces of pasta? Of course. How about the contents of all three bags of the vegetables? Although this would seem like a lot of food (and it is), the high fiber content means that this mass of vegetables contains the same amount of insulin-promoting carbohydrate as the 2 ounces of pasta.

No one in their right mind is going to eat that amount of vegetables, but it does illustrate the differences in insulin-promoting carbohydrate densities of various food sources. Likewise, the other choices (the entire plate of fruit or the massive salad) in Figure 6–2 all contain four blocks of insulin-promoting carbohydrate.

While most people will choose only one protein source per meal, most people will mix and match carbohydrates. Just make sure those carbohydrates don't exceed four blocks. As an example, you could have ¼ cup of cooked pasta, 2 cups of steamed vegetables, and ½ cup of grapes. These are four carbohydrate blocks. Or a large salad a quarter of the size of that shown in Figure 6–2, a cup of steamed vegetables, and half of the fruit plate shown in Figure 6–2. In each case you are simply using blocks to construct the appropriate amount of insulin-promoting carbohydrate to match the amount of low-fat protein to optimize your hormonal carburetor.

If you are thinking hormonally, you know it takes fat to burn fat. So at every meal you want to add some extra fat. You must realize that fat has some very important hormonal consequences. But we want to keep the saturated fat as low as possible on a Zone Diet. That's why high-fat protein choices like the bacon don't make sense. By using low-fat protein choices, you can add monounsaturated fat of your choosing to optimize your hormonal carburetor. A great number of food items contain monounsaturated fat, as shown in Figure 6–3.

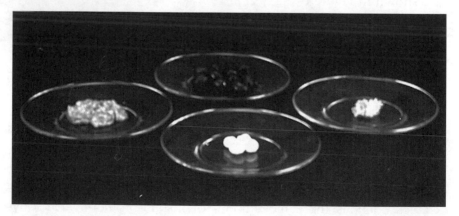

Figure 6-3. Fat Summaries

Each of these fat choices contains four blocks of primarily monounsaturated fat. Remember, fat blocks don't contain that much fat, so you are not talking about adding excessive fat to your meal. Let's start with the world's richest source of monounsaturated fat, macadamia nuts. They are essentially little balls of pure fat. That's why four macadamia nuts equal four fat blocks. Other nuts that are rich in monounsaturated fat are pistachios, cashews, and almonds. That leads us to nut butters like almond butter. Ask many gourmet chefs, and they will tell you that they always cook with almond butter instead of butter. It doesn't burn, and it presents an excellent mouth feel. And two teaspoons of almond butter are equivalent to four fat blocks. If nuts or nut butter are not your cup of tea, try olives. Twelve olives are equivalent to four fat blocks. Or 4 teaspoons of olive oil and vinegar dressing. And finally there is always avocado or my favorite, guacamole. Two tablespoons of guacamole give you four fat blocks.

Let's go back to our figures and construct balanced meals for a person who needs four blocks. It could be fourteen strips of bacon and a single Snickers bar (obviously you don't need to add any extra fat to these choices). Let's try a better choice, like 4 ounces of skinless chicken (four protein blocks), 2 ounces of pasta (four carbohydrate blocks), and four macadamia nuts (four fat blocks). Hormonally it's OK, but your carbohydrate choice isn't too high in vitamins or minerals and there's not much of it on your plate. But if you like pasta that much, then that is all you can have at that meal with that amount of protein. What if we substitute half the fruit plate in Figure 6–2 for half of the pasta? It's still four carbohydrate blocks, but now it represents a better source of vitamins. We're getting there. What if you replaced the remaining pasta with 2 cups of steamed vegetables, and in place of the four macadamia nuts, you add twelve olives to your meal for the monounsaturated fat?

A pretty hearty meal for anyone, yet less than 400 calories, assuming you eat all the vegetables. Can you see why your grandmother told you to eat all your vegetables before you leave the table? If your meal is hormonally balanced every time you eat, then you have to get enough insulin-promoting carbohydrate with each meal to balance off the protein.

What if you are a vegetarian? Simply substitute 12 ounces of firm tofu for the 4 ounces of chicken breast and do a stir fry with the vegetables, layered with twelve split olives. Then have half the fruit plate on the side as dessert. It's easy.

And, as you have seen, you get all the tough science taken care of for you when you work with blocks. All the while you are eating what you like to eat at meals; just remember to maintain the balance of blocks at every meal. Remember, too, that most people will eat a roster of about twenty items at any period in their lives. Just remember the block size of the items you like to eat and will eat. From these twenty items you can construct an infinite number of meals.

Always remind yourself that your protein requirements at a meal dictate the amount of carbohydrate before you get an insulin overload. To make it easier, use the simple one-line table in Figure 6-4.

PROTEIN COURSE	SALAD	ALCOHOL	CARBOHYDRATE MAIN COURSE	DESSERT
_____	_____	_____	_____	_____

Figure 6-4. Simplified Zone Meal Construction Template

Write down the number of protein blocks you plan to eat at your meal. Then start planning the carbohydrate content of your meal. If you want a hearty salad with that meal, then you know that will be equal to one carbohydrate block. If you want some alcohol (wine, beer, or a cocktail) with that meal, then mark down the number of drinks you plan to consume. If you want dessert with that meal, then write down the number of carbohydrate blocks it will contain. Remember that fresh fruit is still the best dessert around.

Add up all the carbohydrate blocks from these side sources of carbohydrates (salad, alcohol, or dessert) and subtract them from the protein blocks. What you have left is the number of carbohydrates remaining for your main course. Obviously if you plan to drink a lot of wine and eat a dessert, there may not be many (if any) carbohydrate blocks left for the main course. But at least you have complete control of how you want to structure a meal.

A slightly more detailed Zone meal construction template was suggested by Jill Sullivan. This template is shown in Figure 6-5 (and can also be found in Appendix D).

	PROTEIN	CARBOHYDRATE	ADDED FAT
Salad			
Protein Course			
Main Carbohydrate Course			
Dessert			
Alcohol			
Total			

Figure 6-5. Detailed Zone Meal Construction Template

For each component of the meal you plan to eat, put in the appropriate number of blocks in the various categories. When you total up all the blocks, they should be in 1:1:1 ratio. Let's say you want to start your meal with a salad. If it is a pretty hearty dinner salad (see Appendix B for some examples), that would be one carbohydrate block. If you plan to add some salad dressing, then simply add the number of fat blocks contained in the dressing in the same category. If you plan to have some alcohol with dinner (like a glass of wine), then put the number of carbohydrate blocks you plan to consume in your total alcohol consumption in its appropriate column. If it's one glass of wine, this will be one carbohydrate block. If it's two glasses of wine, it will be two carbohydrate blocks, and so on. If you plan to have dessert (and fruit is an example of a great dessert), mark down the number of carbohydrate blocks it will contain.

Your protein course will usually consist of your protein requirement. Let's assume that you are having 6 ounces of salmon. That would be four protein blocks. Finally, what's left is to determine the size of your carbohydrate main course, which usually consists of vegetables or some grains or starches. How much salad and dessert you plan to eat plus the amount of alcohol you plan to consume, subtracted from the amount of protein, will determine the size of your carbohydrate main course.

So let's see how this hypothetical meal with 6 ounces of salmon, a glass of wine, a hearty dinner salad with a teaspoon of olive oil and vinegar dressing, and 1½ cups of steamed broccoli to go with your ¾ cup of fresh blueberries for dessert will look on your Zone meal template.

	PROTEIN	CARBOHYDRATE	ADDED FAT
Salad	0	1	1
Protein Course	4	0	0
Main Carbohydrate Course	0	1	0
Dessert	0	1	0
Alcohol	0	1	0
Total	4	4	1

From your template, you can see that the protein and carbohydrate blocks are balanced, but you are still a little short on the fat. Simply add 3 teaspoons of slivered almonds over the salmon. Now all the blocks will be in a 1:1:1 ratio and you have a perfect Zone meal.

Using this simple template, it is virtually impossible not to construct a Zone meal because it prevents you from overconsuming carbohydrates (whatever their source) relative to the amount of protein in that meal, and the template reminds you to add enough extra fat to get the best overall hormonal response for the next four to six hours.

To show you how simple this is, Table 6-1 lists a number of simple Zone meals for a person who needs four protein blocks for each meal.

Table 6-1 Typical Four-Block Zone Meals

PROTEIN	CARBOHYDRATE	ADDED FAT
6 ounces of fish	2 cups of steamed vegetables 1 piece of fruit	4 teaspoons of slivered almonds (mixed with the vegetables)
4 ounces of chicken breast	1 large salad with two tomatoes and two peppers 1 cup of steamed vegetables 1 piece of fruit	4 teaspoons of olive oil and vinegar dressing
2 soybean hamburger patties	2 cups of steamed vegetables 1 piece of fruit ¼ cup of cooked pasta	2 tablespoons of guacamole
1 cup of low-fat cottage cheese	1⅓ cups of cooked oatmeal	four macadamia nuts
Omelette consisting of 6 egg whites and 1 ounce nonfat cheese	¼ cantaloupe 1 cup strawberries 1 cup grapes	1⅓ teaspoons of olive oil (added to the omelette)

The carbohydrates in each of these five meals can be modified infinitely, either by changing the composition of the main carbohydrate course, or by reducing the amount of the main carbohydrate course by adding salads, alcoholic beverages, or dessert. Each of these basic meals can be modified with your Zone meal template. As an example, let's look at the first meal in Table 6-1, with the number of blocks in parentheses.

Table 6-2 Typical Four-Block Meal
Using the Zone Meal Template

	PROTEIN	CARBOHYDRATE	ADDED FAT
Salad	-	-	-
Main Protein Course	6 ounces of fish (4)	-	-
Main Carbohydrate Course	-	2 cups of steamed vegetables (2)	4 teaspoons of slivered almonds (4)
Dessert	-	1 piece of fruit (2)	-
Alcohol	-	-	-
Total	4	4	4

Using the Food Block guides in Appendix B, making substitutions is easy. Furthermore, these five meals in Table 6-1 can be used for breakfast, lunch, or dinner. In fact, it is rare for an individual to eat more than ten different meals at home. Just take the meals you like to eat, determine their block sizes, and then readjust them with the Zone Meal template in Appendix D so that they are in the Zone.

And what about Zone snacks? Typical snacks might include the following:

- 2 ounces of low-fat cottage cheese (¼ cup or approximately 4 tablespoons), ½ piece of fruit, and three sliced olives
- 1 ounce of sliced turkey breast, 1 cup of fruit, and three almonds
- 3 ounces of firm tofu mixed with dry onion soup mix and ⅓ teaspoon of olive oil, and 2 cups of chopped raw vegetables
- 4 ounces of wine with 1 ounce of sliced cheese

That last snack sounds pretty interesting to most people. I'll let you in on a little secret: The French are actually pretty good Zone cooks (as I will explain further in Chapter 12). And the little smidgen of saturated fat in the 1 ounce of cheese is not going to kill you. I have always said, the Zone Diet is a very flexible diet. More importantly, a Zone Diet is real food!

Finally, I want to give you a couple of quick tips as you begin to construct Zone meals and snacks. Try to make all your protein choices low in fat. This will supply adequate levels of essential fatty acids to your body, while reducing your total intake of saturated fat. Make sure most of your carbohydrates come from favorable, low-glycemic and low-density carbohydrates like fruits and vegetables. Finally, when you add fat blocks, make sure they are primarily monounsaturated fat.

Don't get bogged down with attaining absolute precision when you're starting out. Simply ask yourself how you feel for the next four to six hours after a meal. If you have good mental focus and no hunger, then you were in the Zone. So instead of being obsessive about the construction of a Zone meal, pay *very* close attention to how you feel after a Zone meal. How you feel tells you whether that meal was a hormonal winner. If it was, put it into your hormonal winning cookbook that you can go back to over and over again for the same hormonal benefits, just like a drug.

But like your car, sometimes you need a tune-up or adjustment of your hormonal carburetor because not everyone is exactly the same. And here lies the power of the Zone Diet: It can be adjusted with great precision for every individual if you have the rules of how to do it. In the next chapter, I will show you how to become a master mechanic.

7

ADJUSTING YOUR
HORMONAL CARBURETOR

Here's a radical thought: No two people are the same. At least this appears to be a radical thought in certain nutritional circles. The Zone Diet is based on an individual's needs, an individual's likes and tastes. More important, the Zone Diet is based on mathematics (even if it is simple math using blocks) so that it can be adjusted to a particular individual's genetics.

I say genetics because not everyone is genetically the same, especially in the insulin response to a defined intake of carbohydrates. Those genetically lucky ones (about 25 percent of the population) who have a lower insulin response to carbohydrates have a greater "slop factor." They can tolerate more carbohydrates in a meal than the average person before they move out of the Zone. On the other hand, those individuals who have a very high insulin response to carbohydrates have to watch their carbohydrate intake like a hawk.

These genetic variations to the insulin response caused by carbohydrates may be found when you look at various blood groups. For much of human evolutionary time, people were not exposed to high-density carbohydrates, such as grains. Since it takes about 10,000 to 20,000 years for even subtle genetic adaptations to take place in a population, it is not too surprising that individuals with the oldest blood groups are simply not genetically designed to handle high-density carbohydrates.

The oldest blood group is type O, which includes many native tribes such as Australian aborigines, native Hawaiians, and American

Indians. It also includes many people of Northern European ancestry. Individuals with this blood group tend to be very insulin sensitive to carbohydrates, and a high-carbohydrate diet (especially if it is rich in high-gluten grains, like wheat, used to make bread and pasta) tends to be a hormonal disaster for them.

Blood groups AB and B represent more recent genetic variations, and therefore these individuals may have a slightly diminished insulin reaction to carbohydrates. But they are not out of the woods by a long shot if they continue to consume excessive levels of carbohydrates. Finally, individuals with type A blood may represent the genetically lucky ones who can tolerate larger amounts of carbohydrates without severe overproduction of insulin. Maybe 20,000 years from now everyone will be genetically lucky, but not yet.

So how do you begin to adjust your hormonal carburetor? First by knowing when it is in tune. If you have eaten a hormonally correct meal, you won't be hungry for the next four to six hours because you will be maintaining blood sugar levels. For the same biochemical reason, you will have a very sharp mental focus. And here's the best part: You are simultaneously tapping into your stored fat as a virtually unlimited calorie source.

If your last meal put you clearly in the Zone, then mark the exact proportions of that meal in a mental diary because you can always come back to that meal in the exact same proportions again to achieve the same hormonal effect. It's a hormonal winner and one to enshrine in your personal Zone cookbook.

Great, but what happens when the carburetor is out of tune? The first warning sign is that you get hungry before the end of that four-to six-hour time period. But that symptom alone will not tell you if you have produced too much insulin or not enough insulin with your last meal, because in either case you will get hungry within two to three hours after the meal. Why is that? Well, if you are producing *too much* insulin, then blood sugar levels will be driven down, and your mental alertness drops. In other words, you get a loopy feeling. However, if your insulin levels are *too low*, then there is not enough insulin crossing the blood-brain barrier to interact with the hypothalamus to prevent the synthesis of neuropeptide Y, probably the most potent stimulator of appetite. And here is the irony. Although the brain is getting more than adequate amounts of blood sugar and thus retaining excellent mental acuity, you have a growing hunger due to the increase in neuropeptide Y levels in the brain.

So now you can play food detective to retune your carburetor. If you eat a meal and feel hungry and loopy within two to three hours (if not sooner), then that meal contained *too many* carbohydrates relative to the amount of protein. Make a mental note of the number of carbohydrate blocks you ate, and the next time you eat that same meal, maintain the same level of protein blocks, but decrease the number of carbohydrate blocks by one.

Correspondingly, if you are hungry within two to three hours, but maintain a good mental acuity, you have pushed insulin levels too low. Make a mental note of the number of carbohydrate blocks that you ate, and the next time you eat that same meal, maintain the same level of protein blocks, but increase the amount of carbohydrate blocks by one. Figure 7–1 presents these adjustment parameters in a visual format.

This very simple diagnostic chart can be used to continually fine-tune your hormonal carburetor. Regardless of how poor your last meal was, remember that you are only one meal away from getting back into the Zone by using one of your hormonally winning meals from your personal Zone cookbook.

Another way to approach this fine-tuning process is to treat it as a game. People love to play games, because they have defined rules for winning and losing and playing. The Zone Game is no different. It's a great game to play because the payoff occurs within the next four to six hours. And then it's time to play the game again. The goal of the game? Spend more time in the Zone than out of it.

Unlike most games, the Zone Game is a continuum. No matter at what involvement level you play the game, you are going to get some benefits. So to help you along, I have listed some of the basic rules to play this contest in order of increasing skill and precision. The more of the rules you follow, the better the results. Of course, to play the game well you must begin to do some hormonal thinking, and therefore take dietary responsibility in your own hands. But that's easy because on the Zone Diet you are winning along the way.

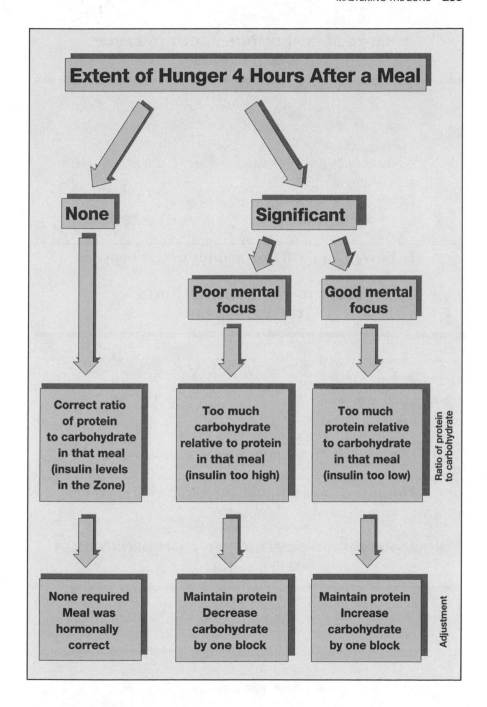

Figure 7-1. Hormonal Adjustment Diagnostic Chart

WHAT-YOUR-GRANDMOTHER-TOLD-YOU RULES
(LEVEL 1: BRONZE)

1. Drink at least 64 ounces of water per day (eight 8-ounce glasses). (Your body is composed of 70 percent water that can be easily lost.)
2. Eat more fruits and vegetables, and less pasta, breads, grains, and starches during the day.
3. Eat more frequent meals with fewer calories.
4. Eat small amounts of low-fat protein at every meal and snack.

The payoff: **You will stop gaining excess body fat.**

BEGIN-TO-PAY-ATTENTION RULES
(LEVEL 2: SILVER)

1. Determine how much protein you require per day and consume that amount.
2. Use the eyeball method to control your ratio of protein to carbohydrate at every meal.
3. Add some extra monounsaturated fat to every meal.
4. Drink 8 ounces of water thirty minutes before a meal.

The payoff: **You are going to start losing excess body fat.**

NOW-I-HAVE-TO-DO-SOME-HORMONAL-THINKING RULES
(LEVEL 3: GOLD)

1. Make sure most of your carbohydrates come from fruits and vegetables, and use grains, starches, pasta, and breads as condiments. Try to keep grains, starches, pasta, and bread to no more than 25 percent of the total carbohydrate consumed at a meal.
2. Never let more than five hours go by without eating a Zone meal or snack.
3. Always eat a Zone breakfast within one hour of rising.

4. Always have a small Zone snack before you go to bed.
5. Always have a small Zone snack thirty minutes before you exercise.

The payoff: **You're in the Zone, and you have done everything possible to achieve SuperHealth.**

Once you know how to tune up your hormonal carburetor, and decide which level of the Zone Game you want to play, then you have complete control of the quality of your life. The better the quality of life you want, the more you have to pay attention to what you eat. Although this may seem like a revelation to most people, it was pretty obvious to your grandmother.

If you put all rules into a simple graphical picture, what you get is the Zone pyramid of eating, which is shown in Figure 7-2.

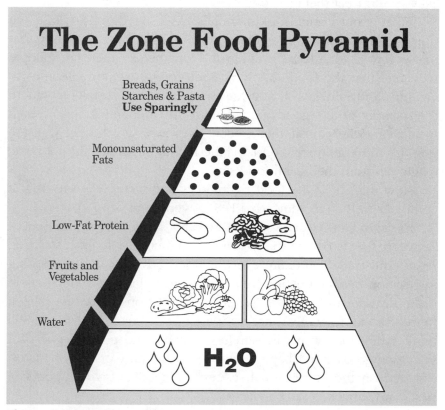

Figure 7-2. Zone Pyramid

You notice the base of the Zone pyramid is water. Your body is 70 percent water, and you need lots of it every day to maintain adequate hydration, especially on a Zone Diet in which you are burning stored body fat instead of incoming carbohydrates for energy. Water is the world's cheapest nutrient, and nobody in America drinks enough of it.

The next step of the Zone pyramid contains fruits and vegetables (the carbohydrates your grandmother told you to eat). The next rung up is low-fat protein. Notice I didn't say meat, just low-fat protein. This category includes tofu or soybean imitation meat products as well as low-fat animal sources. The next rung of the Zone pyramid is monounsaturated fat. This is hormonally neutral fat, and will have no effect on insulin. And finally at the top of the Zone pyramid to be used in moderation are grains, starches, breads, and pasta. The Zone Diet doesn't forbid these items, just asks you to treat them as condiments.

What about vitamins and minerals? As I stated in *The Zone,* the only supplement that is essential on the Zone Diet (and any diet that is low in total fat) is vitamin E. Nonetheless, there are people who feel that the food supply is compromised when it comes to vitamins and minerals. If you feel strongly about supplementation, then simply add a good multivitamin and mineral tablet at each meal. It's a cheap insurance policy. But never let the tail wag the dog. It's the Zone pyramid that is the key to SuperHealth, not some magic pill from the health food store.

Now that the Zone food pyramid is complete, let's see how it compares to the recommended U.S. government's food pyramid.

As you can clearly see, there are some major differences between the two, especially when it comes to grains, starches, pasta, and bread. Virtually every major study has found a strong association between eating fruits and vegetables and reductions in heart disease and cancer. No such correlations have ever been found for eating grains, starches, pasta, and bread. And if you still think eating lots of grains, starches, breads, and pasta is good for you, then go back to Chapter 3 and ask a mummy or read the latest research on the correlation between eating excessive amounts of pasta and cancer.

Now, if you think the rules to the Zone Game are still too hard

The Zone Food Pyramid vs. The USDA Food Pyramid

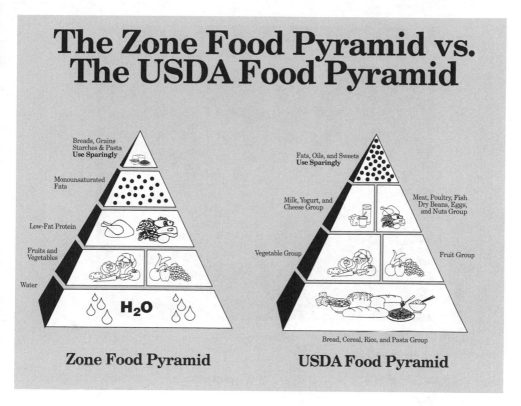

Zone Food Pyramid

Breads, Grains
Starches & Pasta
Use Sparingly

Monounsaturated
Fats

Low-Fat Protein

Fruits and
Vegetables

Water

H₂O

USDA Food Pyramid

Fats, Oils, and Sweets
Use Sparingly

Milk, Yogurt, and
Cheese Group

Meat, Poultry, Fish
Dry Beans, Eggs,
and Nuts Group

Vegetable Group

Fruit Group

Bread, Cereal, Rice, and Pasta Group

Figure 7-3. Zone Food Pyramid versus U.S. Government Food Pyramid

to remember, then simply use your hand and your eye to remind you how to play the Zone Game.

First, look at the palm of your hand and follow these simple steps:

1. Never eat any more low-fat protein than you can fit on the palm of your hand.
2. Let the volume of the low-fat protein you are going to eat determine the volume of the carbohydrates you can eat at the same time. If you're eating unfavorable carbohydrates (grains, starches, pasta, bread, etc.), then you can have the same volume portion as the low-fat protein you're eating. If you're eating favorable carbohydrates (fruits and vegetables), then you can eat double the volume of the low-fat protein portion.

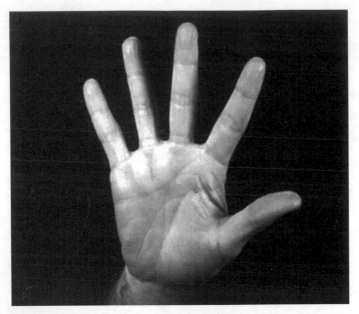

Figure 7-4. Hand Picture

Now look at the fingers on your hand and follow these simple Zone rules:

1. Eat five times a day, divided into three meals and two snacks.
2. Never let more than five hours go by without eating a Zone meal or Zone snack.
3. Try not to eat more than five blocks of any macronutrient (protein, carbohydrate, or fat) per meal.
4. Make sure that the number of carbohydrate blocks on the fingers of one hand is balanced by the number of protein blocks on the other hand at every meal or snack.

FURTHER HELPFUL HINTS

The Zone Game is simple, it's fun to play, and you get an immediate payoff if you win. It's like going to Las Vegas and playing the slot machines. Unlike Las Vegas, where you usually lose but have a good time, you try to win the Zone Game all the time and have a great time. And that's why I want to give you even more helpful tips on how to play this game.

1. Identify your personal Protein Prescription. The foundation for preparing every Zone meal and snack starts with the amount of protein that you decide to put on your plate. Be certain that when your head hits the pillow you have tried your best to consume the entire number of protein blocks that you require for the day.

2. Try having low-fat protein already prepared in your refrigerator. This can be in the form of tuna salad, sliced turkey breast, hard-boiled egg whites, low-fat cottage cheese, or a dip using firm or extra-firm tofu. It's always easy to find carbohydrates for meals or snacks, but a little advance preparation will ensure that you can always find some protein at the same time.

3. Regardless of your protein needs, never consume less than eight protein blocks per day if you're an adult.

4. Map out your daily protein requirements based on the number of protein blocks you need as determined by your Protein Prescription. Plan your Protein Prescription based on your wake-up time. Remember, *try* to eat within one hour after waking—this starts the Zone clock running. Now determine those time points throughout the day when it is necessary to refuel the body. You should never let more than five hours go by without eating, whether you're hungry or not, to maintain and sustain yourself within the Zone. In fact, the best time to eat is when you're not hungry.

5. Use the Food Block guide in Appendix B as a valuable reference tool to reduce the task of meal planning to a simple, easy-to-follow program, which allows you to create an infinite variety of Zone meals and snacks based on foods that you like to eat. Remember, you need only to match the number of protein blocks you consume at any meal or snack with the same number of carbohydrate and fat blocks to get your hormonal carburetor going.

6. Whether you have entered the Zone is ultimately not a question of percentages, totals, amounts, or the glycemic index—it's based

solely on your personal response to a meal. You don't have to be obsessive about constructing Zone meals, but pay very careful attention to how you respond to the meals you do have. Keep a mental diary of your last meal, and look for the following parameters during the next four- to six-hour cycle to determine if that meal puts you in the Zone:

- Lack of hunger.
- Lack of carbohydrate cravings.
- Good mental focus and clarity.
- Good physical energy and performance.

These are all excellent indicators that you're in the Zone. In general, two or more blocks of protein with the correct balance of carbohydrate and fat blocks should generate the desired four- to six-hour response. A one-block snack is good for two to three hours before your next meal or snack. If you're hungry after a meal, then it means you have to readjust the protein-to-carbohydrate ratio of that same meal until it generates the desired responses.

7. After the first two to three days on the Zone Diet, if you sense that you're not experiencing the benefits described earlier during any four- to six-hour interval, you're simply not in the Zone. Remember, you haven't failed, nor has the Zone Diet failed you. It's just that your particular hormonal carburetor may need some fine-tuning. But the protein-to-carbohydrate ratio is usually not to blame. It's often the amount of fat that you're *not* adding back to the diet.

   Remember, dietary fat slows the entry rate of any carbohydrate into the bloodstream. Your success entering the Zone is based on how well you control the entry rates of carbohydrates, both "favorable" and "unfavorable," for the next four- to six-hour interval. View monounsaturated fats in your diet as your ally, not your enemy. If you're having difficulty maintaining the desired four- to six-hour response, then add more monounsaturated fat to your diet at every meal and snack. A block of fat has no effect on insulin levels. Remember, it's insulin, not dietary fat, that makes you fat. This small amount of extra fat will have no effect on your rate of fat loss.

8. Do not forget the critical importance of your late-afternoon snack and especially your late-evening snack. Most people make their

mistakes by not having the late-afternoon snack, thus waiting too long before the evening meal. For example, if you had your afternoon snack at 4:30, and the evening meal is delayed until 8:30, you will begin to exit the Zone before dinner (a one-block snack is good for approximately two to three hours). You are far better off to have a one-block snack at 6:30 to keep you in the Zone until dinnertime, even if you increase the number of total protein blocks that you consume during the day. If you don't have the snack and simply hope for the best at 8:30, you may have completely exited the Zone, and will tend to consume far more carbohydrates than you need, moving you even further away from your goal.

9. Your goal is to spend as many hours of the day as you can in the Zone. Nobody is perfect. If you make a mistake (and we all have bad Zone meals, even bad Zone days), remember you're only four to six hours away from reentering the Zone. This makes the program guilt-free because you realize that you're only one Zone meal or snack away from getting back on track. This is why the late-night snack is so important. Regardless of what happened during the day, your late-night Zone snack will not only nudge you back into the Zone while you sleep, but will literally reset your biochemistry for the next morning.

10. During the first two weeks on the Zone program, try to eat only the favorable carbohydrates (fruits and vegetables). At the end of the first two weeks, reintroduce some of the unfavorable carbohydrates (grains, starches, bread, and pasta), if you desire. It doesn't mean you can't ever eat unfavorable carbohydrates, but they must be consumed in smaller amounts because they are so carbohydrate-dense. If you begin to reintroduce grains and starches and notice a decrease in performance, mental acuity, and appetite suppression, this is a pretty good indicator that you are very carbohydrate sensitive. Grains and starches should never be your primary carbohydrate source at a meal and ideally never more than 25 percent of your total carbohydrate content at a meal. It will be the balance of favorable and unfavorable carbohydrates that determines what volume of carbohydrates can be eaten with the amount of protein you plan to consume at the same meal.

11. Your primary concern is to maintain the desired four- to six-hour response regardless of the carbohydrate source. Learn to play food detective. For example, if you're not hungry before a meal, and then find yourself craving sugars and sweets two hours after a meal, you probably consumed too many carbohydrates or the wrong type of carbohydrate during your last meal.

12. Try to develop a hormonally winning cookbook. Every time you make a meal that leaves you satiated with a good mental focus for the next four to six hours, write it down. You can always come back to that meal in the exact same proportions, like a drug, to get the same hormonal effect in the future. Remember, most people will eat only twenty food items in their entire life, and eat only ten meals repetitively. Take those twenty food items you like to eat to construct an infinite number of hormonally winning Zone meals. Change the effect on your hormonal carburetor of each of your ten favorite meals into hormonal winners. For your favorite recipes like Aunt Millie's succotash, just keep tweaking the composition of that meal until you reach the Zone using the criteria in helpful hint number six. Now you have Aunt Millie's hormonally correct succotash.

13. Eat your protein portion first. Since protein stimulates glucagon, this hormone will cause the release of stored carbohydrate in the liver to keep your brain satisfied, thereby making it easy to control the carbohydrate intake. Furthermore, glucagon depresses insulin secretion, making protein your most powerful tool in controlling insulin levels.

14. Drink an 8-ounce glass of water about thirty minutes before a meal or snack. This not only decreases your hunger, but also is a good way to get the water you need on the Zone diet. Remember, on a fat-burning diet, you will need nearly 50 percent more water than you would have needed on a high-carbohydrate diet. Just as excess insulin makes your body hold on to fat, excess insulin causes water retention. As you lower insulin levels, you need to replace any water that your body is no longer retaining. This means at least eight 8-ounce glasses of water or other suitable beverages per day. Water is the cheapest nutrient on earth, yet no one drinks enough of it.

15. Chew your food thoroughly before swallowing. Does this sound like your grandmother again? Well, she was right. An intricate part of the overall digestive process begins in your mouth with the secretion of enzymes in the saliva. Remember, it's not the amount of food you eat, but the amount that is absorbed. As you age, your digestive capacity will decrease. Therefore, make every use of what you have. Furthermore, by chewing slowly, you are giving the macronutrients time to get into the bloodstream to begin generating some of those hormonal "stop eating" signals.

16. Sit down and eat, just as your grandmother always told you. You're more likely to eat less rapidly, and you might actually engage in some conversation, which allows even more time for the food to enter the bloodstream and more time for those hormonal "stop eating" signals to be sent to the brain.

17. Special Troubleshooting Hint. If all else fails, simply read *The Zone* again. Remember, *The Zone* is your dietary road map, and it takes time to learn its lessons. The principles of the Zone are not obvious. Treat it like a textbook: Mark it up, put comments in the margins, use different colored markers to highlight key passages. The more often you revisit *The Zone,* the easier it is to follow the program on a lifetime basis.

8

A WEEK IN THE ZONE

Now that you know how to spend a day in the Zone and have learned how to make adjustments to your hormonal carburetor, how about spending a week there? Earlier, I said that the Zone Diet is remarkably similar for both average individuals and elite, world-class athletes like Olympians. The only difference between the two populations is that the world-class athletes will require more protein (and therefore more carbohydrates) and significantly *more fat* than average individuals. As you will see, however, the strategy both these groups should use to get into the Zone is almost identical.

To show you how similar, let's compare a week of diets for (1) a typical American female who requires three blocks per meal, (2) a typical American male who requires four blocks per meal, (3) a typical female Olympian who requires five blocks per meal, and (4) a typical male Olympian who requires six blocks per meal. In addition, all these people would be eating two one-block snacks, one as a late-afternoon snack and the other as a late-night snack.

The first thing that should strike you as you read these menus is that they consist of the kinds of everyday foods you already eat. The second thing is that you may find it *hard* to eat all the food. And the third thing is, paradoxically, you may be surprised to know that these meals are all low calorie. They are low calorie because they take advantage of using primarily low-density carbohydrates. As an example, a typical four-block meal contains about 400 calories.

Notice that each of these menus is broken into protein, carbohydrate, and fat blocks so that substitutions can by made by using the Food Block guide in Appendix B. If your own block requirements are slightly different, make a corresponding adjustment either up or down in the proportions. For example, if you need five blocks per meal but like the four-block meal, simply increase the size of each component by about a third. On the other hand, if you need only two blocks but like a three-block meal, then decrease the size of each component in the recipe by about a third.

DAY ONE FOR THE TYPICAL AMERICAN FEMALE (THREE BLOCKS PER MEAL)

Breakfast—Scrambled Eggs

Protein:	4 egg whites or ½ cup egg substitute
	1 ounce nonfat cheese, shredded
Carbohydrate:	1 cup grapes
	½ piece rye toast
Fat:	⅔ teaspoon olive oil
	½ teaspoon fresh-ground or natural peanut butter

Cooking Instructions

Spray nonstick pan with vegetable spray. Beat eggs and shredded nonfat cheese with olive oil and add a little milk if desired. Then scramble.

Lunch—Seafood Salad Sandwich

Protein:	4½ ounces seafood (shrimp, crabmeat, or lobster)
Carbohydrate:	1 small side salad
	1 apple
	½ mini pita pocket
Fat:	1 tablespoon light mayonnaise

Note: For even better results, you can replace the mini pita pocket with a larger salad containing sliced tomatoes, green peppers, and onions (see Food Block guide), or substitute another piece of fruit. This substitution can be made for any meal that contains rye bread or a mini pita pocket. You can also substitute 1 tablespoon olive oil and vinegar dressing for the mayonnaise.

Cooking Instructions

Mix seafood with mayonnaise. Stuff into a mini pita pocket.

Afternoon Snack

> 1 ounce low-fat cheese
> ½ orange

Dinner—Chili

Protein: 4½ ounces lean ground meat
                        (beef or turkey)
                        Sprinkling of shredded nonfat
                        cheese

Carbohydrate: Minced onions, chopped
                        mushrooms, and chopped
                        green bell pepper to taste
                        Chili powder, oregano, and
                        pepper to taste
                        ¼ cup kidney beans
                        1 cup tomatoes, crushed
                        1 peach

Fat: 1 tcaspoon olive oil

Cooking Instructions

Brown meat in the olive oil with onions, mushrooms, green pepper, and spices, stirring often. Add kidney beans and tomatoes. Simmer 30 minutes or until beans are tender, stirring occasionally. Top with shredded cheese. Have the peach for dessert.

Late-Night Snack

> 1 ounce turkey breast, sliced
> 1 cup strawberries
> 6 peanuts

DAY TWO FOR THE TYPICAL AMERICAN FEMALE

Breakfast—Old-Fashioned Oatmeal and Bacon

Protein:	2 tablespoons protein powder (supplying 14 grams of protein)
	1 ounce Canadian bacon
Carbohydrate:	1 cup dry oatmeal plus 2 cups water
	Nutmeg and cinnamon to taste
Fat:	1 tablespoon slivered almonds

Cooking Instructions

Cook oatmeal according to package directions. After cooling, stir in protein powder and spices and top with slivered almonds. Cook Canadian bacon separately.

Lunch—Cheeseburger

Protein:	4½ ounces lean hamburger meat (less than 10 percent fat)
	1 slice reduced-fat cheese
Carbohydrate:	Tomato slice, lettuce leaf, and onion slice
	1 piece rye bread
	½ apple
Fat:	6 peanuts

Cooking Instructions

Broil hamburger to preferred degree of doneness (about 5 minutes per side for medium). Place cheese on top and broil hamburger until cheese is melted. Put cheeseburger together with the tomato, lettuce, and onion. Have the apple and peanuts for dessert.

Afternoon Snack

3 ounces firm tofu mixed with
⅓ teaspoon olive oil and
sprinkling of onion soup mix
1½ cups broccoli and green
peppers, cut for dipping

Dinner—Barbecued Chicken

Protein: 3 ounces skinless chicken
                                 breast
Carbohydrate: Lemon slices
                                 Onion slices
                                 ½ teaspoon barbecue sauce
                                 1½ cups steamed cauliflower
                                 1 spinach salad (see Food
                                 Block guide)
                                 1 cup strawberries for dessert
Fat: 1 tablespoon olive oil and
                                 vinegar dressing

Cooking Instructions

Preheat oven to 450 degrees. Cover the chicken breast with slices of lemon and onion. Bake for 15 minutes. Reduce heat to 350 degrees. Baste with barbecue sauce. Cook for 10–15 minutes or until done.

Late-Night Snack

1 ounce reduced-fat cheese
1 peach
3 olives

DAY THREE FOR THE TYPICAL AMERICAN FEMALE

Breakfast—Fruit Salad

Protein:	¾ cup low-fat cottage cheese
Carbohydrate:	1 cup strawberries
	¾ cup cantaloupe, cubed
	½ cup grapes
Fat:	3 macadamia nuts, crushed

Cooking Instructions
Mix together and enjoy.

Lunch—Chef Salad

Protein:	1½ ounces deli-style ham
	1½ ounces deli-style turkey breast
	1 ounce reduced-fat cheese
Carbohydrate:	1 large tossed green salad (see Food Block guide)
	1 nectarine for dessert
Fat:	1 tablespoon olive oil and vinegar dressing

Afternoon Snack

¼ cup low-fat cottage cheese mixed with ½ cup diced pineapple

Dinner—Foiled Fish

Protein:	4½ ounces fish fillet of your choice (flounder is suggested)
Carbohydrate:	Freshly ground pepper to taste
	Squirt of lemon juice
	Onion to taste, chopped
	1 cup cooked asparagus
	1 tossed salad (see Food Block guide)

	1 plum for dessert
Fat:	1 tablespoon olive oil and
	vinegar dressing
	Sprinkling of Parmesan cheese

Cooking Instructions

Tear off a good-sized piece of foil. Spray the center lightly with vegetable spray. Put the fish in the center of the foil with the onion, pepper, lemon juice, and cheese. Fold foil over the fish, leaving space around the fish. Carefully turn up and seal the sides and the middle so that juices don't leak out. Bake in a 425-degree oven for 18 minutes. When done, carefully open the foil to prevent steam burns.

Late-Night Snack

1 ounce turkey breast, sliced
½ cup grapes
1 macadamia nut

DAY FOUR FOR THE TYPICAL AMERICAN FEMALE

Breakfast—Yogurt and Fruit

Protein:	1 cup plain low-fat yogurt
	1 ounce lean Canadian bacon
Carbohydrate:	1 cup strawberries
Fat:	1 tablespoon slivered almonds

Cooking Instructions

Mix fruit with yogurt and top with slivered almonds. Cook Canadian bacon separately.

Lunch—Grilled Chicken Salad

Protein:	3 ounces grilled chicken
Carbohydrate:	2 cups romaine lettuce
	¼ cup mushrooms, sliced

¼ cup tomatoes, sliced
¼ cup onions, chopped
Lemon juice to taste
Garlic powder
Dash Worcestershire sauce
Pepper to taste
Sprinkling of Parmesan cheese
1 orange

Fat: 1 tablespoon olive oil and
                       vinegar dressing

Cooking Instructions

Prepare the salad. Drizzle salad dressing over the salad. Squeeze the lemon over the salad. Season with garlic powder and Worcestershire sauce, and grind in fresh pepper. Toss until well combined. Place grilled chicken on top and sprinkle cheese. Have the orange for dessert.

Afternoon Snack

1 ounce cheese
½ apple

Dinner—Pork Medallions and Apples

Protein: 3 ounces pork medallions or
                       thinly sliced pork chops

Carbohydrate: ½ apple, sliced
                       Rosemary to taste
                       Dijon mustard to taste
                       1 tablespoon white wine
                       ¼ cup water
                       1½ cups steamed broccoli
                       1 spinach salad (see Food
                          Block guide)

Fat: 1 tablespoon olive oil and
                       vinegar dressing

Cooking Instructions

Put pork into baking dish in a single layer. Top with apple slices, rosemary, and mustard. Pour wine and water around the pork. Bake at 450 degrees for 15 minutes. Baste the pork with pan juices. Reduce heat to 350 degrees and continue cooking for 10–15 minutes or until pork is white, not pink, inside.

Late-Night Snack

> 1 ounce soft cheese
> 4 ounces red wine

DAY FIVE FOR THE TYPICAL AMERICAN FEMALE

Breakfast—French Toast Sticks

Protein:	4 egg whites or ½ cup egg substitute
	1 ounce extra-lean Canadian bacon
Carbohydrate:	1 slice whole grain bread
	1 cup strawberries, sliced
Fat:	1 tablespoon slivered almonds

Cooking Instructions

Cook the Canadian bacon separately. Cut bread into sticks and soak in beaten eggs. (Scramble any egg mixture that remains.) Spray a nonstick pan with vegetable spray. Over medium-low heat, cook breadsticks, turning often, until done. Top with sliced strawberries and slivered almonds.

Lunch—Chicken Salad Sandwich

Protein:	3 ounces cooked chicken breast, shredded
Carbohydrate:	Celery, chopped
	½ cup grapes
	Lettuce
	Tomato slice

1 piece rye bread or 1 mini
pita pocket

Fat: 1 tablespoon light mayonnaise

Cooking Instructions

Mix shredded chicken with mayonnaise, celery, and grapes. Put into mini pita pocket and add lettuce and tomato slice.

Afternoon Snack

½ tablespoon guacamole
wrapped in 1 ounce sliced
turkey
½ cup grapes

Dinner—Meatloaf

Protein: 4½ ounces lean ground beef
(less than 10 percent fat) or
ground turkey
2 tablespoons egg substitute

Carbohydrate: 1 tablespoon ketchup
¼ cup onions, chopped
1 teaspoon bread crumbs
Pepper to taste
Dash Worcestershire sauce
1½ cups cooked zucchini
½ apple
1 tossed salad (see Food Block
guide)

Fat: 1 tablespoon olive oil and
vinegar dressing

Cooking Instructions

Mix ground meat, egg substitute, ketchup, onions, bread crumbs, pepper, and Worcestershire sauce. Form into a shallow loaf and place in microwave-safe dish. Cover with waxed paper. Microwave on medium for 10–15 minutes or until done. Have the zucchini as a side dish and eat the apple for dessert.

Late-Night Snack

1 ounce turkey breast, sliced
1 cup strawberries
3 almonds

DAY SIX FOR THE TYPICAL AMERICAN FEMALE

Breakfast—Skillet Hash

Protein: 3 ounces cooked lean ham,
                            chicken, or beef
Carbohydrate: ⅓ cup cooked potato, diced
                        1 cup tomato, chopped
                        Green bell pepper, onions, and
                            mushrooms to taste,
                            chopped
                        Salt and pepper to taste
                        Dash Worcestershire sauce
                        ¼ cantaloupe
Fat: 1 teaspoon olive oil

Cooking Instructions

In a nonstick pan, sauté green pepper, onions, and mushrooms in olive oil until tender. Add cooked meat, potato, vegetables, spices, and Worcestershire sauce. Cook, stirring, until heated through. Have cantaloupe as side dish.

Lunch—BLT Sandwich

Protein: 2 ounces cooked extra-lean
                            Canadian bacon
                        1 ounce nonfat cheese
Carbohydrate: 1 slice rye bread
                        Lettuce and sliced tomato
                        ½ orange
Fat: 1 teaspoon light mayonnaise
                        6 olives

Afternoon Snack

> 2 ounces low-fat cottage cheese
> ½ cup pineapple, diced
> 1 teaspoon slivered almonds

Dinner—Quick Turkey Dinner

Protein:	4½ ounces deli-style turkey breast or 3 ounces cooked skinless turkey breast
Carbohydrate:	1½ cups steamed broccoli
	½ cup boiled and drained onions
	½ cup cranberries
Fat:	1 tablespoon slivered almonds (sprinkled on the broccoli)

Late-Night Snack

> 1 ounce turkey breast, sliced
> 1 cup strawberries
> 3 olives

DAY SEVEN FOR THE TYPICAL AMERICAN FEMALE

Breakfast—Scrambled Eggs Benedict

Protein:	1 ounce lean Canadian bacon
	4 large egg whites or ½ cup egg substitute
Carbohydrate:	½ English muffin
	½ grapefruit
Fat:	1 teaspoon olive oil

Cooking Instructions

Beat egg whites and olive oil with a little milk if desired. Spray a nonstick pan with vegetable spray and then scramble the eggs. Toast the English muffin. Cook the Canadian bacon, place on the toasted muffin, and top with the eggs.

Lunch—Turkey in a Pocket

Protein: 4½ ounces deli-style turkey
                                 breast or 3 ounces cooked
                                 turkey breast
Carbohydrate: 1 mini pita pocket
                                 ½ green bell pepper, chopped
                                 1 plum
Fat: 1½ tablespoons guacamole

Afternoon Snack

                                 2 hard-boiled egg whites
                                 ½ apple
                                 3 almonds

Dinner—Broiled Salmon

Protein: 4½ ounces salmon fillet
Carbohydrate: Rosemary to taste
                                 Tarragon to taste
                                 Dill to taste
                                 Lemon (optional)
                                 1 cup cooked zucchini
                                 2 tomatoes, split, sprinkled with
                                 Parmesan cheese, and broiled
                                 ½ apple for dessert
Fat: 1 teaspoon olive oil

Cooking Instructions

Rub the fillet with the herbs and then brush with olive oil. Broil for 10 minutes per inch of thickness, turning and basting once. Garnish with lemon if desired. Have the apple for dessert.

Late-Night Snack

                                 1 ounce turkey breast, sliced
                                 1 cup strawberries
                                 ½ tablespoon guacamole

DAY ONE FOR THE TYPICAL AMERICAN MALE
(FOUR BLOCKS PER MEAL)

Breakfast—Scrambled Eggs

Protein:	6 egg whites or ¾ cup egg substitute
	1 ounce nonfat cheese, shredded
Carbohydrate:	1 cup grapes
	1 piece rye toast
Fat:	1 teaspoon olive oil
	½ teaspoon fresh-ground or natural peanut butter

Cooking Instructions

Spray a nonstick pan with vegetable spray. Beat the eggs and shredded nonfat cheese with the olive oil and add a little milk if desired. Then scramble. Spread peanut butter on the toast.

Lunch—Seafood Salad Sandwich

Protein:	6 ounces seafood (shrimp, crabmeat, or lobster)
Carbohydrate:	1 small side salad
	1 apple
	1 piece whole rye bread or 1 mini pita pocket
Fat:	1 tablespoon light mayonnaise
	3 olives, chopped

Note: For even better results, you can replace the rye bread or mini pita pocket with a larger salad containing sliced tomatoes, green bell peppers, and onions (see Food Block guide), or substitute another piece of fruit. This substitution can be made for any meal that contains rye bread or a mini pita pocket. You can also substitute 1 tablespoon olive oil and vinegar dressing for the mayonnaise.

Cooking Instructions

Mix seafood with mayonnaise. Stuff into a mini pita pocket.

Afternoon Snack

1 ounce turkey breast
½ orange
3 almonds

Dinner—Chili

Protein: 6 ounces lean ground meat
                        (beef or turkey)
                        Sprinkling of shredded nonfat
                        cheese
Carbohydrate: Minced onions, chopped
                        mushrooms, and chopped
                        green bell pepper to taste
                        Chili powder, oregano, and
                        pepper to taste
                        ½ cup kidney beans
                        1 cup tomatoes, crushed
                        1 peach
Fat: 1⅓ teaspoons olive oil

Cooking Instructions

Brown the meat in the olive oil with onions, mushrooms, green pepper, and spices, stirring often. Add kidney beans and tomatoes. Simmer 30 minutes or until the beans are tender, stirring occasionally. Top with shredded cheese. Have the peach for dessert.

Late-Night Snack

1 ounce turkey breast, sliced
1 cup strawberries
6 peanuts

DAY TWO FOR THE TYPICAL AMERICAN MALE

Breakfast—Old-Fashioned Oatmeal and Bacon

Protein:	3 tablespoons protein powder (supplying 21 grams of protein)
	1 ounce Canadian bacon
Carbohydrate:	1 cup dry oatmeal plus 2 cups water
	¼ cup unsweetened applesauce
	Nutmeg and cinnamon to taste
Fat:	4 teaspoons slivered almonds

Cooking Instructions

Cook oatmeal according to package directions. After cooling, stir in protein powder, applesauce, and spices, and top with slivered almonds. Cook the Canadian bacon separately.

Lunch—Cheeseburger

Protein:	6 ounces lean hamburger meat (less than 10 percent fat)
	1 slice reduced-fat cheese
Carbohydrate:	Tomato slice, lettuce leaf, and onion slice
	1 piece rye bread
	1 apple
Fat:	4 macadamia nuts

Cooking Instructions

Broil hamburger to preferred degree of doneness (about 5 minutes per side for medium). Place cheese on top and broil hamburger until cheese is melted. Put cheeseburger together with the tomato, lettuce, and onion. Have the apple and nuts for dessert.

Afternoon Snack

3 ounces firm tofu mixed with
⅓ teaspoon olive oil and
sprinkling of onion soup mix
1½ cups broccoli and green
peppers, chopped

Dinner—Barbecued Chicken

Protein: 4 ounces skinless chicken
                    breast
Carbohydrate: Lemon slices
                    Onion slices
                    ½ teaspoon barbecue sauce
                    1½ cups steamed cauliflower
                    1½ cups steamed zucchini
                    1 tossed salad (see Food Block
                    guide)
                    1 cup strawberries for dessert
Fat: 4 teaspoons olive oil and
                    vinegar dressing

Cooking Instructions

Preheat oven to 450 degrees. Cover the chicken breast with slices of lemon and onion. Bake for 15 minutes. Reduce heat to 350 degrees. Baste with barbecue sauce. Cook for 10–15 minutes or until done.

Late-Night Snack

1 ounce nonfat cheese
1 peach
3 olives

DAY THREE FOR THE TYPICAL AMERICAN MALE

Breakfast—Fruit Salad

Protein:	1 cup low-fat cottage cheese
Carbohydrate:	1 cup strawberries
	¾ cup cantaloupe, cubed
	1 cup grapes
Fat:	4 macadamia nuts, crushed

Cooking Instructions
   Mix together and enjoy.

Lunch-Chef Salad

Protein:	1½ ounces deli-style ham
	3 ounces deli-style turkey breast
	1 ounce reduced-fat cheese
Carbohydrate:	1 large tossed green salad (see Food Block guide)
	1 nectarine and 1 plum for dessert
Fat:	4 teaspoons olive oil and vinegar dressing

Afternoon Snack

¼ cup low-fat cottage cheese
½ cup pineapple, diced
1 teaspoon slivered almonds

Dinner—Foiled Fish

Protein:	6 ounces fish fillet of your choice (flounder is suggested)
Carbohydrate:	Freshly ground pepper to taste
	Squirt of lemon juice

	Onion to taste, chopped
	2 cups cooked asparagus
	1 tossed salad
	1 cup strawberries, sliced, for dessert
Fat:	Sprinkling of Parmesan cheese
	4 teaspoons olive oil and vinegar dressing

Cooking Instructions

Tear off a good-sized piece of foil. Spray the center lightly with vegetable spray. Put the fish in the center of the foil with the onion, pepper, lemon juice, and cheese. Fold foil over the fish, leaving space around the fish. Carefully turn up and seal the sides and the middle so that juices don't leak out. Bake in a 425-degree oven for 18 minutes. When done, carefully open the foil to prevent steam burns.

Late-Night Snack

1 ounce turkey breast, sliced
½ cup grapes
1 macadamia nut

DAY FOUR FOR THE TYPICAL AMERICAN MALE

Breakfast—Yogurt and Fruit

Protein:	1½ cups plain low-fat yogurt
	1 ounce lean Canadian bacon
Carbohydrate:	1 cup strawberries, sliced
Fat:	4 teaspoons slivered almonds

Cooking Instructions

Mix fruit with yogurt and top with slivered almonds. Cook the Canadian bacon separately.

Lunch—Grilled Chicken Salad

Protein:	4 ounces grilled chicken
Carbohydrate:	3 cups romaine lettuce
	½ cup mushrooms, sliced
	½ cup tomatoes, sliced
	½ cup onions, chopped
	Lemon juice to taste
	Sprinkling of garlic powder
	Dash Worcestershire sauce
	Pepper to taste
	Sprinkling of Parmesan cheese
	1 breadstick
	1 apple
Fat:	4 teaspoons olive oil and
	vinegar dressing

Cooking Instructions

Prepare the salad. Drizzle salad dressing over the salad. Squeeze the lemon over the salad. Season with garlic powder and Worcestershire sauce, and grind in fresh pepper. Toss until well combined. Place grilled chicken on top and sprinkle with cheese and crumbled breadstick. Have the apple for dessert.

Afternoon Snack

1 ounce nonfat cheese
½ apple
6 peanuts

Dinner—Pork Medallions and Apples

Protein:	4 ounces pork medallions or
	thinly sliced pork chops
Carbohydrate:	1 apple, sliced
	Rosemary to taste
	Dijon mustard to taste
	1 tablespoon white wine
	¼ cup water

$1\frac{1}{2}$ cups steamed broccoli

1 spinach salad (see Food
Block guide)

Fat: 4 teaspoons olive oil and
vinegar dressing

Cooking Instructions

Put pork into baking dish in a single layer. Top with apple slices, rosemary, and mustard. Pour wine and water around the pork. Bake at 450 degrees for 15 minutes. Baste the pork with pan juices. Reduce heat to 350 degrees and continue cooking for 10–15 minutes or until pork is white, not pink, inside.

Late-Night Snack

1 ounce soft cheese

4 ounces red wine

DAY FIVE FOR THE TYPICAL AMERICAN MALE

Breakfast—French Toast Sticks

Protein: 6 egg whites or $\frac{3}{4}$ cup egg
substitute

1 ounce extra-lean Canadian
bacon

Carbohydrate: 1 slice whole grain bread

1 cup strawberries, sliced

$\frac{1}{4}$ cantaloupe, cubed

Fat: 4 teaspoons slivered almonds

Cooking Instructions

Cook the Canadian bacon separately. Cut bread into sticks and soak in beaten eggs. (Scramble any egg mixture that remains.) Spray a nonstick pan with vegetable spray. Over medium-low heat, cook breadsticks, turning often until done. Top with sliced strawberries and slivered almonds. Have the cantaloupe as a side dish.

Lunch—Chicken Salad Sandwich

Protein:	4 ounces cooked chicken breast, shredded
Carbohydrate:	Celery, chopped
	1 cup grapes
	Lettuce
	Tomato slice
	1 piece rye bread or 1 mini pita pocket
Fat:	4 teaspoons light mayonnaise

Cooking Instructions

Mix shredded chicken with mayonnaise, celery, and grapes. Put into mini pita pocket and add lettuce and tomato slice.

Afternoon Snack

1 tablespoon guacamole wrapped in 1 ounce sliced turkey

½ cup grapes

Dinner—Meatloaf

Protein:	3 ounces lean ground beef (less than 10 percent fat)
	3 ounces ground turkey
	2 tablespoons egg substitute
Carbohydrate:	1 tablespoon ketchup
	½ cup onions, chopped
	1 teaspoon bread crumbs
	Pepper to taste
	Dash Worcestershire sauce
	1½ cups cooked zucchini
	1 apple
	1 tossed salad
Fat:	4 teaspoons olive oil and vinegar dressing

Cooking Instructions

Mix ground meat, egg substitute, ketchup, onions, bread crumbs, pepper, and Worcestershire sauce. Form into a shallow loaf and place in microwave-safe dish. Cover with waxed paper. Microwave on medium for 10–15 minutes or until done. Have the zucchini as a side dish and eat the apple for dessert.

Late-Night Snack

> 1 ounce turkey breast, sliced
> 1 cup strawberries
> 6 peanuts

DAY SIX FOR THE TYPICAL AMERICAN MALE

Breakfast—Skillet Hash

Protein:	4 ounces cooked lean ham, chicken, or beef
Carbohydrate:	⅓ cup cooked potato, diced
	1 cup tomato, chopped
	Green bell pepper, onions, and mushrooms to taste, chopped
	Salt and pepper to taste
	Dash Worcestershire sauce
	½ cantaloupe
Fat:	1⅓ teaspoons olive oil

Cooking Instructions

In a nonstick pan, sauté green pepper, onions, and mushrooms in olive oil until tender. Add cooked meat, potato, tomato, spices, and Worcestershire sauce. Cook, stirring, until heated through. Have cantaloupe as side dish.

Lunch—BLT Sandwich

Protein:	3 ounces cooked extra-lean Canadian bacon
	1 ounce nonfat cheese

Carbohydrate: 1 slice rye bread
                             Lettuce and sliced tomato
                             1 orange
Fat: 1 teaspoon light mayonnaise
                             3 macadamia nuts

Afternoon Snack

2 ounces low-fat cottage cheese
½ cup pineapple, diced
3 olives, chopped

Dinner—Quick Turkey Dinner

Protein: 6 ounces deli-style turkey
                                breast or 4 ounces cooked
                                skinless turkey breast
Carbohydrate: 1½ cups steamed broccoli
                             1 cup boiled and drained
                                onions
                             ½ cup cranberries
Fat: 4 teaspoons slivered almonds

Late-Night Snack

1 ounce turkey breast, sliced
1 cup strawberries
6 peanuts

DAY SEVEN FOR THE TYPICAL AMERICAN MALE

Breakfast—Scrambled Eggs Benedict

Protein: 2 ounces lean Canadian bacon
                             4 large egg whites or ½ cup
                                egg substitute
Carbohydrate: ½ English muffin
                             1 orange
Fat: 1⅓ teaspoons olive oil

Cooking Instructions

Beat egg whites and olive oil with a little milk if desired. Spray a nonstick pan with vegetable spray and then scramble the eggs. Toast the English muffin. Cook the Canadian bacon, place on the toasted muffin, and then top with the eggs.

Lunch—Turkey in a Pocket

Protein:	6 ounces deli-style turkey breast or 4 ounces cooked turkey breast
Carbohydrate:	1 mini pita pocket
	1 green bell pepper, chopped
	1 tomato, sliced
	2 plums
Fat:	2 tablespoons guacamole

Afternoon Snack

2 hard-boiled egg whites
½ apple
1 celery stick stuffed with
    ½ teaspoon fresh-ground
    or natural peanut butter

Dinner—Broiled Salmon

Protein:	6 ounces salmon fillet
Carbohydrate:	Rosemary to taste
	Tarragon to taste
	Dill to taste
	Lemon (optional)
	1½ cups cooked zucchini
	2 tomatoes, split and sprinkled with Parmesan cheese
	1 apple for dessert
Fat:	1⅓ teaspoons olive oil

Cooking Instructions

Rub the fillet with the herbs, and then brush with olive oil. Broil for 10 minutes per inch of thickness, turning and basting once. Garnish with lemon if desired. Have the apple for dessert.

Late-Night Snack

> 1 ounce turkey breast, sliced
> 1 cup strawberries
> 1 teaspoon slivered almonds

DAY ONE FOR THE TYPICAL AMERICAN FEMALE OLYMPIC ATHLETE (FIVE BLOCKS PER MEAL)

Breakfast—Scrambled Eggs

Protein:	6 egg whites or ¾ cup egg substitute
	2 ounces nonfat cheese, shredded
Carbohydrate:	1½ cups grapes
	1 piece rye toast
Fat:	2 teaspoons olive oil
	2 teaspoons fresh-ground or natural peanut butter

Cooking Instructions

Spray a nonstick pan with vegetable spray. Beat the eggs and shredded nonfat cheese with the olive oil and add a little milk if desired. Then scramble. Spread peanut butter on the toast.

Lunch—Seafood Salad Sandwich

Protein:	7½ ounces seafood (shrimp, crabmeat, or lobster)
Carbohydrate:	1 small side salad
	½ apple
	1 orange

	1 piece whole rye bread or mini pita pocket
Fat:	5 teaspoons light mayonnaise
	5 macadamia nuts

Note: For even better results, you can replace the rye bread or mini pita pocket with a larger salad containing sliced tomatoes, green peppers, and onions (see Food Block guide), or substitute another piece of fruit. This substitution can be made for any meal that contains rye bread or a mini pita pocket. You can also substitute 5 teaspoons olive oil and vinegar dressing for the mayonnaise and serve the seafood on top of the salad.

Cooking Instructions

Mix seafood with mayonnaise. Stuff into a mini pita pocket.

Afternoon Snack

1 ounce low-fat cheese
½ orange
12 peanuts

Dinner—Chili

Protein:	6 ounces lean ground meat (beef or turkey)
	1 ounce nonfat cheese, shredded
Carbohydrate:	Minced onions, chopped mushrooms, and chopped green bell pepper to taste
	Chili powder, oregano, and pepper to taste
	½ cup kidney beans
	1 cup tomatoes, crushed
	1 nectarine
Fat:	3 teaspoons olive oil
	3 olives

Cooking Instructions
  Brown the meat in the olive oil with onions, mushrooms, green pepper, olives, and spices, stirring often. Add kidney beans and tomatoes. Simmer 30 minutes or until beans are tender, stirring occasionally. Top with shredded cheese. Have the nectarine for dessert.

Late-Night Snack

> 1 ounce turkey breast, sliced
> 1 cup strawberries
> 1 tablespoon guacamole

DAY TWO FOR THE TYPICAL AMERICAN FEMALE OLYMPIC ATHLETE

Breakfast–Old-Fashioned Oatmeal and Bacon

Protein:	4 tablespoons protein powder (providing 21 grams of protein)
	2 ounces Canadian bacon
Carbohydrate:	1⅓ cups dry oatmeal plus 2½ cups water
	Nutmeg and cinnamon to taste
	¼ cantaloupe
Fat:	2 tablespoons slivered almonds
	1⅓ teaspoons olive oil

Cooking Instructions
  Cook oatmeal according to package directions. After cooling, stir in protein powder, spices, and olive oil and top with slivered almonds. Cook the Canadian bacon separately. Have the cantaloupe as a side dish.

Lunch—Cheeseburger

Protein:

7½ ounces lean hamburger
meat (less than 10 percent fat)
1 slice reduced-fat cheese

Carbohydrate:

Tomato slice, lettuce leaf, and
onion slice
1 piece rye bread
1 pear
1 kiwi

Fat:

1 teaspoon reduced-fat
mayonnaise
9 macadamia nuts

Cooking Instructions

Broil the hamburger to preferred degree of doneness (about 5 minutes per side for medium). Put cheese on hamburger and broil until melted. Have the pear, kiwi, and macadamia nuts for dessert.

Afternoon Snack

3 ounces firm tofu mixed with
⅔ teaspoon olive oil and
sprinkling of onion soup mix
2 cups broccoli and green
peppers, chopped

Dinner—Barbecued Chicken

Protein:

5 ounces skinless chicken
breast

Carbohydrate:

Lemon slices
Onion slices
1 teaspoon barbecue sauce
1½ cups steamed cauliflower
¼ cup cooked rice
1 tossed salad (see Food Block
guide)
2 cups strawberries for dessert

Fat: 3 tablespoons olive oil and
                                                   vinegar dressing
                                              6 peanuts, crushed

Cooking Instructions

Preheat oven to 450 degrees. Cover chicken breast with slices of lemon and onion. Bake for 15 minutes. Reduce heat to 350 degrees. Baste with barbecue sauce. Cook for 10–15 minutes or until done. Sprinkle peanuts on top of the salad.

Late-Night Snack

1 ounce reduced-fat cheese
1 peach
6 olives

DAY THREE FOR THE TYPICAL AMERICAN FEMALE OLYMPIC ATHLETE

Breakfast—Fruit Salad

Protein:	1¼ cups low-fat cottage cheese
Carbohydrate:	2 cups strawberries
	¾ cup cantaloupe, cubed
	1 cup grapes
Fat:	10 macadamia nuts, crushed

Cooking Instructions

Mix together and enjoy.

Lunch—Chef Salad

Protein:	3 ounces deli-style ham
	3 ounces deli-style turkey breast
	1 ounce reduced-fat cheese
Carbohydrate:	1 large tossed green salad

	2 nectarines for dessert
Fat:	3 tablespoons olive oil and vinegar dressing
	1 teaspoon slivered almonds

Afternoon Snack

2 ounces low-fat cottage cheese
½ cup pineapple, diced
2 teaspoons slivered almonds

Dinner—Foiled Fish

Protein:	7½ ounces fish fillet of your choice (flounder is suggested)
Carbohydrate:	Freshly ground pepper to taste
	Squirt of lemon juice
	1 onion, chopped
	2 cups cooked asparagus
	¼ cup cooked pasta
	1 tossed salad
Fat:	3 tablespoons olive oil and vinegar dressing
	Sprinkling of Parmesan cheese
	3 almonds

Cooking Instructions

Tear off a good-sized piece of foil. Spray the center lightly with vegetable spray. Put the fish in the center of the foil with the onion, pepper, lemon juice, and cheese. Fold foil over the fish, leaving space around the fish. Carefully turn up and seal the sides and the middle so that juices don't leak out. Bake in a 425-degree oven for 18 minutes. When done, carefully open the foil to prevent steam burns.

Late-Night Snack

1 ounce turkey breast, sliced
½ cup grapes
2 macadamia nuts

DAY FOUR FOR THE TYPICAL AMERICAN FEMALE OLYMPIC ATHLETE

Breakfast—Yogurt and Fruit

Protein:	Roughly ⅓ ounce protein powder (providing 7 grams of protein)
	1½ cups plain low-fat yogurt
	2 ounces lean Canadian bacon or 6 turkey bacon strips
Carbohydrate:	¾ cup cantaloupe, cubed
	½ cup blueberries
Fat:	5 teaspoons slivered almonds
	5 macadamia nuts, crushed

Cooking Instructions

Mix fruit and protein powder with yogurt and top with slivered almonds and crushed macadamia nuts. Cook the Canadian bacon separately.

Lunch—Grilled Chicken Salad

Protein:	5 ounces grilled chicken
Carbohydrate:	3 cups romaine lettuce
	½ cup mushrooms, sliced
	¾ cup tomatoes, sliced
	½ cup onions, chopped
	Lemon juice to taste
	Sprinkling of garlic powder
	Dash Worcestershire sauce
	Pepper to taste
	1 apple
	½ cup grapes
	1 breadstick
Fat:	3 tablespoons olive oil and vinegar dressing
	1 teaspoon slivered almonds
	Sprinkling of Parmesan cheese

Cooking Instructions

Prepare the salad. Drizzle salad dressing over the salad. Squeeze the lemon over the salad. Season with garlic powder and Worcestershire sauce, and grind in fresh pepper. Toss until well combined. Place grilled chicken on top, and sprinkle with slivered almonds and Parmesan cheese.

Afternoon Snack

1 ounce nonfat cheese
½ apple
12 peanuts

Dinner—Pork Medallions and Apples

Protein:	5 ounces pork medallions or thinly sliced pork chops
Carbohydrate:	1 apple, sliced
	Rosemary to taste
	Dijon mustard to taste
	1 tablespoon white wine
	¼ cup water
	1½ cups steamed broccoli
	1 spinach salad (see Food Block guide)
	½ orange as dessert
Fat:	3 tablespoons olive oil and vinegar dressing
	6 peanuts

Cooking Instructions

Put pork into baking dish in a single layer. Top with apple slices, rosemary, and mustard. Pour wine and water around the pork. Bake at 450 degrees for 15 minutes. Baste the pork with pan juices. Reduce heat to 350 degrees and continue cooking for 10–15 minutes or until pork is white, not pink, inside.

Late-Night Snack

1 ounce soft cheese
4 ounces red wine

DAY FIVE FOR THE TYPICAL AMERICAN FEMALE OLYMPIC ATHLETE

Breakfast—French Toast Sticks

Protein:	6 egg whites or ¾ cup egg substitute
	2 ounces extra-lean Canadian bacon
Carbohydrate:	1½ slices whole grain bread
	2 cups strawberries, sliced
Fat:	2 tablespoons slivered almonds
	1⅓ teaspoons olive oil

Cooking Instructions

Cut bread into sticks and soak in beaten eggs. (Scramble any egg mixture that remains.) Spray a nonstick pan with vegetable spray. Over medium-low heat, cook breadsticks, turning often, until done. Top with sliced strawberries and slivered almonds. Sauté Canadian bacon in olive oil.

Lunch—Chicken Salad Sandwich

Protein:	5 ounces cooked chicken breast, shredded
Carbohydrate:	Celery, chopped
	1 cup grapes
	Lettuce
	Tomato slice
	1 piece rye bread or 1 mini pita pocket
	1 plum
Fat:	3 tablespoons light mayonnaise
	3 almonds

Cooking Instructions

Mix shredded chicken with mayonnaise, celery, and grapes. Put into mini pita pocket and add lettuce and tomato slice.

Afternoon Snack

1 tablespoon guacamole
  wrapped in 1 ounce sliced
  turkey
½ cup grapes

Dinner—Meatloaf

Protein: 7½ ounces lean ground beef
                          (less than 10 percent fat) or
                          ground turkey
                        2 tablespoons egg substitute
Carbohydrate: 1 tablespoon ketchup
                        ¼ cup onions, chopped
                        1 teaspoon bread crumbs
                        Pepper to taste
                        Dash Worcestershire sauce
                        2 cups green beans
                        1 apple as dessert
                        1 tossed salad (see Food Block
                          guide)
Fat: 3 tablespoons olive oil and
                          vinegar dressing
                        3 olives, chopped

Cooking Instructions

Mix ground meat, egg substitute, ketchup, onions, bread crumbs, pepper, and Worcestershire sauce. Form into a shallow loaf and place in microwave-safe dish. Cover with waxed paper. Microwave on medium for 15 minutes or until done. Steam green beans as a side dish. Have the apple for dessert.

Late-Night Snack

1 ounce turkey breast, sliced
1 cup strawberries
2 macadamia nuts

DAY SIX FOR THE TYPICAL AMERICAN FEMALE OLYMPIC ATHLETE

Breakfast—Skillet Hash

Protein:	5 ounces cooked lean ham
Carbohydrate:	½ cup cooked potato, diced
	2 cups tomato, chopped
	Green bell pepper, onions, and mushrooms to taste, chopped
	Salt and pepper to taste
	Dash Worcestershire sauce
	½ cantaloupe
Fat:	3 teaspoons olive oil
	6 peanuts

Cooking Instructions

In a nonstick pan, sauté green pepper, onions, and mushrooms in olive oil until tender. Add cooked meat, potato, tomato, spices, and Worcestershire sauce. Cook, stirring, until heated through. Have cantaloupe as side dish.

Lunch—BLT Sandwich

Protein:	3 ounces cooked extra-lean Canadian bacon
	2 ounces nonfat cheese
Carbohydrate:	2 slices rye bread
	Lettuce and sliced tomato
	½ orange
Fat:	1 teaspoon light mayonnaise
	9 macadamia nuts

Afternoon Snack

	1 ounce low-fat cottage cheese
	½ cup pineapple, diced
	12 peanuts

Dinner-Quick Turkey Dinner

Protein:	7½ ounces deli-style turkey breast or 5 ounces cooked skinless turkey breast
Carbohydrate:	3 cups steamed broccoli 1 cup boiled and drained onions ¼ cup cooked cranberries 1 cup steamed string beans
Fat:	5 teaspoons slivered almonds

Cooking Instructions
Cook the slivered almonds with the string beans.

Late-Night Snack

1 ounce turkey breast, sliced
1 cup strawberries
6 olives

DAY SEVEN FOR THE TYPICAL AMERICAN FEMALE OLYMPIC ATHLETE

Breakfast—Scrambled Eggs Benedict

Protein:	2 ounces lean Canadian bacon 6 large egg whites or ¾ cup egg substitute
Carbohydrate:	1 English muffin ½ grapefruit
Fat:	2 tablespoons olive oil 3 almonds

Cooking Instructions
Beat egg whites and olive oil with a little milk if desired. Spray nonstick pan with vegetable spray and then scramble the eggs. Toast the English muffin. Cook the Canadian bacon, place on the toasted muffin, and top with the eggs.

Lunch—Turkey in a Pocket

Protein: 7½ ounces deli-style turkey
                              breast or 5 ounces cooked
                              turkey breast
Carbohydrate: 1 mini pita pocket
                              1 green bell pepper, chopped
                              1 tomato, sliced
                              1 cup strawberries
                              1 orange
Fat: 5 tablespoons guacamole

Afternoon Snack

                              2 hard-boiled egg whites
                              ½ apple
                              6 almonds

Dinner—Broiled Salmon

Protein: 7½ ounces salmon fillet
Carbohyrate: Rosemary to taste
                              Tarragon to taste
                              Dill to taste
                              Lemon (optional)
                              3 cups cooked zucchini
                              2 tomatoes, split, sprinkled
                                with Parmesan cheese,
                                and broiled
                              1 apple for dessert
Fat: 2 teaspoons olive oil
                              4 macadamia nuts

Cooking Instructions

Rub the fillet with the herbs, and then brush with olive oil. Broil for 10 minutes per inch of thickness, turning off and basting once. Garnish with lemon if desired. Have the apple for dessert.

Late-Night Snack

1 ounce turkey breast, sliced
1 cup strawberries
6 olives

DAY ONE FOR THE TYPICAL AMERICAN MALE OLYMPIC ATHLETE (SIX BLOCKS PER MEAL)

Breakfast—Scrambled Eggs

Protein: 8 egg whites or 1 cup egg
                        substitute
                        2 ounces nonfat cheese, shredded
                        1 ounce lean Canadian bacon
Carbohydrate: 1 cantaloupe
                        1 piece rye toast
Fat: 1½ teaspoons fresh-ground or
                        natural peanut butter
                        3 tablespoons olive oil

Cooking Instructions

Spray a nonstick pan with vegetable spray. Beat the eggs and shredded nonfat cheese with the olive oil and add a little milk if desired. Then scramble. Spread peanut butter on the toast.

Lunch—Seafood Salad Sandwich

Protein: 9 ounces seafood (shrimp,
                        crabmeat, or lobster)
Carbohydrate: 1 small side salad
                        1 orange
                        2 pieces whole rye bread or ½
                        regular-sized pita pocket
Fat: 2 tablespoons light mayonnaise
                        2 tablespoons olive oil and
                        vinegar dressing

Note: For even better results, you can replace half of the rye bread or pita pocket with a larger salad containing sliced tomatoes, green pep-

pers, and onions (see Food Block guide), or substitute another piece of fruit. This substitution can be made for any meal that contains rye bread or a mini pita pocket.

Cooking Instructions

Mix seafood with mayonnaise. Stuff into a pita pocket.

Afternoon Snack

> 1 ounce low-fat cheese
> ½ orange
> 2 macadamia nuts

Dinner—Chili

Protein:	7½ ounces lean ground meat (beef or turkey)
	1 ounce nonfat cheese, shredded
Carbohydrate:	Minced onions, chopped mushrooms, and chopped green bell pepper to taste
	Chili powder, oregano, and pepper to taste
	¾ cup kidney beans
	1 cup tomatoes, crushed
	2 peaches
Fat:	4 teaspoons olive oil

Cooking Instructions

Brown the meat in olive oil with onions, mushrooms, green pepper, and spices, stirring often. Add kidney beans and tomatoes. Simmer 30 minutes or until beans are tender, stirring occasionally. Top with shredded cheese. Have the peaches for dessert.

Late-Night Snack

> 1 ounce turkey breast, sliced
> 1 cup strawberries
> 6 olives

DAY TWO FOR THE TYPICAL AMERICAN MALE OLYMPIC ATHLETE

Breakfast—Old-Fashioned Oatmeal and Bacon

Protein:	3 tablespoons protein powder (providing 21 grams of protein)
	3 ounces Canadian bacon
Carbohydrate:	1⅓ cups dry oatmeal plus 2½ cups water
	Nutmeg and cinnamon to taste
	½ cantaloupe
Fat:	4 tablespoons slivered almonds

Cooking Instructions

Cook oatmeal according to package directions. After cooling, stir in protein powder and spices, and top with slivered almonds. Cook the Canadian bacon separately.

Lunch—Cheeseburger

Protein:	7½ ounces lean hamburger meat (less than 10 percent fat)
	1 ounce reduced-fat cheese
Carbohydrate:	Tomato slice, lettuce leaf, and onion slice
	2 pieces rye bread
	1 apple
Fat:	12 macadamia nuts

Cooking Instructions

Broil hamburger to preferred degree of doneness (about 5 minutes per side for medium). Put cheese on hamburger and broil until melted. Have the apple and macadamia nuts for dessert.

Afternoon Snack

3 ounces firm tofu
⅔ teaspoon olive oil
Sprinkling of onion soup mix
1½ cups broccoli and green bell
pepper, chopped

Dinner—Barbecued Chicken

Protein:	6 ounces skinless chicken breast
Carbohydrate:	Lemon slices
	Onion slices
	1 teaspoon barbecue sauce
	3 cups steamed cauliflower
	1 apple
	1 cup strawberries for dessert
	1 tossed salad (see Food Block guide)
Fat:	4 tablespoons olive oil and vinegar dressing

Cooking Instructions

Preheat oven to 450 degrees. Cover the chicken breast with slices of lemon and onion. Bake for 15 minutes. Reduce heat to 350 degrees. Baste with barbecue sauce. Cook for 10–15 minutes or until done.

Late-Night Snack

1 ounce reduced-fat cheese
1 peach
6 olives

DAY THREE FOR THE TYPICAL AMERICAN MALE
OLYMPIC ATHLETE

Breakfast—Fruit Salad

Protein:	1½ cups low-fat cottage cheese
Carbohydrate:	1 cup strawberries
	1 cup honeydew melon, cubed
	1 cup mandarin oranges
Fat:	12 macadamia nuts, crushed

Cooking Instructions
   Mix together and enjoy.

Lunch—Chef Salad

Protein:	3 ounces deli-style ham
	3 ounces deli-style turkey breast
	2 ounces reduced-fat cheese
Carbohydrate:	1 large tossed green salad (see Food Block guide)
	2 nectarines and 1 plum for dessert
Fat:	4 tablespoons olive oil and vinegar dressing

Afternoon Snack

2 ounces low-fat cottage cheese
½ cup pineapple, diced
6 almonds

Dinner—Foiled Fish

Protein:	9 ounces fish fillet of your choice (flounder is suggested)
Carbohydrate:	Freshly ground pepper to taste
	Squirt of lemon juice

	Onion to taste, chopped
	2 cups cooked asparagus
	½ cup cooked pasta
	1 spinach salad (see Food Block guide)
	1 tangerine
Fat:	Sprinkling of Parmesan cheese
	4 tablespoons olive oil and vinegar dressing

Cooking Instructions

Tear off a good-sized piece of foil. Spray the center lightly with vegetable spray. Put the fish in the center of the foil with the onion, pepper, lemon juice, and cheese. Fold foil over the fish, leaving space around the fish. Carefully turn up and seal the sides and the middle so that juices don't leak out. Bake in a 425-degree oven for 18 minutes. When done, carefully open the foil to prevent steam burns.

Late-Night Snack

1 ounce turkey breast, sliced
½ cup grapes
2 macadamia nuts

DAY FOUR FOR THE TYPICAL AMERICAN MALE OLYMPIC ATHLETE

Breakfast—Yogurt and Fruit

Protein:	1½ cups plain low-fat yogurt
	3 ounces lean Canadian bacon
Carbohydrate:	1½ cups pineapple, cubed
Fat:	4 tablespoons slivered almonds

Cooking Instructions

Mix fruit with yogurt and top with slivered almonds. Cook the Canadian bacon separately.

Lunch—Grilled Chicken Salad

Protein:	6 ounces grilled chicken
Carbohydrate:	3 cups romaine lettuce
	1 cup mushrooms, sliced
	2 cups tomatoes, sliced
	1 cup onions, chopped
	1 ounce croutons
	Lemon juice to taste
	Sprinkling of garlic powder
	Dash Worcestershire sauce
	Pepper to taste
	Sprinkling of Parmesan cheese
	1 pear
	1 apple
Fat:	4 tablespoons olive oil and
	vinegar dressing

Cooking Instructions

Prepare the salad. Drizzle salad dressing over the salad. Squeeze the lemon over the salad. Season with garlic powder and Worcestershire sauce, and grind in fresh pepper. Toss until well combined. Place grilled chicken on top. Sprinkle with cheese. Have the pear and the apple for dessert.

Afternoon Snack

1 ounce cheese
½ apple
6 olives

Dinner—Pork Medallions and Apples

Protein:	6 ounces pork medallions or
	thinly sliced pork chops
Carbohydrate:	1 apple, sliced
	Rosemary to taste
	Dijon mustard to taste

1 tablespoon white wine
¼ cup water
1½ cups steamed broccoli
1 spinach salad
1 orange as dessert

Fat: 4 tablespoons olive oil and
       vinegar dressing

Cooking Instructions

Put pork into baking dish in a single layer. Top with apple slices, rosemary, and mustard. Pour wine and water around the pork. Bake at 450 degrees for 15 minutes. Baste pork with pan juices. Reduce heat to 350 degrees and continue cooking for 10–15 minutes or until pork is white, not pink, inside.

Late-Night Snack

1 ounce soft cheese
4 ounces red wine

DAY FIVE FOR THE TYPICAL AMERICAN MALE OLYMPIC ATHLETE

Breakfast—French Toast Sticks

Protein: 8 egg whites or 1 cup egg
           substitute
           2 ounces lean Canadian bacon

Carbohydrate: 2 slices of whole grain bread
                2 cups strawberries, sliced

Fat: 4 tablespoons slivered almonds

Cooking Instructions

Cut bread into sticks and soak in beaten eggs. (Scramble any egg mixture that remains.) Spray a nonstick pan with vegetable spray. Over medium-low heat, cook breadsticks, turning often, until done. Top with sliced strawberries and slivered almonds. Cook the Canadian bacon as a side dish.

Lunch—Chicken Salad Sandwich

Protein:	6 ounces cooked chicken breast, shredded
Carbohydrate:	Celery, chopped
	1 cup grapes
	Lettuce
	Tomato slice
	2 pieces rye bread or 1 mini pita pocket
Fat:	4 tablespoons light mayonnaise

Cooking Instructions

Mix shredded chicken with mayonnaise, celery, and grapes. Put into mini pita pocket and add tomato slice and lettuce.

Afternoon Snack

1 tablespoon guacamole wrapped in 1 ounce sliced turkey
½ cup grapes
2 macadamia nuts

Dinner—Meatloaf

Protein:	9 ounces lean ground beef (less than 10 percent fat) or ground turkey
	4 tablespoons egg substitute
Carbohydrate:	1 tablespoon ketchup
	¼ cup onions, chopped
	1 teaspoon bread crumbs
	Dash Worcestershire sauce
	Pepper to taste
	2 cups cooked zucchini
	1 apple
	1 orange
	1 tossed salad

Fat: 4 tablespoons olive oil and
                                            vinegar dressing

Cooking Instructions

Mix ground meat, egg substitute, ketchup, onions, bread crumbs, pepper, and Worcestershire sauce. Form into shallow loaf and place in microwave-safe dish. Cover with waxed paper. Microwave on medium for 10–15 minutes or until done. Have the apple and orange for dessert.

Late-Night Snack

                                        1 ounce turkey breast, sliced
                                        1 cup strawberries
                                        1 tablespoon guacamole

DAY SIX FOR THE TYPICAL AMERICAN MALE OLYMPIC ATHLETE

Breakfast—Skillet Hash

Protein: 6 ounces cooked lean meat
                                            (chicken, ham, or beef)

Carbohydrate: ⅔ cup cooked potato, diced
                                        2 cups tomato, chopped
                                        Green bell pepper, onions, and
                                            mushrooms to taste, chopped
                                        Salt and pepper to taste
                                        Dash Worcestershire sauce
                                        ½ cantaloupe

Fat: 4 tablespoons olive oil

Cooking Instructions

In nonstick pan, sauté green pepper, onions, and mushrooms in olive oil until tender. Add cooked meat, potato, tomato, spices, and Worcestershire sauce. Cook, stirring, until heated through. Have cantaloupe as side dish.

Lunch—BLT Sandwich

Protein:	3 ounces cooked extra-lean Canadian bacon
	1½ ounces deli-style turkey (added to salad)
	2 ounces nonfat cheese
	Lettuce and sliced tomato
	½ pear
	1 tossed salad (see Food Block guide)
Carbohydrate:	2 slices rye bread
Fat:	1 tablespoon light mayonnaise
	3 tablespoons olive oil and vinegar dressing

Afternoon Snack

2 ounces low-fat cottage cheese
½ cup pineapple, diced
6 olives, sliced

Dinner—Quick Turkey Dinner

Protein:	9 ounces deli-style turkey breast or 6 ounces cooked skinless turkey breast
Carbohydrate:	3 cups steamed broccoli
	1 cup boiled and drained onions
	¼ cup cranberries
	1 nectarine for dessert
Fat:	1 tablespoon slivered almonds
	9 macadamia nuts

Late-Night Snack

1 ounce turkey breast, sliced
1 cup strawberries
6 almonds

DAY SEVEN FOR THE TYPICAL AMERICAN MALE
OLYMPIC ATHLETE

Breakfast—Scrambled Eggs Benedict

Protein:	2 ounces lean Canadian bacon
	8 large egg whites or 1 cup egg substitute
Carbohydrate:	1 English muffin
	½ grapefruit
	1 cup strawberries
Fat:	4 teaspoons olive oil

Cooking Instructions

Beat egg whites and olive oil with a little milk if desired. Spray a nonstick pan with vegetable spray and then scramble the eggs. Toast the English muffin. Cook the Canadian bacon, place on the toasted muffin, and top with the eggs.

Lunch—Turkey in a Pocket

Protein:	9 ounces deli-style turkey breast or 6 ounces cooked turkey breast
Carbohydrate:	1 mini pita pocket
	1 green bell pepper, chopped
	1 tomato, sliced
	1 cup strawberries
	1 orange
Fat:	6 tablespoons guacamole

Afternoon Snack

2 hard-boiled egg whites
½ apple
6 almonds

Dinner—Broiled Salmon

Protein:	9 ounces salmon fillet
Carbohydrate:	Rosemary to taste
	Tarragon to taste
	Dill to taste
	Lemon (optional)
	1½ cups cooked zucchini
	2 tomatoes, split, broiled, and sprinkled with Parmesan cheese
	1 apple
	1 orange
Fat:	4 teaspoons olive oil
	Sprinkling of Parmesan cheese

Cooking Instructions

Rub the fillet with the herbs, and then brush with olive oil. Broil for 10 minutes per inch of thickness, turning and basting once. Garnish with lemon if desired. Have the apple and orange for dessert.

Late-Night Snack

1 ounce turkey breast, sliced
1 cup strawberries
2 macadamia nuts

9

ZONE RECIPES

If Zone cooking sounds boring, or too mathematical, then this chapter might just change your mind. It contains more than one hundred and fifty great-tasting, easy-to-make meals designed by chef Scott C. Lane that all have the same 1:1:1 block ratio of protein, carbohydrate, and fat that will help get you into and maintain yourself in the Zone.

Zone recipes have to look great, taste great, be easy to prepare, and be hormonally correct. You will find that these Zone recipes are a little different from most recipes in that they are laid out in eight-block segments. This means that each recipe contains eight blocks of protein, eight blocks of carbohydrate, and eight blocks of added fat. Depending on how many blocks you and your family require, simply adjust the recipe size accordingly (as explained in Chapter 8, "A Week in the Zone"). The typical adult female will require two to three blocks per meal, the typical adult male will require three to four blocks, and the typical child will require two blocks per meal. And if you're cooking for one, either cut down the size of the meal or make the entire recipe and freeze the portion you don't plan to eat. You should also note that many of the Zone lunches can also be used for dinners.

These recipes are also designed to be extremely flexible. If you want to serve a hearty salad, then simply subtract one carbohydrate block from the recipe for each salad you plan to make. If you want a glass of wine or cocktail with a meal, then further subtract the amount of alcohol in terms of carbohydrate blocks (see Appendix B for a listing) from the remaining carbohydrate blocks in that recipe. If you want a dessert, then make a further reduction in the remaining carbohydrate blocks found in each recipe. By making the appropriate carbohydrate adjustments for salads, alcohol, or desserts, you will always keep your hormonal carburetor in tune.

Because these meals contain a lot of low-density carbohydrates, like fruits and vegetables, many people will even have trouble eating the entire meal despite the fact that the calorie content of a typical four-block portion of one of the following recipes will be under 400 calories.

Don't think of these as meals, think of them as some of the most powerful drugs you will ever be prescribed. I guarantee you that after a week of Zone meals and snacks, you will never look at a bagel or plate of pasta the same way again.

BREAKFAST

Mexican Omelette

Servings: 2 omelettes (four blocks each)

Block Size:

2 Protein	2 whole eggs*
6 Protein	12 egg whites
2 Carbohydrate	2 cups onion, minced
2 Carbohydrate	½ cup cooked chickpeas
2 Carbohydrate	½ cup cooked kidney beans
⅔ Carbohydrate	1 cup green bell pepper, diced
⅔ Carbohydrate	1 cup red bell pepper, diced
⅔ Carbohydrate	2 cups mushrooms, minced
8 Fat	2⅔ teaspoons olive oil, divided

⅛ teaspoon black pepper
⅛ teaspoon hot sauce (or to taste)
⅛ teaspoon dry mustard
¼ teaspoon turmeric
⅛ teaspoon chili powder
4 garlic cloves, minced, divided

Method:
In a medium nonstick sauté pan, cook onion, garlic, chickpeas, kidney beans, red and green peppers, and mushrooms in ⅔ teaspoon oil until tender. In a mixing bowl, whip together whole eggs, egg whites, black pepper, hot sauce, mustard, turmeric, and chili powder. In a second sauté pan, heat 1 teaspoon oil before adding half the egg mixture. Cook until set and an omelette is formed. Fill omelette with half the vegetable mixture, fold over and serve. Repeat process to make second omelette.

*Note: Eggs used in these recipes are sized as large.

Scrambled Vegetable Delight

Servings: 2 Scrambled Vegetable Delight Dishes (four blocks each)

Block Size:

2 Protein	2 ounces skim milk mozzarella cheese, shredded
4 Protein	8 egg whites
2 Protein	2 whole eggs*
1 Carbohydrate	2 cups broccoli, chopped
1 Carbohydrate	3 cups mushrooms, diced
2 Carbohydrate	3 cups red bell pepper, diced
2 Carbohydrate	2 cups onion, diced
1 Carbohydrate	1 cup yellow squash, diced
1 Carbohydrate	1 cup zucchini, diced
8 Fat	2⅔ teaspoons olive oil
	⅛ teaspoon nutmeg
	¼ teaspoon turmeric
	⅛ teaspoon black pepper
	⅛ teaspoon celery salt

Method:

In a medium nonstick sauté pan, cook vegetables in oil until almost tender. In a mixing bowl, combine whole eggs, egg whites, cheese, nutmeg, and turmeric. Mix egg mixture well until all ingredients are blended together. Pour egg mixture over vegetables and continue cooking while stirring. As the egg mixture starts to cook, it will resemble scrambled eggs. When Scrambled Vegetable Delight is cooked to your liking, divide and place on two warmed serving plates. Lightly sprinkle with black pepper and celery salt and serve.

*Note: Eggs used in these recipes are sized as large.

Breakfast Fruit Salad

Servings: 2 Breakfast Fruit Salad dishes (four blocks each)

Block Size:

8 Protein	2 cups low-fat cottage cheese
1 Carbohydrate	½ cup maraschino cherries
1 Carbohydrate	1 cup strawberries, sliced
2 Carbohydrate	1 cup blueberries
2 Carbohydrate	2 kiwi fruit, peeled and diced
2 Carbohydrate	⅔ cup mandarin orange sections
8 Fat	24 black olives, chopped
	2 tablespoon fresh mint, diced
	⅛ teaspoon banana extract
	⅛ teaspoon parsley flakes

Method:

In a mixing bowl, combine all ingredients and gently blend. Mound on two plates, sprinkle with parsley, and serve immediately, because it does not hold up well after several hours.

Apple-Cinnamon Raisin Omelette

Servings: 2 omelettes (four blocks each)

Block Size:

6 Protein	8 egg whites plus 2 whole eggs*
2 Protein	2 envelopes Knox Unflavored Gelatin
4 Carbohydrate	2 red Delicious apples, cored and sliced
2 Carbohydrate	2 tablespoons raisins
2 Carbohydrate	⅔ cup applesauce
8 Fat	2⅔ teaspoons olive oil
	½ cup water
	½ teaspoon plus ⅛ teaspoon cinnamon
	⅛ teaspoon turmeric

Method:
In a medium nonstick sauté pan, place apples, raisins, and water. Simmer mixture under medium heat for 3–4 minutes until apples soften slightly. In a mixing bowl, add gelatin, applesauce, ⅔ teaspoon oil, and ½ teaspoon cinnamon. Add applesauce mixture to apple-raisin mixture and mix well, simmering an additional 3–4 minutes. Place apple-applesauce mixture aside and keep warm. In a mixing bowl, whip egg whites, whole eggs, and turmeric together. Heat 1 teaspoon oil in a second sauté pan. Pour half the egg mixture into the sauté pan and cook until egg sets and an omelette forms. As the omelette is cooking, lightly sprinkle with a dash (⅛ teaspoon) of cinnamon. When omelette is cooked place half the filling on omelette and fold over. Remove to serving plate and serve immediately. Repeat process to make second omelette.

*Note: Eggs used in these recipes are sized as large.

Italian Breakfast Omelette

Servings: 2 omelettes (four blocks each)

Block Size:

6 Protein	8 egg whites plus 2 whole eggs*
2 Protein	2 ounces skim milk mozzarella cheese
2½ Carbohydrate	3½ cups cooked zucchini, sliced
1 Carbohydrate	3 cups cooked mushrooms, sliced
1½ Carbohydrate	1½ cups onion rings, halved
3 Carbohydrate	1½ cups tomato purée
8 Fat	2⅔ teaspoons olive oil, divided

⅛ teaspoon dried marjoram
⅛ teaspoon dried basil
⅛ teaspoon black pepper
⅛ teaspoon dried oregano
⅛ teaspoon turmeric

Method:

In a medium nonstick sauté pan, cook all vegetables, except tomato puree, in ⅔ teaspoon oil until almost tender. Add tomato puree, marjoram, basil, pepper, and oregano to vegetables and simmer for 3–5 minutes. Keep vegetable mixture warm. In a mixing bowl, whip egg whites, whole eggs, and turmeric together. Heat 1 teaspoon oil in a second sauté pan. Pour half the egg mixture into the sauté pan and cook until egg sets and an omelette forms. When omelette is cooked, place half the vegetable-tomato filling on omelette and fold over. Remove to serving plate, sprinkle omelette with 1 ounce mozzarella cheese and serve immediately. Repeat process to make second omelette.

*Note: Eggs used in these recipes are sized as large.

Pancakes with Strawberry Sauce

Servings: 2 dishes of pancakes (four blocks each)

Block Size:

2 Protein	2 whole eggs
4 Protein and 4 Carbohydrate	1⅓ cups soy flour*
2 Protein and 2 Carbohydrate	2 cups 1 percent milk
2 Carbohydrate	2 cups strawberries, sliced
8 Fat	2⅔ teaspoons olive oil
	3 teaspoons strawberry extract, divided**
	2 tablespoons water

Method:
In a small mixing bowl, combine eggs, soy flour, milk, and 2 teaspoons of strawberry extract to form a thin batter. Heat ⅔ teaspoon oil in a nonstick sauté pan. Pour batter into pan to make small (two-inch) pancakes. Batter will make about 24 silver dollar–sized pancakes. The pancakes will cook to a golden brown in color and will resemble buckwheat pancakes in color and flavor. As pancakes are cooked, place on two serving plates and keep warm. Repeat process until all the batter is used. When you have finished making all the pancakes, add sliced strawberries, water, and ½ teaspoon extract to the sauté pan. Lightly heat strawberries until they are warm. Place strawberry mixture on top of pancakes on both plates and serve.

*Note: Available in some health food stores.

**Note: Strawberry extract is needed in the batter to give it the buckwheat taste and to moderate the strong flavor of the soy flour.

Pancakes with Maple-Cinnamon Sauce

Servings: 2 dishes of pancakes (four blocks each)

Block Size:

2 Protein	2 whole eggs
4 Protein and 4 Carbohydrate	1⅓ cups soy flour*
2 Protein and 2 Carbohydrate	2 cups 1 percent milk
2 Carbohydrate	⅔ cup unsweetened applesauce
8 Fat	2⅔ teaspoons olive oil

2 tablespoons strawberry extract**
2 tablespoons plus ⅛ teaspoon
   maple flavor
2 tablespoons water
⅛ teaspoon cinnamon

Method:

In a small mixing bowl, combine eggs, soy flour, milk, strawberry extract, and ⅛ teaspoon maple flavor to form a thin batter. Heat ⅔ teaspoon oil in a nonstick sauté pan. Pour batter into pan to make small (two-inch) pancakes. Batter will make about 24 silver dollar–sized pancakes. The pancakes will cook to a golden brown color and will resemble buckwheat pancakes in color and flavor. As pancakes are cooked, place on two serving plates and keep warm. Repeat process until all the batter is used. When you have finished making all the pancakes, add applesauce, cinnamon, 2 tablespoons water, and 2 tablespoons maple flavor to the sauté pan. Lightly heat applesauce until warm. Place applesauce mixture on top of pancakes on both plates and serve.

Note: Available in some health food stores.

Note: Strawberry extract is needed in batter to give it the buckwheat taste and to moderate the strong flavor of the soy flour.

Blueberry Pancakes

Servings: 2 dishes of pancakes (four blocks each)

Block Size:

2 Protein	2 whole eggs
4 Protein and 4 Carbohydrate	1⅓ cups soy flour*
2 Protein and 2 Carbohydrate	2 cups 1% milk
2 Carbohydrate	1 cup blueberries
8 Fat	2⅔ teaspoons olive oil
	2 tablespoons strawberry extract**

Method:

In a small mixing bowl, combine eggs, soy flour, milk, strawberry extract, and blueberries to form a thin batter. Heat ⅔ teaspoon oil in a nonstick sauté pan. Pour batter into pan to make small (two-inch) pancakes. Batter will make about 24 silver dollar–sized pancakes. The pancakes will cook to a golden brown color and will resemble buckwheat pancakes in color and flavor. As blueberry pancakes are cooked, place on two serving plates and keep warm. Repeat process until all the batter is used.

*Note: Available in some health food stores.

**Note: Strawberry extract is needed in batter to give it the buckwheat taste and to moderate the strong flavor of the soy flour.

Breakfast Sandwich with Cheese

Servings: 2 sandwiches (four blocks each)

Block Size:

6 Protein	8 egg whites plus 2 whole eggs*
2 Protein	2 ounces skim milk mozzarella cheese, shredded
1 Carbohydrate	2 cups celery, diced fine
2 Carbohydrate	1 cup carrots, diced fine
2 Carbohydrate	2 cups onion, diced fine
3 Carbohydrate	3 cups tomato, chopped
8 Fat	2⅔ teaspoons olive oil, divided

Salt and pepper to taste
2 garlic cloves, minced
⅛ teaspoon marjoram
⅛ teaspoon Worcestershire sauce
¼ teaspoon chives
1 teaspoon parsley
⅛ teaspoon turmeric

Method:

In a medium nonstick sauté pan, cook all vegetables and spices, except turmeric, in ⅔ teaspoon oil until almost tender. Keep vegetable mixture warm. In a mixing bowl, whip egg whites, whole eggs, and turmeric together. Heat ½ teaspoon oil in a second sauté pan. Pour a quarter of the egg mixture into the sauté pan and cook until egg sets and an omelette forms. Repeat process to make three more omelettes. When the four omelettes have been made, place one omelette on each serving plate. Spoon half the vegetable mixture onto each omelette, then place the second omelette on top of vegetable mixture to form a sandwich. Sprinkle shredded cheese on top of each breakfast sandwich and serve.

*Note: Eggs used in these recipes are sized as large.

Ground Turkey Omelette Sandwich

Servings: 2 sandwiches (four blocks each)

Block Size:

2 Protein	3 ounces ground turkey
6 Protein	8 egg whites plus 2 whole eggs*
2 Carbohydrate	½ cup cooked kidney beans
2 Carbohydrate	2 cups onion, diced
2 Carbohydrate	2 cups green beans, chopped
1 Carbohydrate	1½ cups green bell pepper, chopped
1 Carbohydrate	1½ cups red bell pepper, chopped
8 Fat	2⅔ teaspoons olive oil

1 teaspoon Worcestershire sauce
½ teaspoon hot sauce
3 garlic cloves, minced
Salt and pepper to taste
⅛ teaspoon turmeric

Method:
In a medium nonstick sauté pan, cook ground turkey, vegetables, and spices, except turmeric, in ⅔ teaspoon oil until almost tender. Keep turkey-vegetable mixture warm. In a mixing bowl, whip egg whites, whole eggs, and turmeric together. Heat ½ teaspoon oil in a second sauté pan. Pour a quarter of the egg mixture into the sauté pan and cook until egg sets and an omelette forms. Repeat process to make three more omelettes. When the four omelettes have been made, place one omelette on each serving plate. Spoon half the turkey-vegetable mixture onto each omelette, then place the second omelette on top of each turkey-vegetable mixture to form a sand-wich. Serve immediately.

*Note: Eggs used in these recipes are sized as large.

Vegetarian Breakfast Omelette Sandwich

Servings: 2 sandwiches (four blocks each)

Block Size:

8 Protein	10 egg whites plus 2 whole eggs*
2 Carbohydrate	2 cups onion, diced
2 Carbohydrate	2 cups leeks, diced
2 Carbohydrate	1 cup carrots, diced
2 Carbohydrate	6 cups mushrooms, sliced
8 Fat	2⅔ teaspoons olive oil

1 tablespoon parsley
1 clove garlic, minced
Salt and pepper to taste
⅛ teaspoon turmeric

Method:
In a medium nonstick sauté pan, cook all vegetables and spices, except turmeric, in ⅔ teaspoon oil until almost tender. Keep vegetable mixture warm. In a mixing bowl, whip egg whites, whole eggs, and turmeric together. Heat ½ teaspoon oil in a second sauté pan. Pour a quarter of the egg mixture into the sauté pan and cook until egg sets and an omelette forms. Repeat process to make three more omelettes. When the four omelettes have been made, place one omelette on each serving plate. Spoon half the vegetable mixture onto each omelette, then place the second omelette on top of each vegetable mixture to form a sandwich. Serve immediately.

*Note: Eggs used in these recipes are sized as large.

Breakfast Spinach Omelette Pie

Servings: 2 pies (four blocks each)

Block Size:

6 Protein	8 egg whites plus 2 whole eggs*
2 Protein	2 ounces skim milk mozzarella cheese
4 Carbohydrate	1 pound spinach
3½ Carbohydrate	3½ cups onion, diced fine
½ Carbohydrate	½ cup shallots, diced fine
8 Fat	2⅔ teaspoons olive oil
	⅛ teaspoon black pepper
	2 garlic cloves, minced
	½ teaspoon nutmeg
	⅛ teaspoon turmeric

Method:

In a medium nonstick sauté pan, cook all vegetables and spices, except turmeric, in ⅔ teaspoon oil until almost tender. Keep spinach mixture warm. In a mixing bowl, whip egg whites, whole eggs, and turmeric together. Heat 1 teaspoon oil in a second sauté pan. Pour half the egg mixture into the sauté pan and cook until egg sets and an omelette forms. Repeat process to make another omelette. Place omelettes in the bottom of two soup bowls. Spoon half the spinach mixture onto each omelette to form a spinach pie. Top with shredded cheese and serve.

*Note: Eggs used in these recipes are sized as large.

Breakfast Zucchini Omelette Pie

Servings: 2 pies (four blocks each)

Block Size:

6 Protein	8 egg whites plus 2 whole eggs*
2 Protein	2 ounces skim milk mozzarella cheese
4 Carbohydrate	6 cups zucchini, quartered
2 Carbohydrate	2 cups onion, half ring slices
2 Carbohydrate	3 cups green bell pepper, diced
8 Fat	2⅔ teaspoons olive oil

6 garlic cloves, minced
2 tablespoons fresh basil, diced
⅛ teaspoon dried oregano
⅛ teaspoon turmeric

Method:

In a medium nonstick sauté pan, cook all vegetables and spices, except turmeric, in ⅔ teaspoon oil until almost tender. Keep zucchini mixture warm. In a mixing bowl, whip egg whites, whole eggs, and turmeric together. Heat 1 teaspoon oil in a second sauté pan. Pour half the egg mixture into the sauté pan and cook until egg sets and an omelette forms. Repeat process to make another omelette. Place omelettes in the bottom of two soup bowls. Spoon half the zucchini mixture onto each omelette to form a zucchini pie. Top with shredded cheese and serve.

Note: Eggs used in these recipes are sized as large.

Breakfast Mirepoux Omelette Soufflé

Servings: 2 soufflés (four blocks each)

Block Size:

8 Protein	12 egg whites plus 2 whole eggs*
1 Carbohydrate	½ cup carrots
2 Carbohydrate	4 cups celery, diced fine
3 Carbohydrate	3 cups onion, diced fine
1 Carbohydrate	¼ cup cooked or canned kidney beans, chopped
1 Carbohydrate	2 teaspoons granulated sugar
8 Fat	2⅔ teaspoons olive oil
	⅛ teaspoon black pepper
	⅛ teaspoon celery salt
	⅛ teaspoon dried oregano

Method:
In a medium nonstick sauté pan, cook all vegetables and spices in ⅔ teaspoon oil until almost tender. Remove from heat and cool. When vegetable mixture has cooled, add beaten whole eggs and set aside. In a mixing bowl, whip egg whites and sugar to form a meringue (a marshmallowlike consistency). Heat 1 teaspoon oil in a second sauté pan. Gently pour half the meringue mixture into pan. On medium-high heat cook meringue until it has an omelette-like look and will slide around the pan. Carefully pour half the vegetable-egg mixture into the center of meringue. Continue cooking until filling is set. Fold meringue sides onto center to form a trifold. Remove to serving plate. Cut a slice down the middle of each soufflé to reveal the filling. Repeat process to make second soufflé.

*Note: Eggs used in these recipes are sized as large.

Breakfast Asparagus Omelette Soufflé

Servings: 2 soufflés (four blocks each)

Block Size:

8 Protein	12 egg whites plus 2 whole eggs*
2 Carbohydrate	2 cups onion, chopped
3 Carbohydrate	3 cups asparagus, chopped
1 Carbohydrate	2¼ cups green bell pepper, chopped
2 Carbohydrate	4 teaspoons granulated sugar
8 Fat	2⅔ teaspoons olive oil
	⅛ teaspoon dried dill weed
	⅛ teaspoon dried chives
	⅛ teaspoon hot sauce
	⅛ teaspoon celery salt

Method:
In a medium nonstick sauté pan, cook all vegetables and spices in ⅔ teaspoon oil until almost tender. Remove from heat and cool. When vegetable mixture has cooled, add beaten whole eggs and set aside. In a mixing bowl, whip egg whites and sugar to form a meringue (a marshmallowlike consistency). Heat 1 teaspoon oil in a second sauté pan. Gently pour half the meringue mixture into pan. On medium-high heat cook meringue until it has an omelette-like look and will slide around the pan. Carefully pour half the vegetable-egg mixture into the center of meringue. Continue cooking until filling is set. Fold meringue sides onto center to form a trifold. Remove to serving plate. Cut a slice down the middle of each soufflé to reveal the filling. Repeat process to make second soufflé.

Note: Eggs used in these recipes are sized as large.

Breakfast Creole Omelette Soufflé

Servings: 2 soufflés (four blocks each)

Block Size:

8 Protein	12 egg whites plus 2 whole eggs*
1 Carbohydrate	½ cup carrots
2 Carbohydrate	4 cups celery, diced fine
3 Carbohydrate	3 cups onion, diced fine
2 Carbohydrate	4 teaspoons granulated sugar
8 Fat	2⅔ teaspoons olive oil
	⅛ teaspoon black pepper
	⅛ teaspoon celery salt
	⅛ teaspoon dried oregano

Method:

In a medium nonstick sauté pan, cook all vegetables and spices in ⅔ teaspoon oil until almost tender. Remove from heat and cool. When vegetable mixture has cooled, add beaten whole eggs and set aside. In a mixing bowl, whip egg whites and sugar to form a meringue (a marshmallowlike consistency). Heat 1 teaspoon oil in a second sauté pan. Gently pour half the meringue mixture into pan. On medium-high heat cook meringue until it has an omelette-like look and will slide around the pan. Carefully pour half the vegetable-egg mixture into the center of meringue. Continue cooking until filling is set. Fold meringue sides onto center to form a trifold. Remove to serving plate. Cut a slice down the middle of each soufflé to reveal the filling. Repeat process to make second soufflé.

*Note: Eggs used in these recipes are sized as large.

Apple-Cinnamon Crepe

Servings: 2 dishes of crepes (four blocks each)

Block Size:

2 Protein	2 whole eggs
4 Protein	6 ounces deli ham, diced fine
1 Protein and 1 Carbohydrate	⅓ cup soy flour*
1 Protein and 1 Carbohydrate	1 cup 1 percent milk
2 Carbohydrate	2 red Delicious apples, peeled, cored, and roughly chopped
2 Carbohydrate	⅔ cup applesauce
2 Carbohydrate	⅔ cup cooked oatmeal
8 Fat	2⅔ teaspoons olive oil
	¼ teaspoon cinnamon

Method:

In a small mixing bowl, combine eggs, soy flour, and milk to form a batter. This amount of batter will make four crepes. Pour ½ teaspoon oil into a nonstick sauté pan or crepe pan. When the oil is hot add a quarter of the batter to pan. Cover pan with another sauté or crepe pan. Cook on medium-high heat until bottom is set and crepe will move easily in pan. To turn crepe over, securely place second pan over first and turn pan over. The crepe will then be in the second sauté pan. The second side of the crepe should cook for only a minute or so to color it. Transfer crepe to serving plate and repeat process to make three more crepes. (If you need more oil in the crepe pan, omit oil from crepe filling and use it for cooking the crepes.) Place apples, applesauce, oatmeal, ⅔ teaspoon oil, ham, and cinnamon in another sauté pan to form crepe filling. Using low heat, cook mixture until apples are tender. When ready, divide filling among the four crepes by placing it in a line along the center of each crepe. Fold over the sides to make a trifold. Serve immediately, two crepes per plate.

*Note: Available in some health food stores.

Two-Berry Crepe

Servings: 2 dishes of crepes (four blocks each)

Block Size:

2 Protein	2 whole eggs
4 Protein	1 cup low-fat cottage cheese
1 Protein and 1 Carbohydrate	⅓ cup soy flour*
1 Protein and 1 Carbohydrate	1 cup 1 percent milk
3 Carbohydrate	1½ cups blueberries
2 Carbohydrate	2 cups raspberries
1 Carbohydrate	4 teaspoons cornstarch
8 Fat	2⅔ teaspoons olive oil
	1 tablespoon orange extract
	¾ cup water

Method:

In a small mixing bowl, combine eggs, soy flour, and milk to form a batter. This amount of batter will make four crepes. Pour ½ teaspoon oil into a nonstick sauté pan or crepe pan. When the oil is hot, add a quarter of the batter to pan. Cover pan with another sauté or crepe pan. Cook on medium-high heat until bottom is set and crepe will move easily in pan. To turn crepe over, securely place second pan over first and turn pan over. The crepe will then be in the second sauté pan. The second side of the crepe should cook for only a minute or so to color it. Transfer crepe to serving plate and repeat process to make three more crepes. (If you need more oil in the crepe pan, omit oil from crepe filling and use it for cooking the crepes.) In a small bowl, add the cornstarch, orange extract, ⅔ teaspoon oil, and water until cornstarch has dissolved. While the crepes are cooking, place dissolved cornstarch in another nonstick sauté pan to make crepe filling. While stirring constantly, heat dissolved cornstarch until a sauce forms, then add berries and heat through to create filling. When ready, divide filling among the four crepes by placing it in a line along the center of each crepe. Place ¼ cup of cottage cheese on top of filling and fold over the sides to make a trifold. Serve immediately, two crepes per plate.

Note: Available in some health food stores.

Mandarin Orange Crepe

Servings: 2 dishes of crepes (four blocks each)

Block Size:

2 Protein	2 whole eggs
1 Protein and 1 Carbohydrate	⅓ cup soy flour*
1 Protein and 1 Carbohydrate	1 cup 1 percent milk
2 Protein and 2 Carbohydrate	1 cup plain low-fat yogurt
2 Protein	2 envelopes Knox Unflavored Gelatin
1 Carbohydrate	4 teaspoons cornstarch
3 Carbohydrate	1 cup mandarin orange sections
8 Fat	2⅔ teaspoons olive oil
	2 teaspoon orange extract

Method:
In a small mixing bowl, combine eggs, soy flour, and milk to form a batter. This amount of batter will make four crepes. Pour ½ teaspoon oil into a nonstick sauté pan or crepe pan. When the oil is hot, add a quarter of the batter to pan. Cover pan with another sauté or crepe pan. Cook on medium-high heat until bottom is set and crepe will move easily in pan. To turn crepe over, securely place second pan over first and turn pan over. The crepe will then be in

the second sauté pan. The second side of the crepe should cook for only a minute or so to color it. Transfer crepe to serving plate and repeat process to make three more crepes. (If you need more oil in the crepe pan, omit oil from crepe filling and use it for cooking the crepes.) In a small bowl, stir together the yogurt, cornstarch, orange extract, ⅔ teaspoon oil, and gelatin. Transfer mixture to another sauté pan to make crepe filling. Heat mixture on low heat while stirring constantly until heated throughout, then add orange sections and heat through. When ready, divide filling among the four crepes by placing it in a line along the center of each crepe. Fold over the sides to make a trifold. Serve immediately, two crepes per plate.

Note: Available in some health food stores.

Kiwi and Pineapple Crepe

Servings: 2 dishes of crepes (four blocks each)

Block Size:

2 Protein	2 whole eggs
4 Protein	1 cup low-fat cottage cheese
1 Protein and	
1 Carbohydrate	⅓ cup soy flour*
1 Protein and	
1 Carbohydrate	1 cup 1 percent milk
2 Carbohydrate	2 kiwi fruit, peeled and diced
4 Carbohydrate	2 cups pineapple
8 Fat	2⅔ teaspoons olive oil
	⅛ teaspoon cinnamon

Method:

In a small mixing bowl, combine eggs, soy flour, and milk to form a batter. This amount of batter will make four crepes. Pour ½ teaspoon oil into nonstick sauté pan or crepe pan. When the oil is hot add a quarter of the batter to pan. Cover pan with another sauté or crepe pan. Cook on medium-high heat until bottom is set and crepe will move easily in pan. To turn crepe over, securely place second pan over first and turn pan over. The crepe will then be in the second sauté pan. The second side of the crepe should cook for only a minute or so to color it. Transfer crepe to serving plate and repeat process to make three more crepes. (If you need more oil in the crepe pan, omit oil from crepe filling and use it for cooking the crepes.) In a sauté pan, combine kiwi fruit, pineapple, ⅔ teaspoon oil, and cinnamon, and heat until they are tender. When the fruit is hot, divide the filling among the four crepes by placing it in a line along the center of each crepe. Place ¼ cup cottage cheese on top of filling in each crepe and fold over the sides to make a trifold. Serve immediately, two crepes per plate.

Note: Available in some health food stores.

Vegetable Breakfast Crepe

Servings: 2 dishes of crepes (four blocks each)

Block Size:

2 Protein	2 whole eggs
4 Protein	4 ounces skim milk mozzarella cheese, shredded
1 Protein and	
1 Carbohydrate	⅓ cup soy flour*
1 Protein and	
1 Carbohydrate	1 cup 1 percent milk
1 Carbohydrate	4 teaspoons cornstarch
1 Carbohydrate	2 cups broccoli spears, sliced thin
1 Carbohydrate	3 cups mushrooms, diced fine
1 Carbohydrate	1 cup onion, diced fine
2 Carbohydrate	2 cups strawberries, sliced
8 Fat	2⅔ teaspoons olive oil
	¼ teaspoon turmeric
	2 tablespoons water
	⅛ teaspoon sherry

Method:

In a small mixing bowl, combine eggs, soy flour, and milk to form a batter. This amount of batter will make four crepes. Pour ½ teaspoon oil into nonstick sauté pan or crepe pan. When the oil is hot, add a quarter of the batter to pan. Cover pan with another sauté or crepe pan. Cook on medium-high heat until bottom is set and crepe will move easily in pan. To turn crepe over, securely place second pan over first and turn pan over. The crepe will then be in the second sauté pan. The second side of the crepe should cook for only a minute or so to color it. Transfer crepe to serving plate and repeat process to make three more crepes. (If you need more oil in the crepe pan, omit oil from crepe filling and use it for cooking the crepes.) In a small saucepan combine turmeric, cornstarch, 2 tablespoons water, and sherry, and mix well. Add cheese and heat. Stir sauce continuously over moderate heat until a thick cheese sauce forms. Remove from heat and keep warm. In a sauté pan, add ⅔ teaspoon oil and cook broccoli, mushrooms, and onions until tender. When the vegetable mixture is cooked, divide the filling among the four crepes by placing it in a line along the center of each crepe. Fold over the sides to make a trifold. Serve two crepes per plate and top crepes with a small quantity of cheese sauce. Garnish each plate with 1 cup sliced strawberries beside crepe.

Note: Available in some health food stores.

Note: Can also be used as a light brunch dish.

Fresh Fruit with Creamy Sauce

Servings: 2 dishes of fruit and sauce (four blocks each)

Block Size:

8 Protein   2 cups low-fat cottage cheese

1 Carbohydrate   ⅓ cup applesauce
2 Carbohydrate   2 peaches
1 Carbohydrate   ½ cup grapes
1 Carbohydrate   ⅓ cup mandarin orange sections
1 Carbohydrate   1 cup strawberries, sliced
2 Carbohydrate   1 apple, cored and sliced

8 Fat   8 teaspoons almonds, sliced

¼ teaspoon cinnamon
⅛ teaspoon nutmeg

Method:
Combine cottage cheese, cinnamon, and nutmeg in a blender. Blend until smooth. Remove from blender and place in a small mixing bowl, then add fruit and gently blend together. Divide fruit mixture into two serving dishes, top with almonds, and serve.

Sweet and Spicy Peaches

Servings: 2 dishes of peaches (four blocks each)

Block Size:

2 Protein	2 envelopes Knox Unflavored Gelatin
4 Protein	2 ounces protein powder (28 grams of protein)
2 Protein and 2 Carbohydrate	1 cup plain low-fat yogurt, lightly heated
5 Carbohydrate	5 peaches, peeled, pitted, and sliced
1 Carbohydrate	1½ teaspoons brown sugar
8 Fat	8 teaspoons almonds, sliced
	1 tablespoon vanilla extract
	⅛ teaspoon allspice
	½ cup water

Method:

In saucepan gently heat peaches, vanilla extract, allspice, brown sugar, gelatin, and water until hot. In a mixing bowl, combine protein powder with yogurt. Place yogurt and protein powder mixture into two serving bowls, then top with heated fruit and serve.

Strawberry Instant Breakfast

Servings: 2 glasses (four blocks each)

Block Size:

2 Protein	2 envelopes Knox Unflavored Gelatin
2 Protein	½ cup low-fat cottage cheese
2 Protein and 2 Carbohydrate	2 cups 1 percent milk
2 Protein and 2 Carbohydrate	1 cup plain low-fat yogurt
4 Carbohydrate	4 cups strawberries, sliced*
8 Fat	2⅔ teaspoons olive oil

Method:
Place all ingredients in blender to make instant breakfast. Blend until smooth. Pour into two large glasses, garnish with a strawberry, and serve.

*Note: Fresh or frozen strawberries can be used. If using frozen strawberries, use whole or sliced berries without sugar or additives. If using fresh strawberries, use only those that are plump and have a solid color. Always store fresh strawberries covered in the refrigerator.

Scrambled Eggs with Vegetables

Servings: 2 scrambled egg dishes (four blocks each)

Block Size:

8 Protein	12 egg whites plus 2 whole eggs
1 Carbohydrate	4 cups spinach
2 Carbohydrate	2 cups green beans
2 Carbohydrate	2 cups wax beans
2 Carbohydrate	½ cup kidney beans
1 Carbohydrate	1 cup onion, chopped
8 Fat	2⅔ teaspoons olive oil, divided
	¼ teaspoon turmeric

Method:

In a medium nonstick sauté pan, add ⅔ teaspoon oil and all vegetables. Cook vegetables until tender, then remove from stove and keep vegetable mixture warm until scrambled eggs are made. In a mixing bowl, whip egg whites, whole eggs, and turmeric together. Heat 2 teaspoons oil in a second sauté pan. Pour the egg mixture into the sauté pan and stir continuously until scrambled eggs are cooked. Divide the scrambled eggs between two heated serving plates and place an equal amount of vegetables beside scrambled eggs.

Breakfast Pizza Omelette

Servings: 2 pizzas (four blocks each)

Block Size:

6 Protein	8 egg whites plus 2 whole eggs
2 Protein	2 ounces skim milk mozzarella cheese, shredded
1 Carbohydrate	3 cups mushrooms, sliced
1 Carbohydrate	1 cup tomato, diced
1 Carbohydrate	1 cup onion, chopped
2 Carbohydrate	½ cup chickpeas, chopped
1 Carbohydrate	1 cup asparagus, chopped
2 Carbohydrate	1 cup tomato puree
8 Fat	2⅔ teaspoons olive oil, divided
	¼ teaspoon turmeric

Method:

In a nonstick medium sauté pan, add 2 teaspoons oil and all vegetables, except tomato puree. Cook vegetables until tender, then remove from stove and keep vegetable mixture warm. In a mixing bowl, whip egg whites, whole eggs, and turmeric together. Heat ⅔ teaspoon oil in a second sauté pan, until almost hot. Pour egg mixture into second sauté pan and cook mixture until egg sets and an omelette forms. Place omelette in baking dish and spoon vegetable mixture on top, to form a topping. Heat tomato puree in small saucepan and pour over contents of baking dish. Top with shredded cheese and place under broiler until cheese melts and browns slightly. Cut into four wedges and serve two wedges per serving plate.

Sausage and Egg Breakfast with Vegetables

Servings: 2 Sausage and Egg Breakfast dishes (four blocks each)

Block Size:

6 Protein	9 ounces ground turkey
2 Protein	2 whole eggs
2 Carbohydrate	2 cups kale
1 Carbohydrate	1 cup leeks, sliced
1 Carbohydrate	2 cups steamed broccoli florets
1 Carbohydrate	½ cup steamed carrots, half slices
1 Carbohydrate	¾ cup red bell pepper, half rings
1 Carbohydrate	1 cup steamed wax beans, chopped
1 Carbohydrate	½ apple, shredded
8 Fat	2⅔ teaspoons olive oil, divided

⅛ teaspoon sage
⅛ teaspoon paprika
⅛ teaspoon nutmeg
Salt and pepper to taste
Water

Method:
In a saucepan, add vegetables with enough water to cover vegetables. Cook vegetables until tender but not overcooked. In a mixing bowl, combine turkey, apple, sage, paprika, nutmeg, salt, and pepper. Form turkey mixture into two patties and sauté in ⅔ teaspoon oil. Remove patties from pan and set aside. In a nonstick sauté pan, heat 2 teaspoons oil, then cook whole eggs over easy. Place vegetables on two plates along with a turkey sausage patty and an over-easy egg on each plate.

Omelette à la Colorado

Servings: 2 omelettes (four blocks each)

Block Size:

6 Protein	8 egg whites plus 2 eggs
1 Protein	1½ ounces deli-style ham, chopped
1 Protein	1 ounce skim milk mozzarella cheese, shredded
1 Carbohydrate	1 cup onion, diced fine
2 Carbohydrate	2 cups kale
1 Carbohydrate	¼ cup cooked black beans
1 Carbohydrate	¼ cup cooked kidney beans
1 Carbohydrate	¼ cup cooked chickpeas
1 Carbohydrate	1 cup onion, chopped fine
½ Carbohydrate	¾ cup green bell pepper, chopped
½ Carbohydrate	¾ cup red bell pepper, chopped
8 Fat	2⅔ teaspoons olive oil

Method:

In a medium nonstick sauté pan, cook 1 cup diced fine onion, kale, beans, and chickpeas in ⅔ teaspoon oil until hot and crisp. In a mixing bowl, whip together whole eggs, egg whites, chopped peppers, 1 cup chopped fine onions, ham, and cheese. In a second sauté pan, heat 1 teaspoon oil before adding half the egg mixture. Cook until set and an omelette is formed. Repeat process to make second omelette. Fill each omelette with half the vegetable mixture, then fold over and serve.

Eggs Arnold

Servings: 2 egg dishes (four blocks each)

Block Size:

4 Protein	4 egg whites plus 2 whole eggs, separated
2 Protein	2 ounces skim milk mozzarella cheese, shredded
2 Protein	3 ounces deli-style ham
1½ Carbohydrate	4 Portobello mushroom caps*
1 Carbohydrate	¾ cup red bell pepper, thin strips
2 Carbohydrate	½ cup cooked kidney beans
3 Carbohydrate	3 cups asparagus, chopped
½ Carbohydrate	2 teaspoons cornstarch
8 Fat	2⅔ teaspoons olive oil

3 tablespoons water
Dash white wine
¼ teaspoon chili powder
⅛ teaspoon turmeric

Method:
Remove stems from mushrooms, then lightly cook mushroom caps in ⅔ teaspoon oil, 1 tablespoon water, and dash white wine. Using an egg poacher, poach eggs and egg whites separately, then reserve for use. In nonstick sauté pan, cook pepper and kidney beans in 2 teaspoons oil until tender. In a saucepan, add asparagus and enough water to cover. Cook asparagus until tender but not over-cooked. In another small saucepan, combine chili powder, turmer-ic, cornstarch, and 2 tablespoons water. Blend mixture until corn-starch dissolves, then add mozzarella cheese and heat until a sauce forms. Assemble dish by placing two mushroom caps on each serv-ing plate and topping mushrooms with the poached egg whites. Layer ham over mushroom capped egg white on each plate. Place a poached whole egg beside the two mushroom caps on each plate,

then gently pour sauce on top. Divide vegetables in half and place beside eggs on plates.

Note: Portobello mushrooms are large-capped mushrooms with a mild meaty flavor, which work excellently with this recipe. The mushroom stems can be diced and added to the asparagus, or saved for another dish.

Poached Eggs on a Spinach Bed

Servings: 2 egg dishes (four blocks each)

Block Size:

6 Protein	8 egg whites plus 2 whole eggs
1 Protein	¼ cup cottage cheese
1 Protein and 1 Carbohydrate	1 cup 1 percent milk
1 Carbohydrate	3 cups mushrooms, diced fine
2 Carbohydrate	2 cups onion, diced fine
2 Carbohydrate	8 cups spinach
2 Carbohydrate	4 teaspoons cornstarch
8 Fat	2⅔ teaspoons olive oil
	¼ teaspoon nutmeg
	⅛ teaspoon allspice
	⅛ teaspoon chili powder
	⅛ teaspoon paprika

Method:
Using an egg poacher, poach eggs and egg whites separately, then reserve for use. In nonstick sauté pan, cook mushrooms and onions in 2 teaspoons oil until tender, then remove and keep warm. In another sauté pan, add the remaining ⅔ teaspoon oil and cook the spinach until just wilted. Combine cottage cheese, nutmeg, allspice, chili powder, milk, and cornstarch in a blender. Blend until smooth. Remove from blender and place in a small saucepan on medium

heat until a sauce forms. Assemble dishes by forming a bed of spinach on each serving plate. Place half the onion and mushroom mixture on each dish, then place four poached egg whites and 1 poached egg on each dish. Evenly divide sauce by pouring over eggs on each serving plate. Sprinkle with paprika and serve.

Quiche Lorraine

Servings: 2 quiche (four blocks each)

Block Size:

4 Protein	4 egg whites plus 2 whole eggs
1 Protein	1½ ounces deli-style ham, shredded
2 Protein	2 ounces skim milk mozzarella cheese, shredded
1 Protein and 1 Carbohydrate	1 cup 1 percent milk
½ Carbohydrate	½ cup onion, diced fine
2 Carbohydrate	2 cups kale
1 Carbohydrate	1 cup zucchini, diced fine
1 Carbohydrate	1 cup yellow squash, diced fine
1 Carbohydrate	1 cup leeks, diced fine
½ Carbohydrate	¾ cup red bell pepper, diced fine
1 Carbohydrate	1 cup tomato, chopped
8 Fat	2⅔ teaspoons, olive oil
	⅛ teaspoon dry mustard
	⅛ teaspoon black pepper

Method:

In a nonstick sauté pan, cook all vegetables and spices in oil until tender. Let vegetables cool to room temperature. In a mixing bowl, whip together eggs and milk, then add cooled vegetables, ham, and cheese. Place combined ingredients in two circular baking dishes. Bake at 400 degrees for 45–60 minutes, serve immediately when removed from oven.

Asparagus Quiche

Servings: 2 quiches (four blocks each)

Block Size:

5 Protein	6 egg whites plus 2 whole eggs
2 Protein	2 ounces skim milk mozzarella cheese, shredded
1 Protein and 1 Carbohydrate	1 cup 1 percent milk
½ Carbohydrate	½ cup onion, diced fine
2 Carbohydrate	2 cups asparagus, sliced
2 Carbohydrate	2 cups kale
½ Carbohydrate	1½ cups mushrooms, sliced
1 Carbohydrate	½ cup carrots, sliced
1 Carbohydrate	1 cup tomato, chopped
8 Fat	2⅔ teaspoons olive oil
	Salt and pepper to taste
	2 garlic cloves, minced
	⅛ teaspoon chili powder
	⅛ teaspoon dried basil
	¼ teaspoon dried dill

Method:

In nonstick sauté pan, cook all vegetables and spices in oil until tender. Let vegetables cool to room temperature. In a mixing bowl, whip together eggs and milk, then add cooled vegetables and cheese. Place combined ingredients in two circular baking dishes. Bake at 400 degrees for 45–60 minutes, serve immediately when removed from oven.

Vegetable Quiche

Servings: 2 quiches (four blocks each)

Block Size:

5 Protein	6 egg whites plus 2 whole eggs
2 Protein	2 ounces skim milk mozzarella cheese, shredded
1 Protein and 1 Carbohydrate	1 cup 1 percent milk
½ Carbohydrate	½ cup onion, diced fine
1 Carbohydrate	4 cups spinach, stems removed
½ Carbohydrate	1 cup carrots, shredded
2 Carbohydrate	2 cups snow peas
½ Carbohydrate	1½ cups cucumber, peeled, seeded, and diced fine
½ Carbohydrate	¾ cup red bell pepper, diced fine
1 Carbohydrate	1 cup yellow squash, diced fine
1 Carbohydrate	½ cup water chestnuts, chopped
8 Fat	2⅔ teaspoons olive oil
	¼ teaspoon celery salt
	⅛ teaspoon hot curry powder
	4 garlic cloves, minced

Method:

In a nonstick sauté pan, cook all vegetables and spices in oil until tender. Let vegetables cool to room temperature. In a mixing bowl, whip together eggs and milk, then add cooled vegetables and cheese. Place combined ingredients in two circular baking dishes. Bake at 400 degrees for 45–60 minutes, serve immediately when removed from oven.

Tuesday Omelette

Servings: 2 omelettes (four blocks each)

Block Size:

1½ Protein	2¼ ounces deli-style ham, medium dice
6 Protein	12 egg whites
½ Protein and ½ Carbohydrate	¼ cup plain low-fat yogurt
1 Carbohydrate	1 cup onion, chopped
1 Carbohydrate	1¼ cups spinach, cooked
1 Carbohydrate	1¼ cups tomato, chopped
½ Carbohydrate	1 cup celery, chopped
2 Carbohydrate	1 apple, cored and sliced
2 Carbohydrate	1 cup honeydew melon, cubed
8 Fat	2⅔ teaspoons olive oil, divided

Salt and pepper to taste
¼ teaspoon turmeric
¼ teaspoon dried chives
⅛ teaspoon celery salt
⅛ teaspoon chili powder

Method:

In nonstick sauté pan, heat ham, onion, spinach, tomato, and celery in ⅔ teaspoon oil until vegetables are tender. While vegetables are cooking, in a medium mixing bowl combine egg whites, yogurt, and spices. The yogurt will appear curdled when mixed with the egg whites but it is fine. Whip the egg white–yogurt mixture until the yogurt has blended into the mixture and it no longer looks curdled. In a second nonstick sauté pan, heat 1 teaspoon oil before adding half the egg mixture. Cook until set and an omelette is formed. Fill omelette with half vegetable mixture, fold over, and serve with half the fruit arranged around the omelette. Repeat process to make second omelette.

Omelette à la California

Servings: 2 omelettes (four blocks each)

Block Size:

7½ Protein	15 egg whites
½ Protein and ½ Carbohydrate	¼ cup plain low-fat yogurt
1 Carbohydrate	⅓ cup cooked pinto beans, rinsed
1 Carbohydrate	¼ cup cooked black beans, rinsed
1 Carbohydrate	¼ cup cooked kidney beans, rinsed
1 Carbohydrate	1¼ cups tomato, chopped
1 Carbohydrate	1 cup onion, chopped
1 Carbohydrate	1 cup asparagus spears, half-inch pieces
½ Carbohydrate	3 cups spinach
1 Carbohydrate	¼ cup chickpeas
8 Fat	2⅔ teaspoons olive oil, divided
	¼ teaspoon dried dill
	Salt and pepper to taste
	¼ teaspoon dried chives
	¼ teaspoon turmeric
	⅛ teaspoon chili powder
	⅛ teaspoon celery salt

Method:
In nonstick sauté pan, heat beans, tomato, onion, asparagus, spinach, chickpeas, and dill in ⅔ teaspoon oil until vegetables are tender. While the vegetables are cooking, in a medium mixing bowl combine the egg whites, yogurt, and remaining spices. The yogurt will appear curdled when mixed with the egg whites but it is fine. Whip the egg white–yogurt mixture until the yogurt has blended into the mixture and it no longer looks curdled. In a second non-stick sauté pan, heat 1 teaspoon oil before adding half the egg mixture. Cook until set and an omelette is formed. Fill omelette with half the vegetable mixture, fold over, and serve. Repeat process to make second omelette.

LUNCH

Buddhist Vegetable Entrée

Servings: 2 lunch entrées (four blocks each)

Block Size:

8 Protein	24 ounces firm tofu, half-inch dice*
1 Carbohydrate	2½ cups celery, sliced
1 Carbohydrate	1 cup onion, sliced thin
1 Carbohydrate	3 cups cabbage, shredded
1 Carbohydrate	3 cups mushrooms, sliced thin
1 Carbohydrate	1½ cup zucchini, quartered and sliced
1 Carbohydrate	1½ cups bell pepper, sliced thin
1 Carbohydrate	3 cups bean sprouts
1 Carbohydrate	4 teaspoons cornstarch
8 Fat	2⅔ teaspoons olive oil

1 cup cold water
2 tablespoons low-sodium soy sauce
¼ teaspoon hot curry powder
½ teaspoon chili powder
Dash garlic powder
Salt and pepper to taste

Method:
In nonstick sauté pan, cook vegetables in oil until almost tender, then add ½ cup water and cover to steam sauté. In saucepan, add cold water, soy sauce, curry powder, chili powder, garlic powder, and cornstarch to form a sauce. (Mix cornstarch with a little water to dissolve it before adding to saucepan.) Heat sauce to a light simmer while constantly stirring, then add diced tofu to sauce and heat through. Add sauce and tofu to vegetables, stir, and simmer for 2–3 minutes. Divide between two lunch plates and serve at once.

*Note: Tofu has a high water content. To eliminate some of the excess water, place the blocks of tofu in a shallow dish and let stand for half an hour.

Spicy Vegetarian Tofu Primavera

Servings: 2 lunch entrées (four blocks each)

Block Size:

8 Protein	24 ounces extra-firm tofu, cubed*
1 Carbohydrate	½ cup carrots, sliced
1 Carbohydrate	1 cup onion, sliced
2 Carbohydrate	4½ cups green bell pepper, sliced
1 Carbohydrate	3 cups cabbage, shredded
2 Carbohydrate	2½ cups tomato, diced
1 Carbohydrate	4 teaspoons cornstarch
8 Fat	2⅔ teaspoons olive oil

1½ cups cold water
2 tablespoons soy sauce
⅛ teaspoon cayenne pepper
⅛ teaspoon crushed red pepper
2 garlic cloves, minced
Salt and pepper to taste

Method:

In nonstick sauté pan, cook vegetables in oil until almost tender, then add ½ cup water and cover to steam sauté. In saucepan, add the rest of the water, soy sauce, cayenne pepper, crushed red pepper, garlic, and cornstarch to form a sauce. (Mix cornstarch with a little water to dissolve it before adding to saucepan.) Heat sauce to a light simmer, constantly stirring. Add diced tofu to sauce and heat through. Add tofu and sauce to vegetables, stir and simmer for 2–3 minutes. Divide between two lunch plates and serve at once.

Note: Tofu has a high water content. To eliminate some of the excess water, place the blocks of tofu in a shallow dish and let stand for half an hour.

Rich and Hearty Cucumber Stew

Servings: 2 lunch entrées (four blocks each)

Block Size:

6 Protein	6 ounces skim milk mozzarella cheese, shredded
2 Protein	2 hard-boiled eggs, sliced
2 Carbohydrate	1 cup tomato puree
1 Carbohydrate	1¼ cups tomato, diced
2 Carbohydrate	6 cups cucumber, diced
1 Carbohydrate	1½ cups green bell pepper, sliced and quartered
2 Carbohydrate	2 cups onion, diced
8 Fat	24 black olives, sliced

1 clove garlic, minced
White pepper to taste
Dash celery salt
¼ teaspoon salt
1½ teaspoons hot sauce
¼ teaspoon dry dill weed
1 cup water

Method:
Combine all ingredients except cheese and eggs in a large saucepan and bring to a boil. Cover and simmer on medium-high heat for 20–25 minutes, stirring frequently. Just before serving stew, stir in shredded mozzarella cheese, then divide into two soup bowls and garnish with egg slices.

Vegetarian Chili

Servings: 2 lunch entrées (four blocks each)

Block Size:

8 Protein	24 ounces extra-firm tofu, shredded
4 Carbohydrate	1 cup cooked kidney beans*
1 Carbohydrate	1 cup medium onion, diced
½ Carbohydrate	1 cup medium celery, diced
1½ Carbohydrate	1½ cups canned tomato, diced with juice
1 Carbohydrate	½ cup tomato puree
8 Fat	2⅔ teaspoons olive oil

1 cup water
6 garlic cloves, minced
1 teaspoon fresh basil
½ teaspoon hot sauce
4 tablespoons chili powder (or to taste)
Salt and pepper to taste

Method:
In saucepan, heat beans, onion, and celery in oil until tender, then add diced tomato, water, tomato puree, tofu, and spices. Heat entire mixture through until hot. Place an equal amount in two soup bowls and serve.

*Note: When using canned beans, always rinse them off before using.

Mexican Black Bean Stew

Servings: 2 lunch entrées (four blocks each)

Block Size:

8 Protein	8 ounces skinless chicken breast, diced fine
4 Carbohydrate	1 cup cooked black beans*
½ Carbohydrate	½ cup onion, diced
½ Carbohydrate	¾ cup zucchini, diced
2 Carbohydrate	1 cup tomato puree
1 Carbohydrate	½ cup salsa
8 Fat	2⅔ teaspoons olive oil, divided
	⅔ cup water
	Salt and pepper to taste
	2 tablespoons parsley

Method:

In saucepan, heat beans, onion, and zucchini in 2 teaspoons oil until tender, then add tomato puree, water, parsley, and salsa. Continue cooking until entire mixture is hot. While the vegetables are cooking, in a sauté pan heat ⅔ teaspoon oil and stir-fry chicken until cooked. Add chicken to vegetables and simmer for 5 minutes. Place an equal amount in two soup bowls and serve.

*Note: When using canned beans, always rinse them off before using.

Beef Stir-Fry

Servings: 2 lunch entrées (four blocks each)

Block Size:

8 Protein   8 ounces beef eye of round, one-
                             eighth-inch slices, cut in half-inch
                             pieces

2 Carbohydrate   ½ cup cooked kidney beans
2 Carbohydrate   2 cups green beans, chopped
1 Carbohydrate   1 cup onion, diced
1 Carbohydrate   2¼ cups red bell pepper, diced
2 Carbohydrate   1 cup tomato puree

8 Fat   2⅔ teaspoons olive oil

                             1 teaspoon Worcestershire sauce
                             ½ teaspoon hot sauce
                             4 garlic cloves, minced
                             1 cup beef stock
                             Salt and pepper to taste

Method:
In nonstick sauté pan place ⅔ teaspoon oil and beef. Cook beef
until browned and done. While beef is cooking, in another sauté
pan place 2 teaspoons oil, kidney beans, green beans, onion, bell
pepper, Worcestershire sauce, hot sauce, and garlic. Cook until
entire mixture is hot, then add tomato puree, beef stock, and
cooked beef. Cook for 5 minutes until entire stir-fry is hot. Place an
equal amount on two lunch plates and serve.

Herbed Beef and Bean Stew

Servings: 2 lunch entrées (four blocks each)

Block Size:

8 Protein	8 ounces beef eye of round, one-eighth-inch slices, diced
4 Carbohydrate	1 cup cooked kidney beans*
1 Carbohydrate	1 cup onion, diced
1 Carbohydrate	½ cup tomato puree
2 Carbohydrate	1 cup salsa
8 Fat	2⅔ teaspoons olive oil, divided

⅛ teaspoon Worcestershire sauce
½ cup beef stock
½ teaspoon chili powder
⅛ teaspoon dried basil
⅛ teaspoon curry powder
⅛ teaspoon dried oregano
Salt and pepper to taste

Method:
In saucepan, cook beans and onion in 2 teaspoons oil until tender, then add tomato puree, Worcestershire sauce, beef stock, spices, and salsa. Continue cooking vegetable mixture under medium heat until hot. While the vegetables are cooking, in nonstick sauté pan add remaining oil and stir-fry beef until cooked. Add beef to vegetables and simmer for 5 minutes. Place an equal amount in two soup bowls and serve.

*Note: When using canned beans, always rinse them off before using.

Sweet and Sour Tofu

Servings: 2 lunch entrées (four blocks each)

Block Size:

8 Protein	24 ounces extra-firm tofu, cubed
1 Carbohydrate	2 teaspoons sugar
1 Carbohydrate	½ cup tomato puree
1 Carbohydrate	4 teaspoons cornstarch
1 Carbohydrate	½ cup pineapple, diced
4 Carbohydrate	2 cups fruit cocktail (packed in water)
8 Fat	2⅔ teaspoons olive oil
	1 cup water
	6 tablespoons vinegar
	4 tablespoons soy sauce
	⅛ teaspoon banana extract (optional)
	Salt and pepper to taste

Method:
In nonstick sauté pan, heat oil until hot, then add tofu. Cook tofu until browned on all sides. While tofu is cooking under medium heat, in saucepan add water, vinegar, sugar, tomato puree, soy sauce, banana extract, and cornstarch. (Mix cornstarch with a little water so that it is dissolved before being added to saucepan.) Cook over medium heat to form a sauce, stirring constantly. When a sauce has formed, add pineapple and fruit cocktail. Taste sauce; if sauce has too strong a vinegar taste, continue simmering for a few more minutes. The flavor will develop into a sweet and sour sauce as it cooks. Heat until fruit is hot, then add entire mixture to tofu in sauté pan. Simmer for 5 minutes, gently stirring mixture. Spoon onto two lunch dishes and serve immediately.

Chicken Stir-Fry

Servings: 2 lunch entrées (four blocks each)

Block Size:

8 Protein	8 ounces chicken tenderloins (or skinless chicken breast), cut into one-inch pieces
⅔ Carbohydrate	1½ cups red bell pepper, one-inch squares
⅔ Carbohydrate	1½ cups green bell pepper, one-inch squares
⅔ Carbohydrate	1½ cups yellow bell pepper, one-inch squares
2 Carbohydrate	3 cups broccoli florets, or diced fine
1 Carbohydrate	3 cups mushrooms, sliced
2 Carbohydrate	2½ cups tomato, diced fine
1 Carbohydrate	4 teaspoons cornstarch
8 Fat	2⅔ teaspoons olive oil

2 tablespoons cider vinegar
⅛ teaspoon dried basil
⅛ teaspoon dried oregano
Salt and pepper to taste
2 cloves garlic, minced
1 cup chicken stock

Method:
In nonstick sauté pan, place ⅔ teaspoon oil and chicken. Cook chicken until browned and done. While the chicken is cooking under medium heat, in another nonstick sauté pan place 2 teaspoons oil, bell peppers, broccoli, mushrooms, vinegar, garlic, tomato, and spices. Heat vegetables until entire mixture is hot, then add chicken stock, cooked chicken, and cornstarch. Mix cornstarch into chicken stock so it can dissolve before adding to pan. Cook for 5 minutes until entire stir-fry is hot and cornstarch has thickened the dish. Place an equal amount on two lunch plates and serve.

Note: When getting vegetable ingredients ready for a stir-fry dish be sure to cut vegetables as close to the same size as possible. This helps in making the cooking time the same.

Curried Chicken

Servings: 2 lunch entrées (four blocks each)

Block Size:

6 Protein	6 ounces chicken, diced
2 Protein and 2 Carbohydrate	1 cup plain low-fat yogurt
1 Carbohydrate	4 teaspoons cornstarch
2 Carbohydrate	6 cups mushrooms, sliced
1 Carbohydrate	2¼ cups red bell pepper, in strips
2 Carbohydrate	2 cups snow peas, in strips
8 Fat	2⅔ teaspoon olive oil
	⅛ teaspoon white wine
	½ cup chicken stock
	2 teaspoons hot curry powder*
	Salt and pepper to taste

Method:
In nonstick sauté pan, place ⅔ teaspoon oil and diced chicken. Cook chicken until browned and done, then add wine, chicken stock, yogurt, curry powder, and cornstarch. (Mix cornstarch in chicken stock so that it can dissolve before being added to pan.) Stirring constantly, heat until a thick curried sauce forms, then simmer for 5 minutes. While the chicken is cooking, in another sauté pan place 2 teaspoons oil, mushrooms, bell pepper, and snow peas. Cook until mixture is tender. Place an equal amount of cooked snow peas, bell pepper, and mushrooms on two lunch plates, then spoon the chicken curry mixture onto the plates.

*Note: There are a number of brands of curry powder. Each has a slightly different blend of spices and level of heat. Experiment until you find one that fits your family's tastes.

Deviled Snow Peas

Servings: 2 lunch entrées (four blocks each)

Block Size:

2 Protein	6 ounces extra-firm tofu
2 Protein	2 whole eggs
4 Protein and 4 Carbohydrate	2 cups plain low-fat yogurt
3 Carbohydrate	3 cups snow peas, whole
1 Carbohydrate	4 teaspoons cornstarch
8 Fat	2⅔ teaspoons olive oil

4 teaspoons dry mustard
2 garlic cloves, minced
Paprika for garnish
Salt and pepper to taste

Method:

In nonstick sauté pan, place oil and snow peas. Cook snow peas until tender. While the snow peas are cooking, in saucepan add yogurt, mustard, tofu, garlic, and eggs. Cook yogurt-tofu mixture over medium heat for 5–10 minutes until mixture is hot and tofu has broken down. (Mix cornstarch with a little water, then add to saucepan.) Stirring constantly, heat until a thick sauce forms, then add cooked snow peas. Continue simmering for 2–3 minutes. Place an equal amount of the deviled snow peas on two lunch plates, then sprinkle with paprika and serve.

Creamy Dilled Tomatoes

Servings: 2 lunch entrées (four blocks each)

Block Size:

2 Protein	2 whole eggs
2 Protein	6 ounces extra-firm tofu, diced fine
4 Protein and	
4 Carbohydrate	2 cups plain low-fat yogurt
1 Carbohydrate	4 teaspoons cornstarch
3 Carbohydrate	3¾ cups tomato, diced
8 Fat	24 black olives, sliced

2 teaspoons mustard
2 garlic cloves, minced
⅛ teaspoon white wine
2 tablespoons dried dill
Lemon herb seasoning
Salt and pepper to taste

Method:
In nonstick saucepan, add yogurt, mustard, eggs, garlic, wine, and dill. Cook for 5–10 minutes until mixture is hot, then add cornstarch. (Mix cornstarch with a little water, then add to saucepan.) Stirring constantly, heat until a thick sauce forms, then add tomato, black olives, and tofu. Continue simmering for 2–3 minutes. Do not overcook, as tomato and tofu will start to break down. Place an equal amount of the creamy dilled tomatoes on two lunch plates, then sprinkle with lemon herb seasoning and serve.

Turkey Burger Casserole

Servings: 2 lunch entrées (four blocks each)

Block Size:

6 Protein	9 ounces ground turkey
2 Protein	2 whole eggs
2 Carbohydrate	2 cups onion, minced
⅔ Carbohydrate	2 cups mushrooms, minced
2 Carbohydrate	½ cup cooked chickpeas
2 Carbohydrate	½ cup cooked kidney beans
⅔ Carbohydrate	1½ cups green bell pepper, diced
⅔ Carbohydrate	1½ cups red bell pepper, diced
8 Fat	2⅔ teaspoons olive oil

4 garlic cloves, minced, divided
⅛ teaspoon dried basil
⅛ teaspoon dried marjoram
⅛ teaspoon black pepper
⅛ teaspoon chili powder
⅛ teaspoon dried oregano
⅛ teaspoon paprika
⅛ teaspoon cayenne pepper
Salt to taste

Method:
In medium bowl, mix together ground turkey, eggs, onion, mushrooms, garlic, basil, marjoram, and black pepper. Form into two oblong loaf-shaped patties and place in baking pan. The loaf-shaped patties may be very sticky and loose; however, the egg will help the patties firm up as they bake. Bake in a preheated 375-degree oven for 30–35 minutes. While the turkey patties are cooking, add oil to nonstick sauté pan and cook chickpeas, kidney beans, peppers, chili powder, oregano, paprika, and cayenne pepper until hot. Using a large spatula, remove turkey patties from baking pan and place one on each lunch plate. Place an equal amount of vegetables on each plate and serve.

Malaysian Chicken Ball Soup

Servings: 2 lunch entrées (four blocks each)

Block Size:

8 Protein	12 ounces ground chicken
½ Carbohydrate	½ cup onion, diced fine
1½ Carbohydrate	1½ cups onion, sliced into half rings
2 Carbohydrate	2 cups leeks, halved and sliced
2 Carbohydrate	6 cups mushrooms, sliced
2 Carbohydrate	8 teaspoons cornstarch
8 Fat	2⅔ teaspoons olive oil
	12 drops hot sauce
	1 teaspoon parsley
	2 tablespoons grated ginger root*
	4 cups chicken stock
	Salt and pepper to taste

Method:
In a large bowl, combine chicken, diced onion, hot sauce, parsley, and ginger root. Form mixture into small half-inch meatballs. Place meatballs in baking dish brushed with oil and bake in a preheated 375-degree oven for 15 minutes. While the meatballs are cooking, put chicken stock in saucepan and bring to a boil. Add onion, leeks, and mushrooms. Cook vegetables in chicken stock until they are tender, then mix cornstarch with a little water and add to saucepan. Simmer for 3–5 minutes, stirring constantly until thickened. Remove meatballs from oven and add to saucepan. Place an equal amount of soup and meatballs in two soup bowls and serve immediately.

*Note: When a recipe calls for fresh ginger root (available in most supermarkets or in Asian grocery stores), it is not advisable to substitute ground ginger. The flavors are very different.

Mexican Burger

Servings: 2 lunch entrées (four blocks each)

Block Size:

8 Protein	12 ounces ground beef
2 Carbohydrate	1 cup salsa
2 Carbohydrate	½ cup cooked kidney beans
2 Carbohydrate	2½ cups green bell pepper, diced
2 Carbohydrate	1 cup tomato puree
8 Fat	2⅔ teaspoons olive oil

⅛ teaspoon chili powder or to taste
⅛ teaspoon hot sauce or to taste
Salt and pepper to taste

Method:
In a medium bowl, mix together the ground beef and salsa. Form into 2 oblong patties and place under broiler. Cook until browned. While the patties are cooking, add oil to nonstick sauté pan and cook kidney beans and peppers until hot, then add chili powder, hot sauce, and tomato puree. Simmer for 5 minutes, stirring constantly. Remove patties from broiler and place a patty on each lunch plate. Place an equal amount of vegetables on each plate and serve.

Hamburger Pie

Servings: 2 lunch entrées (four blocks each)

Block Size:

8 Protein	12 ounces ground beef
1 Carbohydrate	1 cup cooked turnips, mashed
1 Carbohydrate	1 cup onion, diced
2 Carbohydrate	2 cups mushrooms, diced fine, plus 4 cups mushrooms, diced fine

2 Carbohydrate	2 cups green beans, sliced
1 Carbohydrate	1¼ cups tomato, chopped
1 Carbohydrate	4 teaspoons cornstarch
8 Fat	2⅔ teaspoons olive oil
	3 teaspoons Worcestershire sauce
	¼ teaspoon dried marjoram
	¼ teaspoon dried oregano
	⅛ teaspoon dried thyme
	⅛ teaspoon dried sage
	¼ teaspoon black pepper
	2 garlic cloves, minced
	½ cup beef stock
	Salt to taste

Method:

In saucepan, place turnips in enough water to cover. Cook until tender. Drain water from saucepan, and using a masher, mash turnips to a smooth consistency. In nonstick sauté pan, add ⅔ teaspoon oil, ground beef, Worcestershire sauce, onion, and 2 cups diced fine mushrooms. Cook until ground beef is browned. In another nonstick sauté pan, place remaining oil, 4 cups diced fine mushrooms, green beans, tomato, and spices. Cook until vegetables are tender. While the vegetables are cooking, in a small mixing bowl combine garlic, beef stock, and cornstarch. When the vegetables are cooked, add contents of mixing bowl to vegetables and continue heating until a sauce forms. Evenly coat vegetables with sauce. Layer two small baking dishes with beef mixture, then the vegetables and sauce mixture, and lastly the mashed turnips. Bake in preheated 350-degree oven for 10–15 minutes until the mashed turnips top has browned. Place on two lunch plates and serve immediately.

Louisiana-Style Shrimp

Servings: 2 lunch entrées (four blocks each)

Block Size:

7 Protein	10½ ounces cooked shrimp (20 count)
1 Protein and 1 Carbohydrate	1 cup 1 percent milk
1½ Carbohydrate	3 cups green bell pepper, half rings
1½ Carbohydrate	3 cups red bell pepper, half rings
2 Carbohydrate	2 cups onion, sliced
1 Carbohydrate	2 cups celery
1 Carbohydrate	½ cup tomato puree
1 Carbohydrate	4 teaspoons cornstarch
8 Fat	2⅔ teaspoons olive oil
	2 tablespoons cider vinegar
	1 cup water
	⅛ teaspoon hot sauce (or to taste)
	⅛ teaspoon celery salt
	Black pepper to taste

Method:

In nonstick sauté pan add oil, bell pepper half rings, onion, celery, and vinegar. Cook until vegetables are tender, then add shrimp, milk, water, tomato puree, hot sauce, seasonings, and cornstarch. (Mix cornstarch with a little water before adding it to the sauté pan, so that the cornstarch is dissolved.) Bring mixture slowly to a boil, then simmer for 5–10 minutes. Equally divide between two soup bowls and serve.

Stuffed Curry Peppers

Servings: 2 lunch entrées (four blocks each)

Block Size:

2 Protein	2 whole eggs
6 Protein	18 ounces extra-firm tofu
2 Carbohydrate	2 cups onion, diced fine
1 Carbohydrate	3 cups mushrooms, diced fine
2 Carbohydrate	½ cup cooked kidney beans, chopped
1 Carbohydrate	2¼ cups red bell pepper, diced fine
2 Carbohydrate	4 green peppers
8 Fat	2⅔ teaspoons olive oil

4 garlic cloves, minced
2 teaspoons hot curry powder
½ teaspoon dry mustard
⅛ teaspoon celery salt
⅛ teaspoon cinnamon
⅛ teaspoon black pepper
¼ teaspoon turmeric
⅛ teaspoon chili powder
⅛ teaspoon hot sauce (or to taste)
Salt to taste

Method:

In nonstick sauté pan, add oil, onion, garlic, mushrooms, kidney beans, and red bell pepper. Cook until vegetables are tender, then remove from heat and cool. In a mixing bowl, place cooked vegetable mixture, eggs, tofu, spices, and hot sauce. Mix well until all ingredients have been combined. Cut the stem top off the green peppers and remove the seeds inside, also if necessary cut a little off the bottom of the green pepper to allow the green pepper to stand still without moving. Stuff green peppers with tofu vegetable mixture and place in baking dish. If there is any vegetable mixture left over place around green peppers. Tightly seal baking dish with aluminum foil and bake in a preheated oven at 400 degrees for 1 hour. Remove baking dish from oven and place two stuffed peppers on each lunch plate. Serve immediately.

Thai Green Fish Curry

Servings: 2 lunch entrées (four blocks each)

Block Size:

6 Protein	9 ounces fresh fish fillets, cut in slivers
2 Protein and 2 Carbohydrate	1 cup plain low-fat yogurt
2 Carbohydrate	2 cups snow peas, whole
2 Carbohydrate	2 cups onion, chopped
1 Carbohydrate	1½ cups hot peppers, in rings
1 Carbohydrate	4 teaspoons cornstarch
8 Fat	2⅔ teaspoons olive oil
	4 garlic cloves, minced
	4 teaspoons vinegar
	1½ cups water
	1 teaspoon turmeric
	4 teaspoons hot curry powder
	Salt and pepper to taste

Method:
In nonstick sauté pan add oil, snow peas, onion, garlic, hot peppers, and vinegar. Cook until vegetables are tender, then add fish, yogurt, water, and spices. Cover sauté pan and poach fish in vegetable liquid until cooked through. When the fish is cooked, mix the cornstarch with a little water and add to sauté pan. Bring mixture to a boil, then simmer for an additional 5–10 minutes. Equally divide between two soup bowls and serve.

Vegetarian Franks and Beans

Servings: 2 lunch entrées (four blocks each)

Block Size:

8 Protein	8 soy hot dogs
6 Carbohydrate	1½ cups cooked black beans
1 Carbohydrate	1 cup onion, chopped fine
1 Carbohydrate	½ cup tomato puree
8 Fat	2⅔ teaspoons olive oil
	2 garlic cloves, minced
	1 teaspoon dry mustard
	½ cup water

Method:

In nonstick sauté pan, add oil, black beans, and onion. Cook black beans and onion until hot, then add garlic, mustard, tomato puree, water, and soy hot dogs. Cover sauté pan and simmer for 5–10 minutes until soy hot dogs are hot, occasionally stirring. Equally divide the beans and franks between two lunch plates. Place four soy hot dogs and an equal amount of beans on each plate and serve immediately.

Sweet and Sour Pork and Cabbage

Servings: 2 lunch entrées (four blocks each)

Block Size:

8 Protein	8 ounces pork loin, in half-inch cubes
2 Carbohydrate	6 cups cabbage, shredded
4 Carbohydrate	1 cup cooked chickpeas, chopped
2 Carbohydrate	6 cups mushrooms, sliced
8 Fat	2⅔ teaspoons olive oil
	10 tablespoons cider vinegar
	½ cup water
	Salt and pepper to taste

Method:
Sprinkle pork with salt and pepper, then place in nonstick sauté pan with ⅓ teaspoon oil. Cook until pork is browned. When the pork is cooked, remove it from pan and set aside. Add cabbage, chickpeas, mushrooms, vinegar, and 2 teaspoons oil to sauté pan and cook vegetable mixture for about 10–15 minutes, until vegetables are almost tender. Add water and cooked pork to vegetables in sauté pan. Cover sauté pan and braise mixture for 5–10 minutes, stirring occasionally. Divide between two lunch plates and serve.

Beef Chop Suey

Servings: 2 lunch entrées (four blocks each)

Block Size:

8 Protein   8 ounces beef eye of round, one-
                                   eighth-inch slices

1 Carbohydrate   3 cups cabbage, shredded
1 Carbohydrate   2 cups celery, willow leaf cut*
½ Carbohydrate   1½ cups mushrooms, sliced
½ Carbohydrate   1½ cups bean sprouts
1 Carbohydrate   ½ cup water chestnuts
½ Carbohydrate   ½ cup onion, chopped

8 Fat   2⅔ teaspoons olive oil

                                   2 tablespoons cider vinegar
                                   1 tablespoon low-sodium soy sauce
                                   ½ cup beef stock
                                   2 teaspoons Worcestershire sauce

Method:
In nonstick sauté pan, place ⅔ teaspoon oil and beef. Cook beef
until browned and done. While the beef is cooking, in another nonstick sauté pan place 2 teaspoons oil, cabbage, celery, mushrooms,
bean sprouts, water chestnuts, vinegar, and onion. Cook until entire
mixture is hot, then add soy sauce, beef stock, beef, and
Worcestershire sauce. Cover sauté pan and cook for 5–10 minutes,
stirring occasionally to blend flavors. Place an equal amount on two
lunch plates and serve.

*Note: Willow leaf cut means that the celery is cut at approximately
a 45-degree angle. Also, there is no need to add any salt to this dish,
because celery is naturally high in sodium.*

Vegetarian Hot Dog Casserole

Servings: 2 lunch entrées (four blocks each)

Block Size:

8 Protein	8 soy hot dogs, sliced
2 Carbohydrate	6 cups cabbage, shredded
2 Carbohydrate	6 cups mushrooms, sliced
2 Carbohydrate	½ cup cooked chickpeas, chopped
2 Carbohydrate	½ cup carrots, willow leaf cut*
8 Fat	2⅔ teaspoons olive oil

2 garlic cloves, minced
6 tablespoons cider vinegar
2 teaspoons fresh mint, chopped
½ cup water

Method:
In nonstick sauté pan, add oil, cabbage, mushrooms, chickpeas, and carrots. Cook vegetable mixture until hot, then add garlic, vinegar, mint, water, and soy hot dogs. Cover sauté pan and simmer for 5–10 minutes until soy hot dogs are hot, occasionally stirring. Equally divide the cooked vegetables and franks between two lunch plates. Place four soy hot dogs and an equal amount of vegetables on each plate and serve immediately.

Note: Willow leaf cut means that the carrots are cut at approximately a 45-degree angle.

Veal Stew

Servings: 2 lunch entrées (four blocks each)

Block Size:

8 Protein	8 ounces veal, one-inch cubes
1 Carbohydrate	3 cups mushroom caps
2 Carbohydrate	2 cups pearl onion
2 Carbohydrate	2 cups cherry tomato
2 Carbohydrate	2 cups turnips, cut Parisienne style*
1 Carbohydrate	4 teaspoons cornstarch
8 Fat	2⅔ teaspoons olive oil

2 garlic cloves, minced
1 cup beef stock
6 whole peppercorns
¼ teaspoon dried oregano
2 teaspoons fresh basil, chopped
Salt and pepper to taste

Method:
Coat bottom of medium-sized casserole dish with oil. Place all ingredients (veal, vegetables, and spices) in casserole dish, except basil and cornstarch. Tightly cover casserole dish with aluminum foil and place in preheated oven at 400 degrees for 20 minutes. Mix the cornstarch and basil together with a little water to form a paste. After 20 minutes, remove casserole dish from oven and stir in cornstarch-basil paste. Continue stirring meat and vegetables until they have been coated. Re-cover and cook an additional 5–10 minutes. Place equal amount of veal pieces on two lunch plates and top with vegetables and sauce.

Note: Use a small melon ball cutter on turnips to form small balls.

Tuna Fruit Salad

Servings: 2 lunch entrées (four blocks each)

Block Size:

7 Protein	7 ounces chunk light tuna, drained*
1 Protein and 1 Carbohydrate	½ cup plain low-fat yogurt
2 Carbohydrate	1 cup blueberries
2 Carbohydrate	2 cups strawberries, sliced
2 Carbohydrate	⅔ cup mandarin orange sections
1 Carbohydrate	6 cups romaine lettuce, chopped
8 Fat	8 teaspoons slivered almonds
	½ teaspoon parsley flakes
	½ teaspoon dried dill
	⅛ teaspoon onion powder
	⅛ teaspoon nutmeg
	⅛ teaspoon paprika
	Salt and pepper to taste

Method:

In a small mixing bowl, combine tuna (without liquid), yogurt, parsley, dill, onion powder, and nutmeg to form a tuna salad. In another mixing bowl, combine blueberries, strawberries, and orange sections to form a fruit salad. When the tuna salad and fruit salad are made, take two lunch plates and arrange a bed of lettuce on each plate. In the center of the plate on the bed of lettuce place a mound of tuna salad. Place the fruit salad around the tuna salad and sprinkle with paprika and slivered almonds. Chill and serve.

*Note: Use tuna packed in water only.

Chicken Salad Mexicana

Servings: 2 lunch entrées (four blocks each)

Block Size:

8 Protein	8 ounces chicken tenderloins, diced (or skinless chicken breast)
1 Carbohydrate	2 cups celery, diced
2 Carbohydrate	½ cup cooked chickpeas, chopped
2 Carbohydrate	½ cup cooked kidney beans, chopped
2 Carbohydrate	1 cup salsa*
1 Carbohydrate	6 cups romaine lettuce
8 Fat	2⅔ teaspoons olive oil

⅛ teaspoon chili powder
2 garlic cloves, minced
⅛ teaspoon Worcestershire sauce
Onion powder
Salt and pepper to taste

Method:
In nonstick sauté pan, add oil, diced chicken, celery, chili powder, garlic, and Worcestershire sauce. Cook until chicken is browned, then add chickpeas, kidney beans, and salsa. Simmer for 10–15 minutes until heated through and beans have softened. The kidney beans should have a soft consistency like refried beans. While the chicken and vegetables are cooking, take two lunch plates and arrange a bed of lettuce on both plates. Remove sauté pan from stove and let chicken and vegetable mixture cool for 2–3 minutes. Spoon chicken and vegetable mixture into the center of both plates on each bed of lettuce. Sprinkle with onion powder and serve.

*Note: Salsa comes with different levels of heat. Choose one that best fits your family's tastes.

Thousand Island Salad

Servings: 2 lunch entrées (four blocks each)

Block Size:

2 Protein	2 whole hard-boiled eggs, chopped
2 Protein	2 ounces skim milk mozzarella cheese, shredded
1 Protein	1½ ounces deli-style turkey breast, diced
1 Protein	1½ ounces deli-style ham, diced
2 Protein and 2 Carbohydrate	1 cup plain low-fat yogurt
2 Carbohydrate	8 teaspoons sweet pickle relish
1 Carbohydrate	1 head iceberg lettuce
1 Carbohydrate	1 cup cherry tomato, halved
½ Carbohydrate	½ cup onion, diced fine
½ Carbohydrate	1 cup radishes, sliced
1 Carbohydrate	½ cup tomato puree
8 Fat	24 green olives, chopped
	⅛ teaspoon chili powder
	⅛ teaspoon Worcestershire sauce
	Salt and pepper to taste

Method:

In a small mixing bowl, add yogurt, hard-boiled eggs, tomato puree, relish, olives, chili powder, and Worcestershire sauce. Blend together with a wire whip to create the dressing for the salad. When the dressing has been made, take two large oval plates and arrange a bed of lettuce on each plate. On each bed of lettuce, place an equal amount of tomato, onion, radishes, cheese, turkey, and ham. Equally divide the dressing and pour over salad ingredients on both plates. Sprinkle with salt and pepper and serve immediately.

Hot Spinach Salad

Servings: 2 lunch entrées (four blocks each)

Block Size:

8 Protein	12 ounces lean ground pork
1 Carbohydrate	1 cup onion, diced fine
1 Carbohydrate	4 teaspoons cornstarch
2 Carbohydrate	8 cups fresh spinach, stems removed and chopped*
4 Carbohydrate	1 cup cooked chickpeas, diced fine
8 Fat	2⅔ teaspoons olive oil

8 tablespoons cider vinegar
2 garlic cloves, minced
1 cup beef stock
½ teaspoon dry mustard
2 tablespoons red bell pepper, diced fine
Salt and pepper to taste

Method:
In nonstick sauté pan, add oil, pork, onion, vinegar, and garlic. Cook until pork is browned, stirring the pork as it cooks to break the pork up. When the pork has browned, add beef stock, mustard, and cornstarch. (Blend cornstarch and mustard with a little water to dissolve them before adding to sauté pan.) Bring pork mixture to a boil, stirring constantly until thickened and it develops into the hot spinach dressing. On two lunch plates, place 4 cups of cleaned raw spinach per plate. Equally divide hot spinach dressing (pork mixture) between both serving plates by spooning over spinach. Sprinkle each plate with chopped chickpeas and red bell pepper and serve.

*Note: Fresh spinach needs to be cleaned very well, because of sand, so be sure to soak spinach in water to remove any sand or dirt before using.

Shrimp with Tri-Bean Salad

Servings: 2 lunch entrées (four blocks each)

Block Size:

8 Protein   12 ounces shrimp

2 Carbohydrate   ½ cup cooked kidney beans
2 Carbohydrate   ½ cup cooked chickpeas
2 Carbohydrate   2 cups green beans, diagonal cut
1 Carbohydrate   1 cup onion, chopped
1 Carbohydrate   6 cups romaine lettuce, diced

8 Fat   2⅔ teaspoons olive oil

2 tablespoons cider vinegar
2 tablespoons dried chives
⅛ teaspoon dried basil
⅛ teaspoon black pepper
⅛ teaspoon white wine
4 bay leaves
⅛ teaspoon parsley
Salt to taste

Method:
In a small mixing bowl, combine, oil, vinegar, chives, basil, black pepper, kidney beans, chickpeas, green beans, and onion to form a Tri-Bean Salad. Place mixing bowl in refrigerator to allow vegetables to marinate. In saucepan, poach shrimp in boiling water with wine and bay leaves until cooked. Remove shrimp from saucepan and cool. Arrange a bed of lettuce on two large plates. In the center of the plates on the lettuce place a mound of salad. Place the shrimp around the salad and sprinkle with parsley. Chill and serve.

Herbed Cottage Cheese and Asparagus Salad with Fruit

Servings: 2 lunch entrées (four blocks each)

Block Size:

8 Protein	2 cups low-fat cottage cheese
2 Carbohydrate	2 cups cooked asparagus, cut in one-inch pieces
2 Carbohydrate	2 peaches, sliced
2 Carbohydrate	⅔ cup mandarin orange sections
1 Carbohydrate	1 cup strawberries
1 Carbohydrate	6 cups romaine lettuce
8 Fat	2⅔ teaspoons olive oil
	⅛ teaspoon dried oregano
	2 teaspoons fresh basil, diced fine
	⅛ teaspoon black pepper
	⅛ teaspoon parsley
	Salt to taste

Method:

In a mixing bowl, combine cottage cheese, asparagus, oil, oregano, basil, and black pepper. In another mixing bowl, combine peaches, orange sections, and strawberries to form a fruit salad. When the herbed cottage cheese and fruit salad are made, take two lunch plates and arrange a bed of lettuce on each plate. In the center of the plate on the lettuce place a mound of herbed cottage cheese. Place the fruit salad around the herbed cottage cheese and sprinkle with parsley. Chill and serve.

Stuffed Tomato with Chicken Farce

Servings: 2 lunch entrées (four blocks each)

Block Size:

8 Protein	12 ounces ground chicken
2 Carbohydrate	4 tomatoes, crowned and cut in half
2 Carbohydrate	2 cups onion, diced fine
1 Carbohydrate	3 cups mushrooms, diced fine
1 Carbohydrate	½ cup carrots, diced fine
2 Carbohydrate	½ cup cooked chickpeas, chopped
8 Fat	2⅔ teaspoons olive oil
	Salt and pepper to taste
	4 teaspoons parsley
	2 garlic cloves, minced

Method:

Using a knife, cut tomatoes in half in a crown pattern. To crown a tomato, cut a zigzag line around the middle of the tomato with a sharp paring knife. When the two halves are separated, the top and bottom form bases that create the appearance of a crown. After the tomatoes have been cut, carefully cut out or scoop out the inside of the tomato to create a tomato shell. Sprinkle the insides of the tomato shells with salt and pepper. Dice tomato pulp into small chunks. In nonstick sauté pan add oil, onion, mushrooms, carrots, chickpeas, tomato pulp, parsley, garlic, and ground chicken. Cook until mixture is tender and chicken is browned (about 10 minutes). (This mixture is known as a duxell-farce. A *duxell-farce* is finely cooked vegetables and meat used to stuff another item.) When the duxell-farce is cooked, set aside to cool. Stuff crowned tomatoes with duxell-farce, then place in a baking dish. Tightly cover baking dish with aluminum foil and place in preheated oven at 350 degrees for 10–15 minutes to soften the tomatoes. Remove baking dish from oven and place four stuffed tomatoes on both lunch plates. Sprinkle with salt and pepper and serve immediately.

Barbecue Beef with Onions

Servings: 2 lunch entrées (four blocks each)

Block Size:

8 Protein	8 ounces beef eye of round, one-eighth-inch slices
4 Carbohydrate	2 cups tomato puree
4 Carbohydrate	4 cups onion, in half rings
8 Fat	2⅔ teaspoons olive oil

1 teaspoon Worcestershire sauce
1 teaspoon cider vinegar
½ teaspoon chili powder
⅛ teaspoon dried oregano
¼ teaspoon minced garlic
2 tablespoons beef stock
2 tablespoons white wine vinegar

Method:

In nonstick sauté pan, add ⅔ teaspoon oil and beef. Cook beef until browned. When the beef has browned, add tomato puree, Worcestershire sauce, cider vinegar, chili powder, oregano, and garlic. Cover and simmer for 5 minutes until a sauce forms. While the beef is simmering, in another nonstick sauté pan add remaining oil and onion. Cook onion until tender, then add the onion, beef stock, and white wine vinegar to beef. Cover sauté pan and cook 10 minutes, stirring occasionally to blend flavors. Place an equal amount on two lunch plates or in soup bowls and serve.

Creole Shrimp

Servings: 2 lunch entrées (four blocks each)

Block Size:

8 Protein	12 ounces cooked shrimp
1 Carbohydrate	1 cup onion, quarter-inch dice
1 Carbohydrate	2¼ cups green bell pepper, quarter-inch dice
1 Carbohydrate	2½ cups celery, quarter-inch dice
3 Carbohydrate	1½ cups tomato puree
2 Carbohydrate	2 peaches
8 Fat	2⅔ teaspoons olive oil

2 garlic cloves, minced
Hot sauce to taste
½ cup water
⅛ teaspoon celery salt
½ teaspoon dried thyme, crushed
⅛ teaspoon black pepper

Method:

In nonstick sauté pan, add oil, onion, pepper, celery, garlic, and hot sauce. Cook until vegetables are tender, then add shrimp, tomato puree, water, celery salt, thyme, and black pepper. Bring mixture to a boil, then simmer for 5–10 minutes. Equally divide Creole Shrimp between two lunch plates and serve. Serve peaches on the side as a dessert.

Herbed Pork and Bean Stew

Servings: 2 lunch entrées (four blocks each)

Block Size:

8 Protein	12 ounces ground pork
4 Carbohydrate	1 cup cooked kidney beans
2 Carbohydrate	2 cups green beans, diagonal cut
1 Carbohydrate	1 cup onion, chopped
1 Carbohydrate	4 teaspoons cornstarch
8 Fat	2⅔ teaspoons olive oil

4 garlic cloves, minced
2 teaspoons cider vinegar
2 teaspoons Worcestershire sauce
1 cup chicken stock
⅛ teaspoon dried basil
½ teaspoon dried marjoram

Method:
In nonstick saucepan, cook kidney beans, green beans, garlic, and onion in 2 teaspoons oil until tender, then add vinegar, Worcestershire sauce, chicken stock, spices, and cornstarch. (Mix cornstarch with a little water to dissolve it before adding to sauté pan.) Continue cooking under medium heat until entire mixture is hot, stirring constantly. While the vegetables are cooking, in another nonstick sauté pan add remaining oil and stir-fry pork until cooked. When the pork is cooked, add it to the vegetables and simmer for an additional 5 minutes. Place an equal amount in two soup bowls and serve.

Fruity Chicken Salad

Servings: 2 lunch entrées (four blocks each)

Block Size:

8 Protein	8 ounces chicken tenderloins, diced (or skinless chicken breast)
4 Carbohydrate	1 cantaloupe
1 Carbohydrate	½ cup blueberries
1 Carbohydrate	¾ cup maraschino cherries
1 Carbohydrate	1 kiwi fruit, peeled and diced
1 Carbohydrate	1 cup raspberries
8 Fat	2⅔ teaspoons olive oil

Method:

In nonstick sauté pan, add oil and chicken. Cook chicken until browned. Remove chicken from sauté pan and let cool. Using a knife, cut cantaloupe in half in a crown pattern. To crown a cantaloupe, cut a zigzag line around the middle of the cantaloupe with a sharp paring knife. When the two halves are separated, the top and bottom form bases that create the appearance of a crown. After the cantaloupe has been cut, carefully cut out or scoop out the inside of the cantaloupe using a melon baller. Create a cavity inside the melon, leaving about a half inch of the melon on the rind. In a small mixing bowl, combine cantaloupe balls, blueberries, cherries, diced kiwi fruit, raspberries, and diced chicken to make a chicken-fruit salad. Divide chicken-fruit salad equally and fill the two cantaloupe halves, place on two lunch plates, and serve.

Beef and Lentil Stew

Servings: 2 lunch entrées (four blocks each)

Block Size:

8 Protein   8 ounces beef eye of round, diced
                                   in one-eighth-inch squares

1 Carbohydrate   ½ cup tomato puree
1 Carbohydrate   ½ cup carrots, diced fine
1 Carbohydrate   1 cup onion, diced fine
1 Carbohydrate   2½ cups celery, diced fine
4 Carbohydrate   ½ cup dry lentils

8 Fat   2⅔ teaspoons olive oil

                                   4 peppercorns, crushed
                                   4 garlic cloves, minced
                                   ⅛ teaspoon dried marjoram
                                   ⅛ teaspoon dried basil
                                   1 teaspoon parsley
                                   4 cups beef stock

Method:
Combine all ingredients in large saucepan. Bring to a boil, then simmer for 35–40 minutes. Divide between two soup dishes and serve.

Spanish Chicken and Lentil Soup

Servings: 2 lunch entrées (four blocks each)

Block Size:

6 Protein	6 ounces chicken tenderloins, diced fine (or skinless chicken breast)
2 Protein and 2 Carbohydrate	1 cup plain low-fat yogurt
4 Carbohydrate	1 cup cooked lentils
1 Carbohydrate	½ cup tomato puree
½ Carbohydrate	½ cup onion, chopped fine
½ Carbohydrate	3 cups fresh spinach, shredded
8 Fat	2⅔ teaspoons olive oil
	⅛ teaspoon dried parsley
	⅛ teaspoon dried thyme
	⅛ teaspoon dried basil
	⅛ teaspoon dried rosemary
	1 cup chicken stock

Method:

In a large nonstick sauté pan, add ⅔ teaspoon oil and chicken. Cook chicken over medium heat until browned, then add cooked lentils, tomato puree, onion, spinach, spices, and chicken stock. Continue cooking until entire mixture is hot and has come to a boil. Simmer for 5 minutes, remove from heat, and stir in yogurt. Place an equal amount in two soup bowls and serve.

Beef Ratatouille

Servings: 2 lunch entrées (four blocks each)

Block Size:

8 Protein	12 ounces lean ground beef
2 Carbohydrate	3 cups zucchini, quartered
2 Carbohydrate	2 cups onion, half-ring slices
2 Carbohydrate	2½ cups tomato, half slices
2 Carbohydrate	4½ cups red bell pepper, diced
8 Fat	2⅔ teaspoons olive oil
	6 garlic cloves, minced
	2 tablespoons dried basil
	⅛ teaspoon dried oregano
	½ cup beef stock

Method:

In nonstick sauté pan, place ⅔ teaspoon oil and beef. Cook beef until browned and done. In another sauté pan, place 2 teaspoons oil, zucchini, onion, tomato, bell pepper, garlic, basil, and oregano. Cook until entire mixture is hot, then add beef stock and cooked beef. Cover sauté pan and cook for 5–10 minutes, stirring occasionally to blend flavors. Place an equal amount on two lunch plates and serve.

Cinnamon-Chicken Meatballs with Fruit Sauce

Servings: 2 lunch entrées (four blocks each)

Block Size:

8 Protein	12 ounces ground chicken
1 Carbohydrate	1 cup onion, diced fine
1 Carbohydrate	2 cups celery, diced fine, divided
2 Carbohydrate	½ cup kidney beans, chopped fine
1 Carbohydrate	4 teaspoons cornstarch
2 Carbohydrate	1 cup fruit cocktail
1 Carbohydrate	¾ cup maraschino cherries, halved
8 Fat	2⅔ teaspoons olive oil
	⅛ teaspoon black pepper
	1 teaspoon cinnamon plus ⅛ teaspoon
	1½ cups chicken stock
	½ teaspoon orange extract

Method:

In a large bowl, combine ground chicken, onion, 1 cup celery, finely chopped kidney beans, olive oil, black pepper, and 1 teaspoon cinnamon. Form mixture into 32 one-inch meatballs. Place meatballs in baking dish and bake in a preheated 375-degree oven for 15 minutes. While the meatballs are cooking, in a small saucepan combine fruit cocktail, cherries, 1 cup celery, chicken stock, ⅛ teaspoon cinnamon, orange extract, and cornstarch. (Mix cornstarch with chicken stock so that it can dissolve before adding to saucepan.) Simmer lightly until sauce forms, stirring constantly. Remove meatballs from oven and place meatballs in sauce, gently spooning the sauce over the meatballs. Place an equal amount of meatballs on two lunch plates with sauce and serve.

Greek Chicken Stew

Servings: 2 lunch entrées (four blocks each)

Block Size:

8 Protein	8 ounces chicken tenderloins, diced fine (or skinless chicken breast)
2 Carbohydrate	2 cups onion, sliced thin
2 Carbohydrate	1 cup tomato puree
2 Carbohydrate	2 cups fresh green beans, chopped
1 Carbohydrate	½ cup carrots, chopped
1 Carbohydrate	1 cup turnips, one-eighth-inch cubes
8 Fat	24 pitted black olives, sliced (or similar type)
	2 garlic cloves, minced
	2 cups chicken stock*
	⅛ teaspoon red wine
	⅛ teaspoon celery salt
	⅛ teaspoon pepper
	½ teaspoon cinnamon

Method:
Combine all ingredients except olives in a large saucepan. Bring to a boil, then simmer for 30–35 minutes, stirring occasionally, until all vegetables are tender. Add olives and divide between two soup dishes and serve.

*Note: If more chicken stock is needed or a more liquid stew is desired, add additional stock as necessary.

Rich and Hearty Minestrone Soup

Servings: 2 lunch entrées (four blocks each)

Block Size:

8 Protein	8 ounces beef eye of round, diced in one-eighth-inch squares
1 Carbohydrate	2½ cups celery, diced fine
1 Carbohydrate	1 cup onion, diced fine
1 Carbohydrate	3 cups cabbage, diced fine
1 Carbohydrate	½ cup tomato puree
1 Carbohydrate	⅛ cup cooked black beans
1 Carbohydrate	⅛ cup cooked chickpeas
1 Carbohydrate	¼ cup cooked elbow macaroni
8 Fat	2⅔ teaspoons olive oil
	2 garlic cloves, minced
	3 cups beef stock
	Salt and pepper to taste
	½ teaspoon dried basil

Method:

Combine all ingredients except macaroni in a large saucepan. Bring to a boil, then simmer for 30–35 minutes, stirring occasionally, until all vegetables are tender. While the soup is cooking, add macaroni to boiling water and cook. When macaroni is cooked, remove from water and cool until it is time to add the macaroni to the soup. Add macaroni and simmer for an additional 5 minutes. Divide between two soup dishes and serve.

Home-Style Beef-Vegetable Soup

Servings: 2 lunch entrées (four blocks each)

Block Size:

8 Protein	12 ounces lean ground beef
1 Carbohydrate	2½ cups celery, diced fine
2 Carbohydrate	1 cup carrots, diced fine
2 Carbohydrate	2 cups onion, diced fine
2 Carbohydrate	2½ cups tomato, chopped
1 Carbohydrate	½ cup tomato puree
8 Fat	2⅔ teaspoons olive oil

3 cups beef stock
Salt and pepper to taste
4 green peppercorns
2 garlic cloves, minced
⅛ teaspoon marjoram
⅛ teaspoon Worcestershire sauce
¼ teaspoon chives
1 teaspoon parsley
⅛ teaspoon oregano

Method:
Combine all ingredients in a large saucepan. Bring to a boil, then simmer for 35–40 minutes, stirring occasionally, until all vegetables are tender. Divide between two soup dishes and serve.

Variations:

Vegetable Soup Brunoise
Cut vegetable in a fine dice (one-eighth-inch cubes).

Vegetable Soup Paysanne
Means peasant style; the vegetables are cut in a coarse cut (one-quarter-inch cubes).

Thick Old-Fashioned Cabbage Soup

Servings: 2 lunch entrées (four blocks each)

Block Size:

8 Protein   8 soy hot dogs, sliced

1 Carbohydrate   2 cups celery, diced fine
2 Carbohydrate   1 cup carrots, diced fine
2 Carbohydrate   2 cups onion, diced fine
1 Carbohydrate   1¼ cups tomato, diced fine
1 Carbohydrate   3 cups cabbage, shredded
1 Carbohydrate   3 cups mushrooms, diced

8 Fat   2⅔ teaspoons olive oil

                     3 cups chicken stock
                     ⅛ teaspoon caraway seeds
                     2 garlic cloves, minced
                     4 tablespoons cider vinegar
                     Salt and pepper to taste

Method:
Combine all ingredients in a large saucepan. Bring to a boil, then simmer for 35–40 minutes, stirring occasionally until all vegetables are tender. Divide between two soup dishes and serve.

Broiled Tuna Steak with Dill Sauce and Fruit

Servings: 2 lunch entrées (four blocks each)

Block Size:

7 Protein	12 ounces tuna steak
1 Protein and	
1 Carbohydrate	½ cup plain low-fat yogurt
½ Carbohydrate	½ teaspoon sugar
½ Carbohydrate	2 teaspoons cornstarch
2 Carbohydrate	1 cup pineapple, cubed
1 Carbohydrate	½ cup blueberries
2 Carbohydrate	⅔ cup mandarin oranges
1 Carbohydrate	¾ cup maraschino cherries, halved
8 Fat	2⅔ teaspoons olive oil
	2 teaspoons dried dill
	2 teaspoons white wine
	Salt and pepper to taste

Method:
Coat the bottom of a baking dish with oil, then place two 6-ounce pieces of tuna in bottom of baking dish. Sprinkle with 1 teaspoon of the dill, then tightly seal baking dish and bake in preheated oven at 375 degrees for 25–30 minutes. While the tuna is baking, in saucepan combine yogurt, sugar, the rest of the dill, and wine to make a dill sauce. Add a little water to the cornstarch and then add it to dill sauce. Stirring constantly, heat sauce through but do not bring sauce to a boil. In a mixing bowl, combine pineapple, blueberries, orange sections, and cherries to make a fruit salad. Equally divide fruit salad between two lunch plates, then remove baking dish from oven. Using a large spatula, scoop out tuna and place one piece of tuna on each plate. Pour an equal amount of dill sauce over each piece of tuna and serve immediately.

Crabmeat Maryland

Servings: 2 lunch entrées (four blocks each)

Block Size:

8 Protein	12 ounces crabmeat, cut into half-inch pieces
1 Carbohydrate	2 cups celery, cut in matchstick-sized pieces (one-eighth-inch by one-eighth-inch by two inches)
1 Carbohydrate	1 cup onion, sliced in thin half rings
1 Carbohydrate	1 cup shallots, sliced in thin half rings
2 Carbohydrate	1 cup carrots, cut in matchstick-sized pieces (one-eighth-inch by one-eighth-inch by two inches)
1 Carbohydrate	1 cup tomato, diced fine
1 Carbohydrate	2¼ cups red bell pepper, in thin pieces
1 Carbohydrate	½ cup tomato puree
8 Fat	2⅔ teaspoons olive oil

4 garlic cloves, minced
1 cup chicken stock or fish stock
⅛ teaspoon red wine
⅛ teaspoon dried dill
⅛ teaspoon black pepper
⅛ teaspoon dried basil
Salt to taste

Method:

In nonstick sauté pan, add 2 teaspoons oil, celery, onion, shallots, carrots, diced tomato, garlic, and bell pepper. Cook until vegetables are tender, then add tomato puree, stock, red wine, and spices. Simmer for 10 minutes. While the vegetables are simmering, in another sauté pan add ⅔ teaspoon oil and crabmeat. Gently cook crabmeat until done, then add crabmeat to vegetable mixture and simmer an additional 5 minutes. Divide between two lunch plates and serve immediately.

Spicy Mexicali Beef

Servings: 2 lunch entrées (four blocks each)

Block Size:

8 Protein	10 ounces lean ground beef
1 Carbohydrate	¼ cup corn kernels
2 Carbohydrate	1 cup salsa
2 Carbohydrate	½ cup cooked white kidney beans, rinsed
2 Carbohydrate	½ cup cooked black beans, rinsed
1 Carbohydrate	1 cup tomato, seeded and diced fine
5 Fat	1⅔ teaspoons olive oil
3 Fat	9 black olives, diced
	1 tablespoon chili powder
	⅛ teaspoon celery salt
	½ teaspoon onion powder
	⅛ teaspoon cayenne pepper
	½ teaspoon garlic, minced

Method:
In nonstick sauté pan, add ground beef and ⅔ teaspoon oil. When the beef has browned, add all remaining ingredients and cook for 10–15 minutes until hot. Place the mixture in two small bowls and serve.

Chicken Florida

Servings: 2 lunch entrées (four blocks each)

Block Size:

8 Protein	8 ounces chicken tenderloins, diced (or skinless chicken breast)
1 Carbohydrate	1 cup onion, chopped
1 Carbohydrate	1½ cups cooked spinach

1 Carbohydrate	2 cups red bell pepper, sliced and quartered
½ Carbohydrate	1½ cups mushrooms, sliced
½ Carbohydrate	1 cup broccoli florets
½ Carbohydrate	1½ cups cauliflower florets
1 Carbohydrate	1 cup asparagus spears, half-inch pieces
½ Carbohydrate	2 teaspoons cornstarch
2 Carbohydrate	½ cup cooked rotini pasta
8 Fat	2⅔ teaspoons olive oil, divided
	½ cup chicken stock
	¼ teaspoon black pepper
	¼ teaspoon chives, dried
	¼ teaspoon garlic, minced
	⅛ teaspoon tarragon, dried
	⅛ teaspoon thyme, dried
	⅛ teaspoon chili powder
	⅛ teaspoon celery salt

Method:

In a medium-sized nonstick sauté pan, add ⅔ teaspoon oil, onion, and spinach. Cook onion and spinach until spinach is wilted. In another nonstick sauté pan, add remaining oil, chicken, bell pepper, mushrooms, broccoli, cauliflower, and asparagus. Cook chicken and vegetables until done. In a small saucepan, combine chicken stock, spices, and cornstarch and stir until cornstarch has dissolved. Heat chicken stock until it has formed a sauce, then add rotini pasta to saucepan. On two lunch plates, place a mixture of onions and spinach, then place chicken mixture on top. Pour sauce over entire chicken-vegetable mixture and serve.

DINNER

Spinaci Chicken alla Italiana

(Spinach and Chicken Sautéed with Onion and Garlic)

Servings: 2 dinner entrées (four blocks each)

Block Size:

8 Protein	8 ounces skinless chicken breast, half-inch dice
4 Carbohydrate	1 pound fresh spinach, washed
3½ Carbohydrate	3½ cups onion, sliced thin
½ Carbohydrate	½ cup shallots, medium dice*
8 Fat	2⅔ teaspoons olive oil, divided

2 garlic cloves, minced (1 teaspoon)
⅛ teaspoon black pepper
½ teaspoon nutmeg
Fresh parsley sprigs
Salt to taste

Method:
In nonstick sauté pan, cook spinach, onion, garlic, and shallots in 2 teaspoons oil until tender. Just before the vegetables are finished cooking, add black pepper and nutmeg, remove pan from heat and set aside. In another nonstick sauté pan, cook diced chicken in ⅔ teaspoon olive oil until lightly browned, then add spinach mixture into diced chicken and heat through. Simmer entire mixture for 3–5 minutes. Place on two dinner plates and serve garnished with fresh parsley.

*Note: Shallots are available in most supermarkets and have a purple-white appearance. Shallots provide dishes with both an onion and a garlic flavor.

Hawaiian Sweet and Sour Chicken
with Snow Peas

Servings: 2 dinner entrées (four blocks each)

Block Size:

8 Protein	8 ounces skinless chicken breast, half-inch dice
1 Carbohydrate	½ cup tomato puree
1 Carbohydrate	2 teaspoons sugar
2 Carbohydrate	1 cup pineapple, diced
1 Carbohydrate	¾ cup maraschino cherries, quartered
1 Carbohydrate	4 teaspoons cornstarch
2 Carbohydrate	2 cups snow peas
7 Fat	2⅓ teaspoons olive oil
1 Fat	1 teaspoon slivered almonds
	8 tablespoons vinegar
	4 tablespoons water
	2 tablespoons soy sauce
	1 cup chicken stock

Method:

In nonstick sauté pan, cook chicken in 2 teaspoons oil until done. While the chicken is cooking, in another nonstick sauté pan add vinegar, tomato puree, ⅓ teaspoon oil, water, soy sauce, sugar, pineapple, cherries, chicken stock, and cornstarch. (Mix cornstarch into chicken stock and stir well until cornstarch has dissolved before adding to saucepan.) While stirring continuously, heat pineapple and cherry mixture under medium heat until a thick sauce forms. Add chicken to pineapple and cherry mixture and simmer for 10 minutes for the flavors to blend. Taste sauce; if it has too strong a vinegar taste, continue simmering for a few more minutes. The flavor will develop into a sweet and sour sauce as it cooks. Place snow peas in saucepan with enough water to cover and cook until tender. Serve chicken mixture with peapods arranged on the sides of two dinner plates. Sprinkle almonds over snow peas and serve.

Chicken Fricassee with Garden Vegetables

Servings: 2 dinner entrées (four blocks each)

Block Size:

6 Protein	6 ounces skinless chicken breast, sliced in half-inch by two-inch strips
2 Protein and 2 Carbohydrate	1 cup plain low-fat yogurt
1 Carbohydrate	1 cup onion, sliced
1⅓ Carbohydrate	4 cups mushrooms, quartered
1 Carbohydrate	4 teaspoons cornstarch
1 Carbohydrate	1½ cups broccoli florets
⅔ Carbohydrate	2 cups mushrooms, sliced
8 Fat	8 teaspoons slivered almonds
	1½ cups chicken stock
	⅛ teaspoon lemon juice
	Salt and pepper to taste
	Red bell pepper strips for garnish (optional)

Method:

In saucepan, cook onions, quartered mushrooms, and chicken in chicken stock, until vegetables are tender and chicken is done. Remove saucepan from heat and slowly stir in lemon juice and yogurt, then add cornstarch. (Mix cornstarch with a little water and then add to saucepan.) Lightly simmer chicken mixture 4–5 minutes until mixture thickens. In another saucepan, place broccoli and enough water to cover. Cook broccoli until tender. Place Chicken Fricassee mixture on two serving plates along with an equal amount of cooked broccoli topped with sliced mushrooms and slivered almonds. Garnish with a red pepper strip and serve.

Clams à l'Ancienne

Servings: 2 dinner entrées (four blocks each)

Block Size:

4 Protein	6 ounces clams, chopped
2 Protein	2 whole eggs
2 Protein and 2 Carbohydrate	1 cup plain low-fat yogurt
2 Carbohydrate	4½ cups green bell pepper, chopped
1 Carbohydrate	3 cups mushrooms, diced
1 Carbohydrate	1 cup shallots, diced
2 Carbohydrate	2½ cups tomato, diced
1 Carbohydrate	4 teaspoons cornstarch
8 Fat	2⅔ teaspoons olive oil
	2 teaspoons hot sauce
	¼ teaspoon turmeric
	Salt and pepper to taste

Method:

In nonstick sauté pan, stir-fry all vegetables in hot oil until tender (2–3 minutes), then add clams and continue cooking until mixture is heated throughout. In a small mixing bowl, blend yogurt, eggs, hot sauce, seasonings, and cornstarch. (Mix cornstarch with a little water until it has dissolved before adding to mixing bowl.) After the ingredients in the mixing bowl have been mixed together, pour mixture into the sauté pan over clams and vegetable mixture. Stir well and cook an additional 3–5 minutes to heat through until eggs and yogurt are heated. Divide entrée onto two dinner plates and serve.

Indonesian–Javanese Chicken

Servings: 2 dinner entrées (four blocks each)

Block Size:

6 Protein	6 ounces chicken tenderloins, medium dice (or skinless chicken breast)
2 Protein and 2 Carbohydrate	2 cups 1 percent milk
1 Carbohydrate	1 cup onion, diced fine
⅓ Carbohydrate	½ cup jalapeño pepper, chopped fine
1 Carbohydrate	4 teaspoons cornstarch
2 Carbohydrate	6 cups cabbage, shredded
⅔ Carbohydrate	2 cups red bell pepper, sliced
8 Fat	2⅔ teaspoons olive oil
	6 garlic cloves, minced
	2 teaspoons ginger root, grated
	½ teaspoon turmeric
	1 teaspoon coriander
	½ teaspoon curry powder
	Salt and pepper to taste

Method:

In nonstick sauté pan, combine onion, jalapeño pepper, spices, milk, and chicken. Poach (lightly simmer) chicken in vegetable-milk mixture until cooked. Mix cornstarch with a little water, then add to sauté pan and simmer for 3–5 minutes. In a separate nonstick sauté pan, cook cabbage and red bell pepper in oil until tender. Divide cabbage and pepper between two dinner plates, then with a spoon equally divide chicken-vegetable mixture on the beds of cabbage and peppers. Serve immediately.

Chicken Chasseur

Servings: 2 dinner entrées (four blocks each)

Block Size:

8 Protein	Skinless breast pieces from 1-pound chicken, with the bone (approximately half the weight of this chicken breast is in bone) or 8 ounces skinless breast meat
4 Carbohydrate	5 cups tomato, diced
2 Carbohydrate	6 cups mushrooms, sliced
1 Carbohydrate	1 cup onion, sliced
1 Carbohydrate	4 teaspoons cornstarch
8 Fat	2⅔ teaspoons olive oil
	2 cups beef stock
	2 garlic cloves, minced
	⅛ teaspoon white wine
	Salt and pepper to taste

Method:

In a covered saucepan, poach (lightly simmer) chicken pieces in beef stock until cooked. In nonstick sauté pan, cook vegetables and garlic in oil over medium heat until tender, then add dash of wine. Mix cornstarch with a little water to dissolve it, then stir into beef stock with chicken to form a sauce. When the sauce has thickened, add vegetables and coat both chicken and vegetables with sauce. Simmer chicken and vegetables for 5–8 minutes. Place an equal amount of chicken pieces and vegetables on two dinner plates and serve.

Chicken with Rosemary

Servings: 2 dinner entrées (four blocks each)

Block Size:

6 Protein	6 ounces skinless chicken breast, sliced in half-inch by two-inch strips
2 Protein and 2 Carbohydrate	1 cup plain low-fat yogurt
1 Carbohydrate	4 teaspoons cornstarch
1 Carbohydrate	1½ cups broccoli florets
2 Carbohydrate	2½ cups tomato, sliced
2 Carbohydrate	1 pear, sliced
8 Fat	2⅔ teaspoons olive oil
	2 teaspoons dried rosemary
	1 cup chicken stock
	⅛ teaspoon paprika
	Salt and pepper to taste

Method:

In nonstick sauté pan, cook chicken in oil until lightly browned. When the chicken is cooked, add yogurt, paprika, and rosemary to sauté pan and simmer 3 minutes. Mix cornstarch with chicken stock and then add to sauté pan. Simmer until a sauce forms and the mixture thickens. While the chicken and sauce are simmering, place broccoli in saucepan with enough water to cover. Cook broccoli until tender. Prepare two dinner plates by placing a bed of tomato slices on each plate, topped with cooked broccoli. Place chicken and sauce beside broccoli and tomato slices on each plate. Garnish chicken with pear slices and serve.

Beef Stroganoff

Servings: 2 dinner entrées (four blocks each)

Block Size:

6 Protein	6 ounces beef eye of round, one-eighth-inch-thick slices
2 Protein and 2 Carbohydrate	1 cup plain low-fat yogurt
2 Carbohydrate	6 cups mushrooms, sliced
1 Carbohydrate	1 cup onion, diced fine
1 Carbohydrate	4 teaspoons cornstarch
2 Carbohydrate	2 cups green beans, French cut
8 Fat	2⅔ teaspoons olive oil

⅛ teaspoon red wine
⅛ teaspoon Worcestershire sauce
½ cup beef stock
2 tablespoons red bell pepper, diced fine
Salt and pepper to taste

Method:
In nonstick sauté pan, cook mushrooms, onion, and beef in hot oil for 5–10 minutes. While the beef and vegetables are cooking in saucepan, combine wine, yogurt, Worcestershire sauce, beef stock, and cornstarch together to make a sauce. (Mix cornstarch with beef stock before adding to saucepan, so that the cornstarch can dissolve.) Simmer sauce, stirring occasionally until it has thickened and heated through; however, do not allow sauce to boil. When the sauce is hot, add the sauce to the mushrooms, onions, and beef, then simmer for 5 minutes. While the beef, vegetables, and sauce are simmering, in another saucepan, add green beans and red bell pepper with enough water to cover. Cook until tender. On two dinner plates, place an equal amount of Beef Stroganoff mixture and cooked green beans with red bell pepper. Serve immediately.

Vietnamese–Sweet Pork with Onions

Servings: 2 dinner entrées (four blocks each)

Block Size:

8 Protein	8 ounces pork, diced
8 Carbohydrate	8 cups onion, medium dice
8 Fat	2⅔ teaspoons olive oil

½ cup beef stock
4 tablespoons apple cider vinegar
4 garlic cloves, chopped
Salt and pepper to taste

Method:
In nonstick sauté pan, add diced oil, pork, and onion. Cook pork and onion over medium heat until both are browned. When onions have caramelized to a brown color, add beef stock, vinegar, and garlic. Bring mixture to a boil, then reduce heat and simmer for 30–45 minutes. Place an equal amount of the pork-onion mixture on two dinner plates and serve.

Swiss Steaks Jardiniere

Servings: 2 dinner entrées (four blocks each)

Block Size:

8 Protein	8 ounces beef eye of round, one-eighth-inch slices
2 Carbohydrate	1 cup tomato puree
1 Carbohydrate	2 cups celery, cut in matchstick-sized pieces (one-eighth-inch by one-eighth-inch by two inches)
2 Carbohydrate	2 cups onion, sliced in thin half rings

2 Carbohydrate

1 cup carrots, cut in matchstick-sized pieces (one-eighth-nch by one-eighth-inch by two inches)

1 Carbohydrate

2¼ cups red bell pepper

8 Fat

2⅔ teaspoons olive oil

1 cup beef stock
⅛ teaspoon red wine
4 garlic cloves, minced
⅛ teaspoon dried oregano
⅛ teaspoon black pepper
⅛ teaspoon dried basil
Salt to taste

Method:

In nonstick sauté pan, place ⅔ teaspoon of oil and beef. Cook beef until browned and done. After the beef has browned, add beef stock, tomato puree, and red wine. Continue cooking until a sauce forms and mixture is hot. In a second nonstick sauté pan, place 2 teaspoons oil and vegetables. Sprinkle vegetables with spices and cook until tender, stirring constantly. When the vegetables are cooked, add the beef mixture to the vegetables and simmer the entire mixture for 5 minutes. Place an equal amount of beef and vegetables on two dinner plates and serve.

Sweet and Sour Pork

Servings: 2 dinner entrées (four blocks each)

Block Size:

8 Protein	8 ounces pork, diced
1 Carbohydrate	2 teaspoons sugar
1 Carbohydrate	½ cup tomato puree
1 Carbohydrate	4 teaspoons cornstarch
3 Carbohydrate	1½ cups pineapple, diced
2 Carbohydrate	1 cup fruit cocktail, packed in water
8 Fat	2⅔ teaspoons olive oil

1 cup chicken stock
8 tablespoons vinegar
4 tablespoons water
2 tablespoons soy sauce
4–6 snow peas for garnish (optional)
Salt and pepper to taste

Method:
In nonstick sauté pan, cook pork in hot oil until lightly browned. While the pork is cooking, in a saucepan add chicken stock, vinegar, water, soy sauce, sugar, tomato puree, and cornstarch. (Mix cornstarch with chicken stock to dissolve cornstarch before adding to saucepan.) Simmer mixture in saucepan, stirring continuously, until it has thickened and heated through; however, do not bring mixture to a boil. Taste sauce; if it has too strong a vinegar taste, continue simmering for a few more minutes. The flavor will develop into a sweet and sour sauce as it cooks. When the desired sweet and sour sauce flavor has developed, add pork and fruit to saucepan and simmer for 10–15 minutes to allow flavors to blend and vinegar to tenderize the pork. Place an equal amount of pork and fruit on two dinner plates, garnish with snow peas, if desired, and serve.

Chicken Kabobs

Servings: 2 dinner entrées (four blocks each)

Block Size:

8 Protein	8 ounces chicken tenderloins cut into one-inch pieces (or skinless chicken breast)
2 Carbohydrate	4½ cups red bell pepper, cut in one-inch squares
2 Carbohydrate	3 cups broccoli florets
2 Carbohydrate	6 cups mushrooms, halved
2 Carbohydrate	2½ cups tomato, cubed
8 Fat	2⅔ teaspoons olive oil

2 cups chicken stock
2 tablespoons cider vinegar
⅛ teaspoon dried basil
⅛ teaspoon dried oregano
2 garlic cloves, minced
Salt and pepper to taste

Method:
Combine oil, stock, vinegar, basil, oregano, and garlic in a baking dish to create a marinade. Prepare eight skewers for kabobs. On each skewer place chicken, bell pepper, broccoli, mushrooms, and tomato, repeating the process until all ingredients have been placed on skewers. Place skewers in baking dish and baste with marinade. Tightly seal baking dish with foil. Bake in preheated oven at 350 degrees for 30 minutes. When the kabobs are ready, place four kabobs on each of the two dinner plates and serve.

Note: If you decide to grill the kabobs and are using wooden skewers, be sure to soak the sticks in water for 1 hour beforehand. Otherwise the intense heat will char them.

Chicken Marsala Forestiere

Servings: 2 dinner entrées (four blocks each)

Block Size:

8 Protein	8 ounces skinless chicken breast, diced

1 Carbohydrate	1 cup onion, sliced and halved
4 Carbohydrate	12 cups mushrooms, sliced
2 Carbohydrate	4 lemons, juice and pulp
1 Carbohydrate	4 teaspoons cornstarch

8 Fat	2⅔ teaspoons olive oil

½ cup chicken stock
2 tablespoons fresh basil, chopped
⅛ teaspoon Marsala wine
Salt and pepper to taste

Method:
In nonstick sauté pan, add oil, chicken, onion, and mushrooms. Cook until chicken and vegetables are tender, then add lemon juice and pulp, chicken stock, basil, wine, and cornstarch. (Mix cornstarch with chicken stock so that the cornstarch can dissolve before adding to pan.) Simmer ingredients in a sauté pan for 5–10 minutes, then place an equal amount of chicken and vegetables on two dinner plates and serve.

Gourmet Rock Cornish Hen à l'Orange

Servings: 2 dinner entrées (four blocks each)

Block Size:

8 Protein	1 Rock Cornish game hen, roughly 2 pounds (half of weight is in bone)
1 Carbohydrate	3 cups mushrooms, diced fine
2 Carbohydrate	2 cups onion, diced fine
2 Carbohydrate	⅔ cup mandarin orange sections
½ Carbohydrate	2 teaspoons cornstarch
1 Carbohydrate	1½ cups broccoli spears
1½ Carbohydrate	3 cups red bell pepper, diced
8 Fat	2⅔ teaspoons olive oil, divided

4 garlic cloves, minced
2 tcaspoons parsley
½ teaspoon paprika, divided
½ cup chicken stock
⅛ teaspoon white wine
½ teaspoon orange extract
Salt and pepper to taste

Method:

Using a large sharp knife, slice Rock Cornish hen in half along the backbone. Remove tail and skin and discard, along with gizzards. Set hen aside. In a sauté pan, add ⅔ teaspoon oil, mushrooms, garlic, parsley, and onion. Cook until mixture is translucent (about 10 minutes). (This mixture is known as a *duxell*. A duxell consists of finely cooked vegetables used to stuff another item.) When the duxell is cooked, set aside to cool. Sprinkle each Rock Cornish hen half with ¼ teaspoon paprika and rub it with remaining oil. Form two mounds of duxell in a casserole dish, place hen halves on top, and gently press them into the duxell. Tightly seal the casserole with aluminum foil and place in preheated 400-degree oven for 45 minutes. While the hen halves are cooking, combine stock, wine, orange extract, and orange sections in a small saucepan. Add cornstarch to a little water and then stir into saucepan. Cook over medium heat until the liquid thickens to form a sauce. In another saucepan, add broccoli and bell pepper with enough water to cover. Cook until tender. Remove casserole dish from oven and drain off any juices. Using a large spatula, scoop out duxell and hen halves as one piece and place on two dinner plates. Pour orange sauce over each hen half and add an equal amount of broccoli and bell pepper to each plate. Serve immediately.

Note: This recipe takes some time to make.

Chinese Sautéed Shrimp with Tomato

Servings: 2 dinner entrées (four blocks each)

Block Size:

8 Protein	12 ounces large shrimp, cleaned, deveined, and halved (20 count)
1 Carbohydrate	2¼ cups red bell pepper, cut in quartered rings
2 Carbohydrate	2 cups snow peas, sliced in thirds
1 Carbohydrate	3 cups bean sprouts
2 Carbohydrate	2 cups scallions, chopped
2 Carbohydrate	1 cup tomato puree
8 Fat	2⅔ teaspoons olive oil

4 teaspoons ginger root, diced fine
⅛ teaspoon white wine
4 tablespoons water
2 teaspoons cider vinegar
⅛ teaspoon hot sauce
Salt and pepper to taste

Method:
In a saucepan, place bell pepper, snow peas, and sprouts in enough water to cover. Cook vegetables until they are tender. While the

vegetables are cooking, in nonstick sauté pan add oil, shrimp, and scallions. Heat shrimp and scallions until cooked, then add tomato puree, ginger root, wine, the 4 tablespoons water, vinegar, and hot sauce. Simmer for 5 minutes. On two dinner plates, arrange a bed of sprouts, snow peas, and bell peppers. Place shrimp mixture and sauce on top of vegetable mixture on both plates and serve.

Chicken Apple Pie

Servings: 2 dinner entrées (four blocks each)

Block Size:

8 Protein	8 ounces chicken tenderloins, flattened (or skinless chicken breast)
4 Carbohydrate	1⅓ cup applesauce
2 Carbohydrate	1 cup fruit cocktail, packed in water
2 Carbohydrate	6 cups mushrooms, sliced
8 Fat	2⅔ teaspoons olive oil, divided
	6 tablespoons cider vinegar, divided
	½ teaspoon cinnamon
	⅛ teaspoon parsley
	⅛ teaspoon paprika
	Salt and pepper to taste

Method:
In a sauté pan, add ⅔ teaspoon oil, 4 tablespoons vinegar, and flattened chicken. Cook until chicken is browned, then add applesauce, fruit cocktail, and cinnamon to sauté pan. Simmer for 5–10 minutes to blend flavors. In a second nonstick sauté pan, add 2 teaspoons oil, 2 tablespoons vinegar, and mushrooms. Cook mushrooms until tender. On two dinner plates, place a mound of sautéed mushrooms, topped with the chicken mixture. Sprinkle with parsley and paprika and serve.

Baked Salmon

Servings: 2 dinner entrées (four blocks each)

Block Size:

8 Protein	12 ounces salmon
2 Carbohydrate	2 cups onion, sliced into rings
3 Carbohydrate	3 cups asparagus spears
1 Carbohydrate	2¼ cups red bell pepper, cut in rings
2 Carbohydrate	½ cup cooked chickpeas, chopped
8 Fat	2⅔ teaspoons olive oil

Dried dill
Garlic powder
1 cup water
Dash hot sauce (or to taste)
Dried chives
Black pepper
Celery salt

Method:
Coat bottom of a baking dish with oil, then layer the baking dish with onion rings, asparagus, bell pepper, and chickpeas. Place two fresh 6-ounce pieces of salmon on the vegetable bed in the baking dish. Sprinkle the salmon pieces lightly with dill and garlic powder, then add water and hot sauce to baking dish and seal tightly with aluminum foil. Bake in preheated oven at 350 degrees for 35 minutes. Remove baking dish from oven and drain off cooking liquid. Using a large spatula, scoop out vegetables with salmon and place on two dinner plates. Sprinkle with chives, black pepper, and celery salt, and serve.

Note: The asparagus will bleach out during cooking. If you prefer, it can be cooked separately.

Beef Roulade

Servings: 2 dinner entrées (four blocks each)

Block Size:

8 Protein	8 ounces beef eye of round, one-eighth-inch slices
1 Carbohydrate	1 cup onions, diced fine
1 Carbohydrate	½ cup carrots, diced fine
⅔ Carbohydrate	2 cups mushrooms, diced fine
1 Carbohydrate	1½ cups broccoli florets
1⅓ Carbohydrate	4 cups mushrooms, sliced
2 Carbohydrate	1 cup tomato puree
1 Carbohydrate	4 teaspoons cornstarch
8 Fat	2⅔ teaspoons olive oil
	1½ cups beef stock
	Salt and pepper to taste

Method:

Place beef slices between plastic wrap and flatten out with a mallet or heavy saucepan. In nonstick sauté pan, add oil, onions, carrots, and 2 cups diced fine mushrooms. Cook until mixture is tender. (This mixture is known as a *duxell*. A duxell consists of finely cooked vegetables used to stuff another item.) When the duxell is cooked, set aside to cool. Spoon equal amounts of the duxell mixture onto the pieces of beef and roll them up. Secure each beef roll with a wooden toothpick to form a roulade. Place rolled beef roulades, beef stock, broccoli, sliced mushrooms, tomato puree, and any leftover duxell in a medium sauté pan and cover tightly. Braise meat and vegetables in liquid for 10–15 minutes until cooked. Add a little water to the cornstarch and stir into broccoli, mushrooms, and beef stock. Heat mixture until a sauce forms, then place an equal amount of rolled beef roulades on two dinner plates, topped with vegetables and sauce.

Note: Braising is an old method of cooking that tenderizes the meat as it cooks. Usually the meat is browned in a liquid or in a covered pan on top of the stove.

Dumplings of Fish with Venetian Sauce

Servings: 2 dinner entrées (four blocks each)

Block Size:

2 Protein	4 egg whites
6 Protein	9 ounces boneless whitefish, diced
2 Carbohydrate	2½ cups tomato, diced
2 Carbohydrate	2 cups onion, diced
1 Carbohydrate	4 teaspoons cornstarch
1 Carbohydrate	1½ cups broccoli florets
2 Carbohydrate	⅔ cup applesauce

⅛ teaspoon nutmeg
1 cup water
1 cup white wine vinegar
2 tablespoons dried tarragon
⅛ teaspoon paprika
Salt and pepper to taste

Method:
A blender or food processor is needed for this recipe. Coat the bottom of a casserole dish with oil, then layer the casserole dish with the diced tomato and diced onion. Set aside for use with the fish dumplings. Place egg whites, diced raw fish, and nutmeg in a food processor. Process mixture until it forms a paste. Form fish paste into one-inch dumplings by scooping the paste into a teaspoon and placing it in a saucepan with simmering water. Hold the spoon in the simmering water for 2–3 minutes until dumpling slides off. Repeat process until all the fish paste has been used. Simmer dumpling for 4–5 minutes before removing and placing in casserole dish. In a saucepan, combine water, vinegar, and tarragon. Mix cornstarch with a little water, then add to saucepan. Simmer ingredients in saucepan for 3–5 minutes to create a Venetian sauce. Pour Venetian sauce over fish dumpling in casserole dish. Cover tightly and bake in preheated oven at 350 degrees for 15–20 minutes. While the casserole dish is in the oven, place broccoli in saucepan

with enough water to cover, and cook until tender. Remove casserole dish from oven and spoon the fish dumplings and sauce onto two dinner plates. Serve each dinner plate accompanied an equal amount of cooked broccoli and applesauce. Sprinkle with paprika and serve.

Chicken with Grapes

Servings: 2 dinner entrées (four blocks each)

Block Size:

8 Protein	8 ounces chicken tenderloins, flattened (or skinless chicken breast)
2 Carbohydrate	1½ cups red seedless grapes
2 Carbohydrate	1½ cups green seedless grapes
2 Carbohydrate	⅔ cup applesauce
1 Carbohydrate	4 teaspoons cornstarch
1 Carbohydrate	3 cups mushrooms, sliced
8 Fat	2⅔ teaspoons olive oil, divided
	4 tablespoons cider vinegar, divided
	2 cups plus 4 tablespoons water
	2 teaspoons orange extract
	⅛ teaspoon dried dill
	½ teaspoon cinnamon plus ⅛ teaspoon
	Dash cloves
	Salt and pepper to taste

Method:
In nonstick sauté pan, add ⅔ teaspoon oil, 2 tablespoons vinegar, 2 tablespoons water, and flattened chicken. Cook until chicken is cooked. In a saucepan, place grapes, applesauce, and 2 cups water. Simmer grapes and applesauce until grapes are tender. Combine cornstarch with 2 tablespoons of water, orange extract, dill, ½ teaspoon cinnamon, and cloves to form a spicy sauce thickener. Add

spicy sauce thickener to saucepan with grapes, applesauce, and water. Cook until thickened and a grape sauce forms. Add grape sauce to chicken and simmer for 5–10 minutes to blend flavors. In another nonstick sauté pan, add 2 teaspoons oil, 2 tablespoons vinegar, ⅛ teaspoon cinnamon, and mushrooms. Cook until mushrooms are tender. On two dinner plates, place a mound of sautéed mushrooms, topped with the chicken and grape mixture.

Chicken Cacciatore

Servings: 2 dinner entrées (four blocks each)

Block Size:

8 Protein	1 pound chicken, skinless breast pieces with the bone (approximately half the weight of this chicken breast is in bone)
2 Carbohydrate	2½ cups tomato, diced
1 Carbohydrate	2¼ cups green pepper, diced
1 Carbohydrate	3 cups mushrooms, diced
1 Carbohydrate	1 cup onions, sliced
2 Carbohydrate	1 cup tomato puree
1 Carbohydrate	4 teaspoons cornstarch
8 Fat	2⅔ teaspoons olive oil
	4 garlic cloves, minced
	1 cup chicken stock
	⅛ teaspoon red wine
	1 teaspoon dried basil
	1 teaspoon dried oregano
	Salt and pepper to taste

Method:
In nonstick sauté pan, cook chicken pieces in ⅔ teaspoon oil until lightly browned. Remove chicken and place in baking dish. Using the same sauté pan, add the remaining oil, garlic, and vegetables,

except tomato puree. Cook vegetables over medium heat until tender. In saucepan, combine tomato puree, chicken stock, wine, spices, and cornstarch. (Mix cornstarch with a little water before adding to saucepan.) Cook mixture in saucepan over medium heat until a thickened sauce forms, then add vegetables to form the cacciatore sauce. Simmer sauce for 5 minutes, then place cacciatore sauce on top of chicken in baking dish. Tightly seal baking dish with aluminum foil and bake in preheated oven at 400 degrees for 20 minutes. Remove casserole dish from oven and place an equal amount of chicken on two dinner plates, topped with cacciatore sauce.

Beef à la Mode Parisienne

Servings: 2 dinner entrées (four blocks each)

Block Size:

8 Protein	8 ounces beef eye of round, one-eighth-inch slices
1 Carbohydrate	3 cups mushroom caps
2 Carbohydrate	2 cups pearl onions
2 Carbohydrate	2 cups cherry tomatoes
2 Carbohydrate	2 cups turnips, cut Parisienne style*
1 Carbohydrate	4 teaspoons cornstarch
8 Fat	2⅔ teaspoons olive oil
	2 garlic cloves, minced
	1 cup beef stock
	6 whole peppercorns
	¼ teaspoon dried oregano
	2 teaspoons fresh basil, chopped
	Salt and pepper to taste

Method:
Coat bottom of a casserole dish with oil. Place all ingredients (beef, vegetables, and spices) in medium-sized casserole dish, except basil

and cornstarch. Tightly cover casserole dish with aluminum foil and place in preheated oven at 400 degrees for 20 minutes. Mix the cornstarch and basil together with a little water to form a paste. After 20 minutes, remove casserole dish from oven and stir in cornstarch-basil paste. Continue stirring meat and vegetables until they have been coated. Re-cover and cook an additional 5–10 minutes. Remove casserole dish from oven and place an equal amount of beef on two dinner plates and top with vegetables and sauce.

Note: Use a small melon ball scoop on turnips to form small balls.

Chinese Sautéed Beef and Celery

Servings: 2 dinner entrées (four blocks each)

Block Size:

8 Protein	8 ounces beef eye of round, diced fine
4 Carbohydrate	8 cups celery, willow leaf cut*
1 Carbohydrate	4 teaspoons cornstarch
1 Carbohydrate	1 kiwi fruit, sliced
2 Carbohydrate	⅔ cup mandarin orange sections
8 Fat	2⅔ teaspoons olive oil
	1 cup beef stock
	2 teaspoons red wine
	2 tablespoons low-sodium soy sauce
	2 teaspoons ginger root, diced fine

Method:
In nonstick sauté pan, add ⅔ teaspoon oil and beef. Cook beef until brown, then remove and set aside. Using the same sauté pan, add remaining oil and celery. Cook celery over medium heat until tender. While the celery is cooking, in a saucepan mix together stock, wine, soy sauce, ginger root, and cornstarch. (Mix cornstarch with cold beef stock so that the cornstarch will be dissolved before

adding to saucepan.) Stir ingredients well in the saucepan, bringing to a light boil to form a sauce. Add beef and sauce to celery in sauté pan and simmer mixture for 5–10 minutes while constantly stirring beef and celery until they have been coated with sauce. Place an equal amount of beef and celery on two dinner plates, accompanied by kiwi fruit and orange sections. Serve immediately.

Note: Willow leaf cut means that the celery is cut at approximately a 45-degree angle. Also, there is no need to add any salt to this dish, because celery is naturally high in sodium.

Pizza-Topped Haddock

Servings: 2 dinner entrées (four blocks each)

Block Size:

8 Protein	12 ounces haddock
4 Carbohydrate	2 cups salsa*
4 Carbohydrate	4 cups green beans, French cut**
8 Fat	2⅔ teaspoon olive oil

Method:
Coat bottom of a baking dish with oil, then place two 6-ounce pieces of haddock in the bottom of the baking dish. Place 1 cup salsa on top of each piece of haddock. Tightly seal baking dish and bake in preheated oven at 375 degrees for 25–30 minutes. While the haddock is baking, in a saucepan add green beans and enough water to cover. Cook green beans until tender. Equally divide green beans between two dinner plates, then remove baking dish from oven. Using a large spatula, scoop out haddock and place on top of green beans on both dinner plates and serve.

Note: Salsa come with different levels of heat. Choose one that best fits your family's tastes. Someone who would like more heat than the others can add a dash of hot sauce to the portion.

**Note: If you prefer, snow peas can be substituted for the green beans.*

Salmon with Dill Sauce

Servings: 2 dinner entrées (four blocks each)

Block Size:

7 Protein	10½ ounces salmon, divided into two pieces
1 Protein and 1 Carbohydrate	½ cup plain low-fat yogurt
½ Carbohydrate	½ teaspoon sugar
½ Carbohydrate	2 teaspoons cornstarch
3 Carbohydrate	1½ cups pineapple, cubed
2 Carbohydrate	1½ cups cantaloupe, cubed
1 Carbohydrate	¾ cup maraschino cherries, halved
8 Fat	2⅔ teaspoons olive oil
	3 teaspoons dried dill weed
	2 teaspoons white wine
	Salt and pepper to taste

Method:
Coat bottom of a baking dish with oil, then place two pieces of salmon in the bottom of the baking dish. Sprinkle salmon with 1 teaspoon dill, then tightly seal baking dish and bake in preheated oven at 375 degrees for 25–30 minutes. While the salmon is baking, in a saucepan combine yogurt, sugar, 2 teaspoons dill, and wine to make the dill sauce. Add a little water to the cornstarch and then add it to dill sauce. Stirring constantly, heat sauce through but do not bring sauce to a boil. In a mixing bowl, combine pineapple, cantaloupe, and cherries to make a fruit salad. Equally divide fruit salad between two dinner plates, then remove baking dish from oven. Using a large spatula, scoop out salmon and place one piece of salmon on each dinner plate. Pour an equal amount of dill sauce over each piece of salmon and serve immediately.

Scallops Mornay

Servings: 2 dinner entrées (four blocks each)

Block Size:

6 Protein	9 ounces scallops*
2 Protein and 2 Carbohydrate	1 cup plain low-fat yogurt
3 Carbohydrate	3 cups green beans, French cut
1½ Carbohydrate	3 lemons, juice and pulp
½ Carbohydrate	½ cup onion, minced
1 Carbohydrate	4 teaspoons cornstarch
8 Fat	2⅔ teaspoons olive oil

⅛ teaspoon Worcestershire sauce
2 teaspoons dry mustard
⅛ teaspoon white wine
2 garlic cloves, minced
Paprika for garnish
Salt and pepper to taste

Method:
In nonstick sauté pan, add oil and green beans. Cook green beans until tender. While the green beans are cooking, in another nonstick sauté pan cook scallops in lemon juice with pulp, Worcestershire sauce, onion, mustard, wine, garlic, and yogurt. Cook scallops for 5–10 minutes. Depending on size of scallops, more or less cooking time may be required. Mix cornstarch with a little water and then add to scallops and simmer for 2–3 minutes until a sauce forms, stirring constantly to coat scallops. Equally divide green beans between two dinner plates. Using a serving spoon, place scallops and sauce on plates beside green beans. Serve immediately.

*Note: Small scallops are best for this dish, but if you can't find them in your supermarket or fish store, cut the larger ones into smaller pieces.

Ginger and Peach Chicken

Servings: 2 dinner entrées (four blocks each)

Block Size:

8 Protein   8 ounces chicken tenderloins, flattened (or skinless chicken breast)

4 Carbohydrate   2 cups peaches, sliced
1 Carbohydrate   ½ cup water chestnuts, sliced
1 Carbohydrate   4 teaspoons cornstarch
2 Carbohydrate   2 cups snow peas

8 Fat   2⅔ teaspoons olive oil

4 tablespoons cider vinegar, divided
2 teaspoons powdered ginger*
⅛ teaspoon cinnamon, plus more for sprinkling
2 teaspoons orange extract
⅛ teaspoon dried dill
⅛ teaspoon cloves (scant)
1½ cups plus 4 tablespoons water

Method:
In nonstick sauté pan, add ⅔ teaspoon oil, 2 tablespoons vinegar, 2 tablespoons water, and flattened chicken. Cook until chicken is browned. In a saucepan, place peaches, ginger, and water chestnuts and 1½ cups water. Sprinkle with cinnamon. Simmer peaches until tender. Combine cornstarch with 2 tablespoons water, then add orange extract, dill weed, ⅛ teaspoon cinnamon, and cloves to form a spicy sauce thickener. Add spicy sauce thickener to saucepan with peaches and water. Cook until thickened and a peachy ginger sauce forms. Add peaches and sauce to chicken and simmer for 5–10 minutes to blend flavors and infuse chicken with ginger flavor. In another nonstick sauté pan, add 2 teaspoons oil and snow peas. Cook snow peas until tender. On two dinner plates place a mound of sautéed snow peas, topped with an equal amount of peachy ginger chicken.

*Note: Adjust the amount of ginger flavor by increasing or decreasing the amount in the recipe to taste.

Antipasto Salad

Servings: 2 dinner salads (four blocks each)

Block Size:

2 Protein	2 ounces chunk light tuna*
2 Protein	2 ounces skim milk mozzarella cheese, shredded
2 Protein	3 ounces deli-style turkey, julienne
2 Protein	3 ounces deli-style ham, julienne
1 Carbohydrate	1 head iceberg lettuce, shredded
1 Carbohydrate	2 cups celery, sliced
1 Carbohydrate	½ cup carrots, sliced thin**
1 Carbohydrate	3 cups mushrooms, sliced
1 Carbohydrate	1 cup onion, in half rings
2 Carbohydrate	½ cup cooked chickpeas
1 Carbohydrate	2¼ cups red bell pepper, in half rings
8 Fat	2⅔ teaspoons extra-virgin olive oil
	2 tablespoons white wine vinegar
	⅛ teaspoon Worcestershire sauce
	2 garlic cloves, minced
	2 tablespoons water
	⅛ teaspoon dried marjoram
	⅛ teaspoon black pepper
	⅛ teaspoon dried oregano
	⅛ teaspoon dried basil

Method:

In a small mixing bowl, add oil, vinegar, Worcestershire sauce, garlic, water, and spices. Blend together with a wire whip. When finished, take two large oval plates and arrange a bed of lettuce on each plate. Place on the bed of lettuce, starting in a vertical line from the right side of the plate to the left, celery, carrots, mushrooms, onions, and chickpeas. Then place the tuna, cheese, turkey, and ham on both plates.

Divide the sections with strips of red bell pepper. Again whip herbal dressing and pour over both antipasto salads.

Note: Use water packed tuna.

**Note: Cut carrots in half and then slice thinly.*

Sautéed Beef with Mushroom Sauce

Servings: 2 dinner entrées (four blocks each)

Block Size:

8 Protein	8 ounces beef eye of round, one-eighth-inch slices
3 Carbohydrate	9 cups mushrooms, sliced
1 Carbohydrate	4 teaspoons cornstarch
3 Carbohydrate	3 cups cooked asparagus spears
1 Carbohydrate	2¼ cups red bell pepper, half rings
8 Fat	2⅔ teaspoons olive oil
	1 cup beef stock
	⅛ teaspoon red wine
	2 garlic cloves, minced
	Chopped fresh basil

Method:

In nonstick sauté pan, add ⅔ teaspoon oil and mushrooms. Cook mushrooms until tender. While the mushrooms are cooking, in another nonstick sauté pan add remaining oil and beef. Cook beef until browned, then add mushrooms, beef stock, red wine, garlic, basil, and cornstarch to sauté pan. Mix cornstarch with the beef stock before adding to the sauté pan so that the cornstarch can dissolve. Simmer, stirring frequently, until it reduces and thickens into a sauce and coats the beef. In a saucepan, add asparagus and red bell pepper with enough water to cover both vegetables. Cook until tender. On two dinner plates, equally divide the beef and vegetables. Sprinkle beef with basil and serve.

Veal Goulash

Servings: 2 dinner entrées (four blocks each)

Block Size:

8 Protein	8 ounces veal, in half-inch cubes
3 Carbohydrate	3 cups onions, diced fine
4 Carbohydrate	2 cups tomato puree
1 Carbohydrate	4 teaspoons cornstarch
8 Fat	2⅔ teaspoons olive oil

6 garlic cloves, minced
2 cups beef stock
¼ teaspoon caraway seeds
8 teaspoons paprika
4 teaspoons Worcestershire sauce
½ teaspoon celery salt
Pepper to taste
Fresh basil, roughly chopped

Method:
Coat bottom of a casserole dish with oil. Place all ingredients (veal, vegetables, and spices) in casserole dish, except basil and cornstarch. Tightly cover casserole dish with aluminum foil and place in preheated oven at 400 degrees for 20 minutes. Mix cornstarch and basil together with a little water to form a paste. Remove casserole dish from oven and stir in cornstarch-basil paste. Continue stirring meat and vegetables until they have been coated. Re-cover and cook an additional 5–10 minutes. Place an equal amount of beef pieces on two dinner plates and top with vegetables and sauce.

Mediterranean-Style Chicken

Servings: 2 dinner entrées (four blocks each)

Block Size:

8 Protein	8 ounces chicken tenderloins, flattened (or skinless chicken breast)
4 Carbohydrate	5 cups tomato, diced
4 Carbohydrate	6 cups cooked eggplant*
2 Fat	⅔ teaspoon olive oil
6 Fat	18 black olives, sliced

8 garlic cloves, minced
2 teaspoons dried basil
1 teaspoon dried oregano
4 tablespoons water
2 tablespoons red wine

Method:
In nonstick sauté pan, add ⅔ teaspoon oil and flattened chicken. Cook chicken until lightly browned, then add diced tomato, garlic, basil, oregano, olives, water, and red wine. Simmer, covered, for 10 minutes or until almost all the liquid evaporates. While the chicken is cooking, cut eggplant in one-eighth-inch-thick slices and place in boiling salted water for 10 minutes, or until tender. On two dinner plates place a bed of cooked eggplant, then place the chicken-tomato mixture on top of the eggplant. Serve immediately.

*Note: When you are buying eggplants, look for those that are firm and have a deep purple color. The skin should have a glossy shine and be free of blemishes and discoloration.

Japanese Sweet and Sour Mandarin Shrimp

Servings: 2 dinner entrées (four blocks each)

Block Size:

8 Protein	12 ounces, cooked shrimp
1 Carbohydrate	2½ cups celery, willow leaf cut*
2 Carbohydrate	2 cups onion, rings halved
1 Carbohydrate	3 cups cucumber, peeled, halved lengthwise, and sliced
1 Carbohydrate	½ cup pineapple, diced fine
1 Carbohydrate	4 teaspoons cornstarch
2 Carbohydrate	⅔ cup mandarin orange sections**
8 Fat	2⅔ teaspoons olive oil
	8 tablespoons vinegar
	2 tablespoons soy sauce
	1 cup chicken stock
	Black pepper to taste

Method:
In nonstick sauté pan, add 2 teaspoons oil, celery, and onions. Just before the celery and onions are tender, add the cucumber. Continue cooking until all ingredients are tender. While vegetables are cooking, in small saucepan combine vinegar, soy sauce, chicken stock, shrimp, pineapple, ⅔ teaspoon oil, and cornstarch to form a sweet and sour sauce. (Mix cornstarch with a little water before adding it to saucepan, so that the cornstarch can dissolve.) Stir sweet and sour sauce until it has thickened. When the vegetables in the sauté pan are tender, add them to the sweet and sour sauce. Simmer for 2–3 minutes, then add orange sections. Divide mixture between two dinner plates and serve immediately.

*Note: Willow leaf cut means that the celery is cut at approximately a 45-degree angle. Also, there is no need to add any salt to this dish, because celery is naturally high in sodium.

**Note: Be careful not to overcook cucumber or orange sections because they will break down.

Veal Mozzarella with Italian Vegetables

Servings: 2 dinner entrées (four blocks each)

Block Size:

6 Protein	6 ounces veal scallopini
2 Protein	2 ounces skim milk mozzarella cheese, shredded
2 Carbohydrate	3 cups eggplant, half-inch cubes
2 Carbohydrate	3 cups zucchini, half-inch cubes
2 Carbohydrate	2 cups tomato, half-inch cubes
1 Carbohydrate	1 cup onions, rings halved
1 Carbohydrate	½ cup tomato puree
8 Fat	2⅔ teaspoons olive oil

2 tablespoons plus ⅛ teaspoon dried basil
⅛ teaspoon dried rosemary
½ teaspoon dried marjoram
⅛ teaspoon dried sage
⅛ teaspoon onion powder
⅛ teaspoon salt
⅛ teaspoon pepper
½ teaspoon dried oregano
4 garlic cloves, minced
½ cup plus 2 tablespoons water

Method:
In a sauté pan, add 2 teaspoons oil, spices, and vegetables, except tomato puree. Cook until tender; however, just before the vegetables are tender, add the tomato puree. While the vegetables are cooking, place veal in a second sauté pan with ⅔ teaspoon oil and 2 tablespoons water. Cook veal until browned. While the veal is cooking, sprinkle with onion powder, salt, pepper, and basil. When the veal in the sauté pan is done, divide equally between two dinner plates. Place an equal amount of vegetables on top of the veal. Lightly sprinkle both dishes with shredded mozzarella cheese and serve immediately.

Stuffed Pork Chops with Vegetable Sauce

Servings: 2 dinner entrées (four blocks each)

Block Size:

8 Protein	2 boneless pork chops (4 ounces each), trimmed
½ Carbohydrate	1½ cups mushrooms, diced fine
2 Carbohydrate	½ cup cooked chickpeas, chopped
½ Carbohydrate	½ cup onions, diced fine
1 Carbohydrate	2 cups celery, sliced
1 Carbohydrate	1½ cups broccoli, small florets or diced fine*
1 Carbohydrate	2 cups cauliflower, small florets or diced fine*
1 Carbohydrate	2¼ cups red bell pepper, medium dice
1 Carbohydrate	4 teaspoons cornstarch
8 Fat	2⅔ teaspoons olive oil
	⅛ teaspoon black pepper
	⅛ teaspoon Worcestershire sauce
	⅛ teaspoon dried marjoram
	3 cups chicken stock
	⅛ teaspoon dried basil
	⅛ teaspoon cinnamon
	⅛ teaspoon chili powder
	⅛ teaspoon nutmeg
	Salt to taste

Method:

In a sauté pan, add ⅔ teaspoon oil, mushrooms, chickpeas, black pepper, Worcestershire sauce, marjoram, and onions. Cook until mixture is translucent (about 10 minutes). (This mixture is known as a *duxell*. A duxell consists of finely cooked vegetables used to stuff another item.) When the duxell is cooked, set aside to cool. Cut a pocket in each pork chop and fill with cooled duxell. Secure pockets with toothpicks so that the duxell will not fall out. If there is any duxell left over, then place a mound of duxell in a baking dish and place the pork chops on top of the duxell. Cover the baking dish and bake in preheated oven at 375 degrees for 20–25 minutes. While the pork chops are cooking, in saucepan combine chicken stock, celery, broccoli, cauliflower, bell pepper, basil, cinnamon, chili powder, and nutmeg. Bring to boil and cook for 10 minutes or until vegetables are tender. Mix cornstarch with a little water and add to vegetables. Reduce heat and simmer 5 minutes, until a sauce forms. Remove baking pan from oven and then carefully remove toothpicks. Place a baked pork chop on each of the two dinner plates with an equally divided amount of vegetables and sauce.

Note: Be sure that broccoli and cauliflower are in small florets or diced fine so that the vegetables will cook in the same amount of time.

Belgian Pork Chops

Servings: 2 dinner entrées (four blocks each)

Block Size:

8 Protein	8 ounces thin boneless pork chops, trimmed of fat
4 Carbohydrate	4 cups brussels sprouts*
3 Carbohydrate	3 cups onion rings, halved
1 Carbohydrate	4 teaspoons cornstarch
8 Fat	2⅔ teaspoons olive oil, divided
	2 tablespoons cider vinegar
	2 tablespoons beer
	1 cup chicken stock

Method:

In a saucepan, place brussels sprouts in enough water to cover. Cook brussels sprouts until tender. While the brussels sprouts are cooking, in a sauté pan add oil, onions, and pork chops. Cook pork chops and onions until the onions are tender and pork chops are well browned; just before the pork chops and onions are done, add 2 tablespoons cider vinegar. In another saucepan, combine beer, chicken stock, and cornstarch. (Mix cornstarch with the cold stock before adding to saucepan.) Heat beer, chicken stock, and cornstarch in saucepan until a sauce forms. When sauce has thickened, add to sauté pan with pork chops and onions, then simmer for 5–10 minutes. Place an equal amount of brussels sprouts on two dinner plates and an equal amount of pork chops and onions on each plate. Serve immediately.

Note: Cut a cross (+) in the stem end of each brussels sprout. This helps keep them from breaking apart during the cooking process.

Broiled Lamb Chops with Basil Green Beans

Servings: 2 dinner entrées (four blocks each)

Block Size:

8 Protein	12 ounces lamb chops (approximately 4 ounces will be bone)
4 Carbohydrate	1⅓ cups unsweetened applesauce*
3 Carbohydrate	3 cups green beans
1 Carbohydrate	2¼ cups red bell pepper, quarter rings
8 Fat	2⅔ teaspoons olive oil
	Celery salt
	Onion powder
	Garlic powder
	Black pepper to taste
	1 teaspoon fresh mint, chopped**
	2 garlic cloves, minced
	¼ teaspoon dried basil
	2 teaspoons red bell pepper, diced fine

Method:
Sprinkle chops with celery salt, onion powder, garlic powder, and black pepper. Place them in a baking pan with a little water and broil about four inches from heat. Broil for about 5 minutes (be careful not to overcook). While the lamb chops are broiling, place the applesauce in a small saucepan with mint and heat. In nonstick sauté pan, cook green beans and bell pepper in oil with garlic and basil. Cook until vegetables are tender. Garnish with the diced red pepper. Remove lamb chops from oven and place on two dinner plates. Place applesauce, green beans, and bell pepper beside the lamb chops and serve.

*Note: You may substitute a cored and sliced apple for the applesauce and sprinkle it with the mint.

**Note: Do not use mint extract because it overpowers the applesauce.

Braised Lamb Bretonne

Servings: 2 dinner entrées (four blocks each)

Block Size:

8 Protein	8 ounces lamb medallions, about the size of a silver dollar and one-eighth-inch thick
4 Carbohydrate	1 cup cooked black beans
2 Carbohydrate	1 cup tomato puree
½ Carbohydrate	1 cup celery
1½ Carbohydrate	1½ cups onion, chopped fine
8 Fat	2⅔ teaspoons olive oil

2 garlic cloves, minced
⅛ teaspoon Worcestershire sauce
1 cup beef stock
⅛ teaspoon white wine
⅛ teaspoon dried basil
Salt and pepper to taste

Method:
Combine lamb and all other ingredients in a large saucepan, then cover the saucepan and simmer for 20–30 minutes. Divide between two dinner dishes and serve.

Pork Meatballs with Tomato-Tarragon Sauce

Servings: 2 dinner entrées (four blocks each)

Block Size:

8 Protein	12 ounces lean ground pork
4 Carbohydrate	1 cup cooked lentils
1 Carbohydrate	1 cup onion, diced fine
1 Carbohydrate	1½ cups steamed broccoli
2 Carbohydrate	1 cup tomato puree
8 Fat	2⅔ teaspoons olive oil

¼ teaspoon chili powder
⅛ teaspoon dried basil
⅛ teaspoon dried tarragon
⅛ teaspoon black pepper
⅛ teaspoon dried marjoram
½ cup beef stock
2 teaspoons cider vinegar

Method:
In a large mixing bowl, combine the cooked lentils, pork, diced onion, chili, basil, dash tarragon, pepper, and dash marjoram. Form mixture into 16 one-inch meatballs. Place meatballs in a baking dish brushed with oil. Bake meatballs in a preheated 375-degree oven for 15 minutes. While the meatballs are cooking, in a saucepan add broccoli and enough water to cover. Cook broccoli until tender but not overcooked. In another small saucepan, combine tomato puree, dash tarragon, dash marjoram, beef stock, and vinegar. Simmer 3–4 minutes to heat throughout. Remove meatballs from oven and gently place meatballs in sauce, gently spooning the sauce over meatballs. Place eight meatballs on each dinner plate and equally divide broccoli and serve.

Note: When a recipe calls for a dash or a pinch of an ingredient, it usually means less than ⅛ teaspoon.

Meatloaf with Italian Sauce

Servings: 2 dinner entres (four blocks each)

Block Size:

8 Protein	12 ounces ground chicken breast
1 Carbohydrate	½ cup carrots, diced fine
1 Carbohydrate	2 cups celery, diced fine
3 Carbohydrate	1½ cups tomato puree, divided
1 Carbohydrate	4 teaspoons cornstarch
8 Fat	2⅔ teaspoons olive oil

4 garlic cloves, minced
1 teaspoon dried basil, divided
1 teaspoon dried oregano, divided
Dried thyme
½ teaspoon dried marjoram
1 cup beef stock
⅛ teaspoon onion powder

Method:

In a medium bowl, mix together the chicken, carrots, celery, ½ cup tomato puree, 2 cloves garlic, ½ teaspoon basil, ½ teaspoon oregano, thyme, and marjoram. Form into two oblong meatloaves and place in baking pan. Bake in a preheated 375-degree oven for 30–35 minutes. While meatloaf is cooking, in a small saucepan combine the oil, beef stock, 1 cup puree, ½ teaspoon basil, ½ teaspoon oregano, 2 cloves garlic, onion powder, and cornstarch to make an Italian sauce. (Mix the cornstarch with the cold beef stock before adding it to the saucepan.) Lightly simmer sauce until it thickens. Remove meatloaf from oven and place on two dinner plates. The loaves are very tender. Remove from baking pan with a large spatula that will support the whole loaf. Pour Italian sauce over meatloaves and serve.

Moo Goo Gai Pan

Servings: 2 dinner entrées (four blocks each)

Block Size:

8 Protein	1 pound chicken, skinless breast pieces with the bone (approximately half the weight of this chicken breast is in bone) or 8 ounces skinless breast meat

1 Carbohydrate	3 cups mushrooms, sliced
1 Carbohydrate	1 cup scallions, sliced
1 Carbohydrate	½ cup water chestnuts, sliced
4 Carbohydrate	4 cups snow peas
1 Carbohydrate	4 teaspoons cornstarch

8 Fat	2⅔ teaspoons olive oil

Salt
Black pepper
3 cups chicken stock
2 tablespoons water
½ teaspoon ginger root, diced fine
2 tablespoons low-sodium soy sauce
2 garlic cloves, minced

Method:
Sprinkle chicken with salt and pepper, then place chicken in non-stick sauté pan with 2 teaspoons oil. Cook chicken until browned and flavor has been sealed inside chicken. Place chicken in baking dish and bake in a preheated 375-degree oven for 15–20 minutes. While the chicken is cooking, in the same sauté pan used to cook the chicken, add mushrooms, scallions, and remaining oil. Cook until mushrooms and scallions are almost tender, then add chicken stock, water, water chestnuts, peapods, ginger root, soy sauce, garlic, and cornstarch. (Mix the cornstarch with a little water before adding it to the saucepan.) Heat mixture in saucepan, stirring occasionally until it is thickened. Remove chicken from oven and add

chicken to mushroom-scallion sauce mixture. Coat chicken with sauce and vegetables and simmer for 3–5 minutes. Divide entrée between two dinner plates and serve.

North African Chicken Tangiers

Servings: 2 dinner entrées (four blocks each)

Block Size:

8 Protein	1 pound chicken, skinless breast pieces with the bone (approximately half the weight of chicken breast is in bone)
2 Carbohydrate	2½ cups cooked kale*
1 Carbohydrate	1½ teaspoons honey
1 Carbohydrate	4 teaspoons cornstarch
4 Carbohydrate	1⅓ cups mandarin orange sections
8 Fat	2⅔ teaspoons olive oil

Salt and pepper to taste
2 teaspoons cider vinegar
3 cups chicken stock
⅛ teaspoon red wine
¼ teaspoon ginger root, grated
½ teaspoon orange extract

Method:
Sprinkle chicken with salt and pepper, then place chicken in nonstick sauté pan with 2 teaspoons oil. Cook chicken until browned and flavor has been sealed inside chicken. Place chicken in baking dish and bake in a preheated 375-degree oven for 15–20 minutes. While the chicken is cooking in the oven, place in the nonstick sauté pan used to brown the chicken the remaining ⅔ teaspoon of oil, kale, and vinegar. Cook until kale is almost tender. In small saucepan, blend chicken stock, honey, wine, ginger root, orange extract, and cornstarch. (Mix the cornstarch with a little water before adding it to the

saucepan.) Heat mixture in saucepan, stirring occasionally until it is thickened. Remove chicken from oven and place chicken and orange sections in sauce. Do not allow orange sections to break up from overcooking. Simmer 3–5 minutes, then equally divide kale on two dinner plates and top with an equally divided amount of chicken.

Note: Kale should be just heated through, never overcooked.

Mustard Chicken

Servings: 2 dinner entrées (four blocks each)

Block Size:

6 Protein	12 ounces chicken, skinless breast pieces with the bone (approximately half the weight of chicken breast is in bone)
2 Protein and 2 Carbohydrate	1 cup plain low-fat yogurt
1 Carbohydrate	3 cups mushrooms, sliced
4 Carbohydrate	5 cups cooked kale, thickly shredded*
1 Carbohydrate	4 teaspoons cornstarch
8 Fat	2⅔ teaspoons olive oil
	Salt and pepper to taste
	1 teaspoon dry mustard
	⅛ teaspoon white wine
	½ cup chicken stock

Method:
Sprinkle chicken with salt and pepper, then place chicken in non-stick sauté pan with 2 teaspoons oil. Cook chicken until browned and flavor has been sealed inside chicken. Place chicken in baking dish and bake in a preheated 375-degree oven for 15–20 minutes. While the chicken is cooking in the oven, place in the nonstick

sauté pan used to brown the chicken the remaining ⅔ teaspoon oil, mushrooms, and kale. Cook until mushrooms and kale are almost tender. In a small saucepan, add yogurt, mustard, wine, chicken stock, and cornstarch to make a mustard sauce. (Mix the cornstarch with a little water before adding it to the saucepan.) Heat mixture in saucepan, stirring occasionally until it is thickened. Remove chicken from oven and place chicken in mustard sauce. Simmer 3–5 minutes, then equally divide mushroom-kale mixture on two dinner plates and top with an equally divided amount of chicken and mustard sauce.

Note: Kale should be just heated through, never overcooked.

Fried Deviled Chicken with Asparagus

Servings: 2 dinner entrées (four blocks each)

Block Size:

8 Protein	1 pound chicken, skinless breast pieces with the bone (approximately half the weight of chicken breast is in bone) or 8 ounces skinless breast meat
2 Carbohydrate	½ cup tomato puree
1 Carbohydrate	4 teaspoons cornstarch
2 Carbohydrate	2 cups cooked pearl onions
3 Carbohydrate	3 cups cooked asparagus
8 Fat	2⅔ teaspoons olive oil
	⅛ teaspoon paprika
	⅛ teaspoon dried basil
	⅛ teaspoon onion powder
	⅛ teaspoon garlic powder
	⅛ teaspoon dried oregano
	Salt and pepper to taste
	2 garlic cloves, minced
	1 cup chicken stock

½ teaspoon hot curry powder
¼ teaspoon white pepper
Water

Method:
Sprinkle chicken with paprika, basil, onion powder, garlic powder, oregano, salt, and pepper, then place chicken in nonstick sauté pan with 2 teaspoons oil. Cook chicken until browned and flavor has been sealed inside chicken. Place chicken in baking dish and bake in a preheated 375-degree oven for 15–20 minutes. While the chicken is cooking in the oven, place in the nonstick sauté pan used to brown the chicken the remaining ⅔ teaspoon oil, tomato puree, minced garlic, chicken stock, curry powder, pepper, and cornstarch. Blend cornstarch with a little water before adding to sauté pan. Simmer for 5–10 minutes to blend flavors and allow mixture to thicken into a sauce, then add pearl onions. In a saucepan, add asparagus and enough water to cover. Cook asparagus until tender but not overcooked. Remove chicken from oven and place chicken in sauté pan. Coat chicken with sauce while simmering for an additional 5 minutes. Equally divide asparagus on two dinner plates and place equally divided amount of chicken and devil sauce on plate.

Braised Pork and Cabbage

Servings: 2 dinner entrées (four blocks each)

Block Size:

8 Protein	12 ounces ground pork
3 Carbohydrate	9 cups cabbage, shredded
2 Carbohydrate	½ cup chickpeas, chopped
1 Carbohydrate	3 cups mushrooms, sliced
2 Carbohydrate	4 teaspoons granulated sugar
8 Fat	2⅔ teaspoons olive oil
	¼ teaspoon black pepper
	⅛ teaspoon celery salt

8 tablespoons cider vinegar
1 cup chicken stock
¼ teaspoon marjoram
⅛ teaspoon caraway seed
Paprika

Method:

In a small mixing bowl, sprinkle pork with pepper and celery salt and mix throughout. In a medium-sized nonstick sauté pan, cook pork in ⅔ teaspoon oil over medium-high heat until browned. While the pork is cooking, in another nonstick sauté pan add remaining oil, cabbage, chickpeas, mushrooms, vinegar, sugar, and other spices. Cook vegetable mixture for about 10–15 minutes, until vegetables are almost tender, then add stock and cooked pork to the sauté pan. Braise mixture for 5–10 minutes, until heated through. Divide between two dinner dishes and serve with paprika sprinkled on top.

Chicken Gumbo Creole

Servings: 2 dinner entrées (four blocks each)

Block Size:

8 Protein	8 ounces chicken tenderloins, diced (or skinless chicken breast)
1 Carbohydrate	2 cups celery, diced fine
2 Carbohydrate	2 cups onion, diced fine
1 Carbohydrate	1¼ cups tomato, diced fine
1 Carbohydrate	2¼ cups green peppers, diced fine
1 Carbohydrate	1 cup okra, cut in half-inch slices
2 Carbohydrate	⅔ cup cooked long-grain rice*
8 Fat	2⅔ teaspoons olive oil
	¼ teaspoon tabasco sauce or to taste
	2 garlic cloves, minced
	3 cups chicken stock**

Method:

Combine diced chicken and all ingredients together in a mixing bowl. Mix gently, then place the mixture in a large saucepan. Cover the saucepan and simmer on medium-high heat for 25–30 minutes. Divide into two soup bowls and serve.

*Note: ⅖ cup is approximately halfway between ⅓ and ½ cup.

**Note: If a thinner soup is desired, add 2 more cups stock.

Beefy-Vegetable Stir-Fry

Servings: 2 dinner entrées (four blocks each)

Block Size:

8 Protein	12 ounces lean ground beef
2 Carbohydrate	2 cups onion, sliced and halved
3 Carbohydrate	¾ cup chickpeas, rinsed and chopped
1 Carbohydrate	1½ cups red bell pepper, sliced and quartered
1 Carbohydrate	3 cups cabbage, shredded
1 Carbohydrate	3 cups mushrooms, sliced
8 Fat	2⅔ teaspoon olive oil, divided
	2 tablespoons apple cider vinegar
	¼ teaspoon Worcestershire sauce
	Salt and pepper to taste
	1 tablespoon low-sodium soy sauce

Method:

In nonstick sauté pan, add ground beef, onion, and ⅔ teaspoon oil. Cook ground beef and onion until browned. In another nonstick sauté pan, add 2 teaspoons oil and remaining ingredients, and cook until cabbage is tender. When the cabbage is tender, add cooked beef and onions to the cabbage. Simmer entire mixture for 10–15 minutes. Divide mixture between two dinner plates and serve.

Tangy Chicken and Bean Salad

Servings: 2 dinner entrées (four blocks each)

Block Size:

8 Protein	8 ounces chicken tenderloins, diced (or skinless chicken breast)
1 Carbohydrate	1 cup fresh green beans, half-inch pieces
1 Carbohydrate	¼ cup cooked red kidney beans, rinsed
1 Carbohydrate	1 cup onion, diced fine
1 Carbohydrate	¼ cup chickpeas, rinsed
½ Carbohydrate	½ head lettuce, shredded
1 Carbohydrate	1¼ cups tomato, diced
½ Carbohydrate	1½ cups raw mushrooms, sliced
1 Carbohydrate	1 cucumber, peeled, seeded, diced
1 Carbohydrate	6 cups spinach
8 Fat	2⅔ teaspoons olive oil
	¼ cup water
	¼ cup apple cider vinegar
	⅛ teaspoon dry mustard
	⅛ teaspoon cayenne pepper
	⅛ teaspoon chili powder
	⅛ teaspoon curry powder (Madras hot)
	¼ teaspoon celery salt

Method:

In medium-sized sauté pan, add 2 teaspoons oil, chicken, green beans, kidney beans, onion, and chickpeas. Cook on medium-high heat for 10–15 minutes until the chicken is done and vegetables are crispy-tender. While the chicken and vegetables are cooking, in a saucepan add ⅔ teaspoon oil, water, vinegar, and spices, and heat.

When the mixture in the saucepan has come to a boil, add liquid to the chicken and vegetables and stir to coat the chicken and vegetables. On two large dinner plates, arrange a bed of lettuce, tomato, mushrooms, cucumber, and spinach to form a salad. Top the salad with the chicken mixture and serve.

SNACKS AND DESSERTS

Jellied Fruit Salad with Walnuts

Servings: 4 serving dishes (one block each)

Block Size:

4 Protein	4 envelopes Knox Unflavored Gelatin
1 Carbohydrate	1 kiwi fruit, peeled and diced
1 Carbohydrate	1 cup raspberries
1 Carbohydrate	1 cup strawberries, diced
1 Carbohydrate	½ cup seedless red grapes, halved
4 Fat	4 teaspoons walnuts, chopped
	2 cups water
	1 tablespoon banana extract
	1 tablespoon orange extract
	½ teaspoon strawberry extract
	Mint leaves

Method:

In saucepan, place gelatin and water, stir until dissolved, then add fruit and extracts. Heat to a simmer, stirring gently for 10 minutes until the raspberries dissolve. Pour liquid into eight-inch by eight-inch by two-inch pan and let cool. When Jellied Fruit Salad has set, place in four serving dishes and garnish with mint leaves.

Note: When choosing berries, look for those that are medium-sized and uniform in color. They should also feel solid to the touch and not be leaking juice.

Orange-Yogurt Dessert

Servings: 4 serving dishes (one block each)

Block Size:

1 Protein	1 envelope Knox Unflavored Gelatin
1 Protein	3 ounces extra-firm tofu, mashed
2 Protein and 2 Carbohydrate	1 cup plain low-fat yogurt
2 Carbohydrate	⅔ cup mandarin orange sections
4 Fat	1⅓ teaspoons olive oil

1 teaspoon orange extract
¼ teaspoon cinnamon
Mint leaves

Method:
In saucepan, place gelatin, yogurt, tofu, and oil, stir until gelatin is dissolved, then add fruit, orange extract, and mint leaves. Heat to a simmer, stirring gently, for 10 minutes until orange sections start to break down. Pour into eight-inch by eight-inch by two-inch pan and let cool. When orange-yogurt has set, cut into cubes and place in four serving dishes. Sprinkle orange-yogurt cubes with cinnamon before serving.

Note: When using yogurt in a recipe, be sure not to bring it to a boil. This will cause the yogurt to break down. This can also happen if it is stirred too much.

Apple-Cinnamon Squares

Servings: 4 serving dishes (one block each)

Block Size:

4 Protein

4 envelopes Knox Unflavored
Gelatin

4 Carbohydrate

1⅓ cups applesauce

4 Fat

1⅓ teaspoons olive oil

2 cups water
⅛ teaspoon nutmeg
1 teaspoon cinnamon

Method:

In saucepan, place 2 cups water, gelatin, and oil, stir until gelatin is dissolved, then add applesauce, nutmeg, and cinnamon. Heat to a simmer, stirring gently for 10 minutes. Pour into eight-inch by eight-inch by two-inch pan and let cool. When Apple-Cinnamon Squares have set, cut into cubes and place on four serving dishes.

Melon Wrapped in Ham

Servings: 4 serving dishes (one block each)

Block Size:

4 Protein

6 ounces deli-style ham, cut in strips

4 Carbohydrate

1 cantaloupe, quartered and cubed*

4 Fat

12 black olives

Method:

Wrap ham around melon cubes and secure with a toothpick. Arrange on serving dish and garnish with olives.

*Note: For a more elegant presentation, use a large melon ball scoop instead of cubing the melon.

Dessert Omelette

Servings: 8 serving dishes (one block each)

Block Size:

8 Protein	14 egg whites plus 2 egg yolks (separate egg whites from yolks)
2 Carbohydrate	4 teaspoons granulated sugar
3 Carbohydrate	3 cups strawberries, sliced
3 Carbohydrate	1 cup mandarin orange sections
8 Fat	2⅔ teaspoons olive oil
	Pinch salt

Method:

In a medium-sized mixing bowl, whip egg whites to form a meringue (marshmallowlike consistency). In another bowl, beat egg yolks, sugar, and pinch of salt. Gently pour egg yolks into meringue and fold in with a spatula until it becomes marbleized. Heat oil in a medium sauté pan, then pour the egg mixture into the sauté pan and smooth it out into an even layer. On medium-high heat, cook until the edges of the egg mixture are dry and the center is somewhat creamy. Lift the edge of the omelette in the pan to check the color; it should be a light golden brown color. Remove from heat and place under a broiler until center is set. As soon as the omelette has set, remove from broiler and spoon some of the strawberries in a line along the center. Add the rest of the strawberries and the mandarin oranges to the omelette and fold over the other half. Remove the omelette from the pan and transfer to a plate. Cut the omelette into eight portions and place on serving dishes.

Frozen Peach Yogurt

Servings: 8 serving dishes (one block each)

Block Size:

3 Protein	3 envelopes Knox Unflavored Gelatin
1 Protein	2 egg whites
4 Protein and 4 Carbohydrate	2 cups plain low-fat yogurt
3 Carbohydrate	3 peaches, halved, pitted, and chopped
1 Carbohydrate	2 teaspoons sugar
8 Fat	8 teaspoons slivered almonds
	2 teaspoons vanilla extract
	1/8 teaspoon ginger
	Dash allspice

Method:
In saucepan, place yogurt, gelatin, fruit, spices, and extract. Heat until mixture becomes thoroughly warm, no more than 180 degrees. Cool and set aside. In a mixing bowl, whip egg whites until firm. When the mixture in the saucepan has cooled, combine it with the whipped egg whites and chopped almonds. Place mixture in a pan and place in freezer or add mixture to an ice cream maker and blend. When mixture is frozen, scoop into eight small serving dishes.

Frozen Strawberry Yogurt

Servings: 8 serving dishes (one block each)

Block Size:

3 Protein	3 envelopes Knox Unflavored Gelatin
1 Protein	2 egg whites
4 Protein and 4 Carbohydrate	2 cups plain low-fat yogurt
3 Carbohydrate	3 cups strawberries, diced fine
1 Carbohydrate	2 teaspoons sugar
8 Fat	8 teaspoons almonds, chopped fine
	2 teaspoons imitation strawberry extract

Method:

In saucepan, place yogurt, gelatin, fruit, and extract. Heat until mixture becomes thoroughly warm, no more than 180 degrees. Cool and set aside. In a mixing bowl, whip egg whites and sugar until firm. When the mixture in the saucepan has cooled, combine it with the whipped egg whites and chopped almonds. Place mixture in pan and place in freezer or add mixture to an ice cream maker and blend. When mixture is frozen, scoop into eight small serving dishes.

Frozen Orange Cream

Servings: 8 serving dishes (one block each)

Block Size:

3 Protein	3 envelopes Knox Unflavored Gelatin
1 Protein	2 egg whites
4 Protein and 4 Carbohydrate	2 cups plain low-fat yogurt
3 Carbohydrate	1 cup mandarin orange sections
1 Carbohydrate	2 teaspoons sugar
8 Fat	8 teaspoons almonds, chopped fine
	⅛ teaspoon cinnamon 2 teaspoons orange extract

Method:

In saucepan, place yogurt, gelatin, fruit, cinnamon, and extract. Heat until mixture becomes thoroughly warm, no more than 180 degrees. Cool and set aside. In a mixing bowl, whip egg whites until firm. When the mixture in the saucepan has cooled, combine it with the whipped egg whites and chopped almonds. Place mixture in a pan and place in freezer or add mixture to an ice cream maker and blend. When mixture is frozen, scoop into eight small serving dishes.

Cottage Cheese Pudding

Servings: 8 serving dishes (one block each)

Block Size:

1 Protein	1 envelope Knox Unflavored Gelatin
1½ Protein	1 egg plus 1 egg white
4 Protein	1 cup low-fat cottage cheese
½ Protein and ½ Carbohydrate	¼ cup plain low-fat yogurt
1 Protein and 1 Carbohydrate	1 cup 1 percent milk
1 Carbohydrate	2 teaspoons sugar
1 Carbohydrate	¾ cup maraschino cherries
4½ Carbohydrate	2¼ cups fruit cocktail
8 Fat	8 teaspoons slivered almonds

Method:

In saucepan, combine gelatin, yogurt, milk, egg, and egg white. Heat mixture in saucepan while constantly stirring, until heated to just below boiling. Remove from heat and cool for 5 minutes before stirring in the remaining ingredients. Pour into eight dessert dishes and let set.

Strawberry Soufflé

Servings: 4 serving dishes

Block Size:

1 Protein	1 envelope Knox Unflavored Gelatin
3 Protein	6 egg whites
2 Carbohydrate	2 cups strawberries, pureed* (makes 1 cup)
1 Carbohydrate	1 lemon, pulp and juice
1 Carbohydrate	2 teaspoons sugar
4 Fat	1⅓ teaspoons olive oil
	Cream of tartar

Method:

In a medium-sized mixing bowl, whip egg whites and cream of tartar to form a meringue (marshmallowlike consistency). Place bowl to one side while preparing puree filling. Place strawberries, gelatin, lemon, and sugar in saucepan and heat until hot. Cool strawberry mixture for about 5 minutes, then pour the puree into the whipped egg whites. Gently fold strawberry puree into whipped egg whites until mixture is uniform in color. Spoon the batter into four soufflé dishes that have been brushed with the 1⅓ teaspoons oil. (If you prefer, you can add mixture to a two-quart soufflé dish, and then divide into four serving dishes after it is removed from the oven. However, individual soufflé dishes make a nice presentation.) Level off the top of the batter in the soufflé dishes. When filling the soufflé dishes, fill to only about a quarter inch from rim of dish. This will ensure that the soufflé will form properly. Bake the soufflé dishes in a preheated 375-degree oven for 20 minutes, or until the soufflé is puffed and lightly browned. Serve at once.

*Note: Any berry in season may be substituted.

Fruit Salad

Servings: 4 serving dishes (one block each)

Block Size:

4 Protein	1 cup low-fat cottage cheese
1 Carbohydrate	⅓ cup mandarin orange sections*
1 Carbohydrate	½ apple, peeled, cored, and chopped
1 Carbohydrate	1 kiwi fruit, peeled and chopped*
1 Carbohydrate	1 cup raspberries*
4 Fat	4 crushed macadamia nuts
	Fresh ground black pepper to taste
	Cinnamon

Method:
In a mixing bowl, combine pepper and cottage cheese, blend thoroughly, then place a small mound of peppered cottage cheese on four serving plates. In another mixing bowl, mix all fruits together to form a fruit salad. Place fruit salad around cottage cheese on four serving plates. Sprinkle with crushed macadamia nuts and cinnamon and serve.

*Note: Any other fruits in season can be substituted, as long as the blocks remain the same.

Fruit Curry

Servings: 4 serving dishes (one block each)

Block Size:

4 Protein	1 cup low-fat cottage cheese
¼ Carbohydrate	½ teaspoon granulated sugar
¼ Carbohydrate	¼ teaspoon brown sugar
¼ Carbohydrate	½ lemon, pulp and juice*
½ Carbohydrate	2 teaspoons cornstarch
½ Carbohydrate	¼ cup pineapple, cubed
1 Carbohydrate	¾ cup peaches, chopped
¾ Carbohydrate	¾ kiwi fruit, peeled and chopped
½ Carbohydrate	½ cup strawberries, quartered
3 Fat	1 teaspoon olive oil
1 Fat	1 teaspoon slivered almonds, toasted
	2 tablespoons water
	Dash rum
	¼ teaspoon cinnamon
	¼ teaspoon ginger
	Dash curry
	Dash nutmeg
	Cocoa powder
	Fresh mint leaves, chopped

Method:

In a sauté pan, place 2 tablespoons water, oil, sugars, lemon pulp and juice, rum, cinnamon, ginger, curry, nutmeg, and cornstarch. (Mix cornstarch with a little water and then add to sauté pan.) Cook mixture on medium-high heat, stirring constantly until a saucelike consistency forms. Add fruit and continue cooking for 3–4 minutes. Mound cottage cheese in the center of four serving plates. When the fruit is heated through, spoon fruit around cheese on serving plates. Sprinkle with almonds, cocoa powder, and mint.

*Note: Choose lemons that are a solid yellow color. The skins should be thin and smooth. It is best to store lemons at room temperature.

Yogurt-Sauced Peaches

Servings: 4 serving dishes (one block each)

Block Size:

2 Protein	½ cup cottage cheese
2 Protein and 2 Carbohydrate	1 cup plain low-fat yogurt
2 Carbohydrate	1½ cups peaches, chunks
4 Fat	4 teaspoons almonds, chopped
	⅛ teaspoon cardamom

Method:
Using a blender, combine cottage cheese and cardamom. Blend until mixture is smooth. Fold yogurt into blended cottage cheese to make a spiced yogurt sauce. Divide peaches into four serving dishes. Spoon sauce over peaches and sprinkle with almonds. Chill and serve.

Stuffed Tomato Snacks

Servings: 4 serving dishes (one block each)

Block Size:

4 Protein	1 cup low-fat cottage cheese
3 Carbohydrate	4 tomatoes, halved and pulp removed
1 Carbohydrate	1 cucumber, peeled, seeded, and shredded
4 Fat	4 teaspoons almonds, chopped
	Salt and pepper to taste ⅛ teaspoon dried dill ⅛ teaspoon paprika

Method:
Using a knife, cut tomatoes in half, then carefully cut out the insides of the tomatoes to create tomato shells. Sprinkle insides of tomatoes with salt and pepper. Dice tomato pulp into small chunks. In a mixing bowl, combine cottage cheese, diced tomato chunks, chopped almonds, dill, salt, pepper, and shredded cucumber. Place two tomato shells on each of the four serving plates, then stuff tomatoes with cheese mixture and let any excess cheese mixture overflow tomato shell onto each plate. Sprinkle with paprika and cover dishes with plastic wrap. Chill before serving.

Vegetables with Garden Dip

Servings: 4 serving dishes (one block each)

Block Size:

3 Protein	¾ cup low-fat cottage cheese
1 Protein and 1 Carbohydrate	½ cup plain low-fat yogurt
1 Carbohydrate	1½ cups broccoli florets
1 Carbohydrate	2 cups cauliflower florets
1 Carbohydrate	2 cups celery sticks
4 Fat	4 teaspoons almonds, chopped

⅛ teaspoon garlic powder
1 tablespoon parsley
1 teaspoon chives
1 teaspoon chili powder
1 teaspoon basil
Hot sauce to taste

Method:
In medium bowl, gently combine cottage cheese, yogurt, almonds, and seasonings. Pour blended mixture into four serving bowls on a lunch plate. Place washed raw vegetables on lunch plate around serving bowls and serve.

Sweetened Peaches

Servings: 4 serving dishes (one block each)

Block Size:

4 Protein	1 cup low-fat cottage cheese
1 Carbohydrate	2 teaspoons sugar
3 Carbohydrate	2¼ cups canned peaches, sliced
4 Fat	1⅓ teaspoons olive oil
	5 tablespoons water

Method:
In nonstick sauté pan, heat oil and sugar, continuously stirring until sugar melts. When sugar has melted, add peaches and stir to coat peaches with sugar. Add 3 tablespoons water and stir occasionally to loosen peaches. Cook peaches until they are lightly browned on all sides. While peaches are cooking, place cottage cheese in four serving dishes. Remove peaches from pan and add on top of cottage cheese. Add 2 more tablespoons water to the sauté pan and heat water until it deglazes the pan and forms a thin sauce. Pour over peaches.

Spiced Caramelized Apples

Servings: 4 serving dishes (one block each)

Block Size:

4 Protein	1 cup low-fat cottage cheese
1 Carbohydrate	2 teaspoons sugar
3 Carbohydrate	1½ apples, peeled, cored, and chopped*
4 Fat	1⅓ teaspoons olive oil
	⅛ teaspoon allspice
	¼ teaspoon cinnamon
	Dash nutmeg
	5 tablespoons water

Method:

In a sauté pan, heat oil and sugar, stirring continuously until sugar melts. When sugar has melted, add apples and spices, stir to coat apples. Add 3 tablespoons water and stir occasionally to loosen apples. Cook apples until they are lightly browned on all sides. While apples are cooking, place cottage cheese in four serving dishes. Remove apples from pan and add on top of cottage cheese. Add 2 tablespoons water to the sauté pan. Cook liquid until it forms a thin sauce. Pour over apples.

*Note: To stop apples from turning brown, dip cut apples in a little lemon juice and water mixture.

Strawberry-Yogurt Jelly

Servings: 4 serving dishes (one block each)

Block Size:

2 Protein	2 envelopes Knox Unflavored Gelatin
2 Protein and 2 Carbohydrate	1 cup plain low-fat yogurt
1 Carbohydrate	2 teaspoons granulated sugar
1 Carbohydrate	1 cup strawberries, hulled and pureed
4 Fat	4 macadamia nuts, crushed
	½ cup water

Method:
In saucepan, place gelatin and water, stirring until dissolved. Heat gelatin and water over low heat, bringing mixture to a simmer, then remove from heat and cool to room temperature. In a mixing bowl, combine yogurt, sugar, and strawberries. When the gelatin has cooled to room temperature, add yogurt mixture and stir until uniform. Pour into four serving glasses and refrigerate until set (about two hours). Sprinkle macadamia nuts evenly over the four glasses before serving.

Stuffed Melon

Servings: 4 serving dishes (one block each)

Block Size:

4 Protein	1 cup low-fat cottage cheese
1 Carbohydrate	½ cup melon balls, from two fresh melons*
1 Carbohydrate	¾ cup peach chunks
1 Carbohydrate	¾ cup maraschino cherries
1 Carbohydrate	⅓ cup mandarin orange sections
4 Fat	4 teaspoons slivered almonds

Method:

Cut 2 small melons in half to form four melon bowls. If necessary, cut the ends of the melons so that the melon bowls will sit on a plate without moving. Using a melon baller, remove the flesh by scooping out the melon. Leave a thin border wall inside the melon bowls. Mound cottage cheese in the center of each melon shell. In a mixing bowl combine fruits, then equally divide fruit and spoon on top of cottage cheese in melon bowls. Garnish with almonds and serve.

*Note: Depending on the size of the melon, you may not need all the flesh from two melons, so store the excess or use in another recipe.

Zucchini Dip

Servings: 4 serving dishes (one block each)

Block Size:

4 Protein | 1 cup low-fat cottage cheese

2 Carbohydrate | 2½ cups steamed zucchini, chopped
1 Carbohydrate | 1½ cups broccoli florets
1 Carbohydrate | 2 cups cauliflower florets

1 Fat | 2 teaspoons imitation bacon bits
3 Fat | 3 teaspoons slivered almonds

⅛ teaspoon dried basil
Salt and pepper to taste
Dash garlic powder
⅛ teaspoon nutmeg
⅛ teaspoon chives

Method:
In saucepan, place zucchini and enough water to cover. Cook until tender. Remove from stove and cool. Using a blender, combine cooked zucchini, cottage cheese, and spices. Blend until mixture is smooth, fold in bacon bits and slivered almonds, and scoop into four serving bowls. Arrange an equal amount of washed fresh broccoli and cauliflower florets around dip. Chill and serve.

Tomato-Zucchini Nibbles

Servings: 4 serving dishes (one block each)

Block Size:

4 Protein	1 cup cottage cheese
1 Carbohydrate	1¼ cups zucchini, chopped fine
3 Carbohydrate	3 cups cherry tomatoes
4 Fat	4 teaspoons slivered almonds, chopped
	¼ teaspoon garlic salt
	1 teaspoon snipped chives

Method:

In saucepan, place zucchini and enough water to cover. Cook until tender. Remove from stove and cool. Using a knife, cut the tomatoes in half, then carefully cut out the inside of the tomato or use a small melon baller to scoop out the inside of the tomato to create a tomato shell. If necessary, cut a little off the bottom of the tomatoes so that the tomatoes will sit on a plate without moving. Using a blender, combine cooked zucchini, tomato pulp, cottage cheese, almonds, garlic salt, and chives. Blend until mixture is smooth. Fill tomatoes with cheese mixture by piping it out with a pastry bag. Arrange on serving plates and chill.

Yogurt-Berry Bowl

Servings: 4 serving dishes (one block each)

Block Size:

4 Protein	2 cups plain low-fat yogurt
2 Carbohydrate	1 cup blueberries
1 Carbohydrate	1 cup raspberries
1 Carbohydrate	1 cup strawberries, sliced
4 Fat	4 teaspoons slivered almonds

Method:
In a mixing bowl, combine all ingredients except almonds and gently blend. Equally divide into four portions, sprinkle with almonds, and chill before serving.

Afternoon Fruity–Cottage Cheese Snack

Servings: 4 serving dishes (one block each)

Block Size:

4 Protein	1 cup low-fat cottage cheese
1 Carbohydrate	¾ cup cantaloupe, cubed
1 Carbohydrate	½ cup honeydew melon, cubed
1 Carbohydrate	¾ cup canned peaches, cubed
1 Carbohydrate	½ cup pineapple, cubed
4 Fat	4 teaspoons slivered almonds

Method:
Place ¼ cup cottage cheese in a mound in the center of four serving dishes. Surround the cottage cheese with fruit cubes and sprinkle with almonds.

10

SHOPPING IN
THE WAR ZONE

It's a war out there. In fact, every time you enter the supermarket, consider it a war zone. It's you versus the food industry. And it's not fair. The food manufacturers have the high-tech weapons (e.g., marketing and packaging). You don't. They have the resources (e.g., advertising). You don't. The only thing you have in your favor is knowledge. Put that knowledge to work, and you can win the battle and the war.

First things first. Before you go off to battle, make sure that you're prepared. Eat a Zone snack before you shop. When you get to the store, follow this ideal battle plan: Try to stay on the periphery of the supermarket and never go down the aisles. Once you venture within, it's like a scene from *Moby Dick* in which Ahab is beckoning you to go after all of those neatly packaged carbohydrates and take them home to eat. Although Ahab's crew was powerless to prevent their doom, you don't have to be.

For once, the government is finally on your side in this battle of wits. Those nutritional labels that once seemed so meaningless give you the information you need to make intelligent choices in the trenches. Let's take a close look at what is commonly seen as another government make-work intervention in your life: the nutrition panel label. When people look at a nutrition panel label (see Figure 10-1), most see only one thing: the dreaded grams of FAT.

If you've read this far, you know that fat is not your enemy (and in fact it may be your greatest ally in getting into the Zone). In fact,

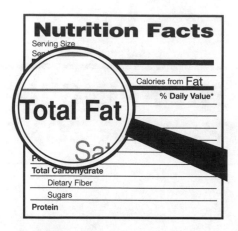

Figure 10-1. Nutritional Panel

within the borders of the nutritional label lies the real information that's going to allow you to win this war. And what is that information? The ratio of protein to carbohydrate in that food product.

That's right, every packaged food in America contains the real information you need to win the Zone war. For every 3 grams of protein, you want about 4 grams of carbohydrate. Let's be frank. It is highly unlikely that you will ever find a single food product in those aisles that has the right protein-to-carbohydrate ratio. The secret is to mix and match foods until you get the right combination. If you are going to do this mixing and matching within the confines of the supermarket, you have to go back to the blocks. Simply convert every label into blocks (divide the number of protein grams per serving by 7 grams and the number of carbohydrate grams per serving by 9 grams) and you can quickly tell what other kinds of food you need to buy to keep a precise balance in your hormonal carburetor.

For example, let's read the label on one of the first convenience foods introduced into America—Grape-Nuts. What seems more all-American than Grape-Nuts? I know this all too well. As a young high school athlete, I lived on Grape-Nuts. Grape-Nuts for breakfast, Grape-Nuts for after-school snacks, Grape-Nuts for dinner (I didn't particularly like vegetables or low-fat protein), Grape-Nuts for a late-night snack. But what was I really eating? Sugar, and lots of it. Let's look at the label. Figure 10-2 shows a Grape-Nuts nutritional label.

Nutrition Facts

Serving Size 1/2 cup
Servings 8

Amount Per Serving

Calories 200   Calories from Fat 10

% Daily Value*

Total Fat 1g

   Saturated Fat 0g

Cholesterol 0mg

Sodium 350mg

Potassium   mg

Total Carbohydrate 47g

   Dietary Fiber 5g

   Sugars 7g

Protein 6g

Figure 10-2. Grape-Nuts Label

A ½-cup serving (2 ounces) has 6 grams of protein and 47 grams of carbohydrate. But since it also has 5 grams of fiber, the total content of insulin-promoting carbohydrate is only 42 grams. Of course, no one ever eats only 1 ounce of Grape-Nuts (more likely about 4 ounces, since that is what it takes to fill a typical bowl). Nonetheless, whether I ate 1 ounce or 4 ounces, the protein-to-carbohydrate ratio, and hence the effect on my hormonal carburetor, would be the same.

Let's assume that I ate my typical 4-ounce serving. In that serving I should be getting 12 grams of protein, but because of the fiber content, I will actually absorb less than that listed amount of protein. Let's assume that only 75 percent is absorbed (which is typical of most nonanimal sources of protein), which means that in a 4-ounce serving, I would actually be getting 9 grams of protein. Take that 9 grams of protein and divide it by 84 grams of carbohydrate, which gives a protein-to-carbohydrate ratio of 0.11. Since you are trying to get 3 grams of protein for every 4 grams of carbohydrate (a protein-to-carbohydrate ratio of 0.75), a bowl of Grape-Nuts is definitely not going to put you in the Zone.

In fact, the protein-to-carbohydrate ratio of Grape-Nuts is actually very similar to a typical candy bar. Even adding a little milk to it would not greatly change the ratio. No wonder I never made it to the NBA.

But a far better way to calculate is to break the Grape-Nuts into blocks. So let's look at the typical 4-ounce bowl of Grape-Nuts in blocks. Nine grams of protein is a little more than one protein block (9 grams of absorbed protein divided by 7 grams of protein per block). Eighty-four grams of total carbohydrate is approximately nine blocks of carbohydrates (84 grams of total carbohydrate divided by 9 grams of carbohydrate per block). What's wrong with this picture? First, the ratio of protein-to-carbohydrate blocks is nowhere near the 1:1 ratio needed for your hormonal carburetor. Second, you are consuming far more carbohydrate blocks than even the largest person would ever want in a meal. Third, there are no fat blocks. Summation, a hormonal disaster, but a correctable hormonal disaster. Simply eat less Grape-Nuts (like 1 ounce, which would give you three carbohydrate blocks) with a little low-fat milk, add another three blocks of low-fat protein (like ¾ cup of nonfat cottage cheese) and three blocks of fat using three macadamia nuts. Now you have the makings of a hormonal winner. Of course, an even better choice would have been to replace the Grape-Nuts completely with one cup of strawberries and an orange. But we're winning the battle.

Let's try looking at a typical 6-ounce can of tuna fish.

Each serving contains 12 grams of protein, 5 grams of fat, and zero grams of carbohydrate. So we have two blocks of protein per serving (12 grams divided by 7 grams equals approximately two blocks), two blocks of internal fat (5 grams divided by the 1.5 grams in one fat block equals approximately three blocks), and zero carbohydrate.

Nutrition Facts

Serving Size 2oz.
Servings 2.5

Amount Per Serving

Calories 95	Calories from Fat 45
	% Daily Value*
Total Fat 5g	
Saturated Fat 2g	
Cholesterol 35mg	
Sodium 250mg	
Potassium mg	
Total Carbohydrate 0g	
Dietary Fiber 0g	
Sugars 0g	
Protein 12g	

Figure 10-3. Label of Canned Tuna Fish

Here's an example of hidden fat found in all low-fat protein sources. Every block of low-fat protein will contain about one block of fat. That internal fat is not quite enough to optimize your hormonal carburetor. To do so, you should add one additional external block of fat for every block of low-fat protein. Now if you add up the internal fat in the low-fat protein and the external fat you plan to add, you will get the appropriate balance of protein, carbohydrate, and fat.

However, nobody eats half a can of tuna, so let's try and decipher the label of a whole can to see that each can contains about three servings. So a whole can of tuna fish would contain six protein blocks, and no carbohydrate. Obviously, if you are going to have a can of tuna for a meal, then you had better find six carbohydrate blocks to add to it and add another six external fat blocks. That could be two slices of bread and one apple with 1 tablespoon of mayonnaise. That's a pretty big sandwich, but when cut in half, it becomes two three-block meals. Or your choice may be a massive salad containing a head of lettuce, three tomatoes, two onions, and three green peppers, with six tablespoons of olive oil and vinegar dressing. Again, splitting this salad into two portions will also give you two three-block meals. And if that seems too much, then reduce the size of the salad and have a piece of fruit. The choice is yours, as long as you maintain your hormonal carburetor.

What about high-fat foods, such as peanuts? Most people think of peanuts as a high-protein food, because they are taught that peanut butter is a great source of protein for young kids. In reality, both peanuts and peanut butter are great sources of fat with a little protein and carbohydrate thrown in. Let's look at a typical label for peanuts.

First, I hope you are not going to eat the entire jar, since one serving of peanuts (unlike tuna fish) is about 1 ounce (fifteen individual nuts). In those fifteen nuts you are going to have 11 grams of fat, 6 grams of protein, and 7 grams of carbohydrate. Breaking this down to blocks would give nine fat blocks (11 grams divided by 1.5 grams equals nine blocks), one protein block (6 grams divided by 7 grams equals approximately one block), and one carbohydrate block (7 grams divided by 9 grams equals approximately one block). So while the peanuts (and other seeds and nuts) have an

Nutrition Facts
Serving Size 1oz.
Servings 16

Amount Per Serving

Calories 150   Calories from Fat 90

% **Daily Value***

Total Fat 11g
    Saturated Fat 1.5g
Cholesterol 0mg
Sodium 115mg
Potassium 180mg
Total Carbohydrate 7g
    Dietary Fiber 2g
    Sugars 0g
Protein 6g

Figure 10-4. Label for Peanuts

appropriate protein-to-carbohydrate ratio, they are essentially all fat as far as the Zone is concerned. But they *can* be used to add extra fat to other meals that are too low in fat, to optimize your hormonal carburetor (and this is especially true of fresh-ground or natural peanut butter, which contains no additives, only ground peanuts).

Now that you are understanding how to break down food labels into blocks, let's take the next step and find a typical frozen dinner to see how it stacks up. Figure 10-5 shows the food labeling for a typical low-fat meal: Weight Watchers Ravioli Florentine.

Nutrition Facts
Serving Size 1
Servings 1

Amount Per Serving

Calories 220   Calories from Fat 15

% **Daily Value***

Total Fat 2g
    Saturated Fat 0g
Cholesterol 5mg
Sodium 450mg
Potassium   mg
Total Carbohydrate 43g
    Dietary Fiber 4g
    Sugars 10g
Protein 9g

Figure 10-5. Label for Low-Fat Ravioli

The first thing you see is that the meal is low-fat (because you're still focusing on the fat content), with a total of 2 grams. In fact, the back of the box says, "How can it be so low in fat . . . and so delicious?" But 2 grams of fat is approximately one fat block (2 grams divided by 1.5 grams equals approximately one block). Now go to the carbohydrate content, and notice we have 43 grams. But bear in mind what is important is the insulin-promoting carbohydrate content. Since the meal has 4 grams of fiber, we should subtract this amount from the total of 43 grams of carbohydrate, leaving 39 grams of insulin-promoting carbohydrate. This translates into four carbohydrate blocks (39 grams divided by 9 grams equals approximately four blocks). So what about the protein? Well, it has only 9 grams of protein, which equals about one block of protein (9 grams divided by 7 grams is approximately one block). This ratio of four carbohydrate blocks to one protein block is just about the same as a Hershey's Chocolate Bar with Almonds—no wonder it's so delicious.

So before you eat this frozen dinner, how can you make it hormonally correct? First, it needs more protein. Since the frozen dinner contains four blocks of carbohydrate, we need to add another three blocks of protein to give it a total of four protein blocks. So go into your refrigerator and get 3 ounces of turkey breast or tuna fish to eat with this frozen dinner. But you're still not quite there. You need three more blocks of fat, and we are going to make this monounsaturated fat. The easiest way to do this is add three macadamia nuts or 3 teaspoons of slivered almonds. Now we have a hormonal winner, even though it started out as a hormonal loser. And the total calories with all these extra protein and fat additions? 365! The hormonal winner is also low-calorie. Not nearly as appetizing as the hundreds of Zone meals in Chapter 9, but at least it's a relatively fast meal that won't take you out of the Zone.

The best thing to do is to shop for fresh stuff and make it yourself. After all, who wants to eat frozen meals when they can enjoy family recipes handed down over the generations? People eat maybe ten favorite meals at home, because they tend to like the same meals over and over again. So why not take each of these ten favorite family meals and transform them into hormonal winners, just as we did for the Weight Watchers Ravioli Florentine, to be eaten and enjoyed again and again.

11

EATING OUT
IN THE ZONE

Who actually eats in the Zone? Surprisingly, the French and Northern Italians come close without trying. These two cultures and cuisines are noted for being incredibly refined and sophisticated.

Think about the very posh four-star French restaurant. For fifty dollars you get a glass of great wine, a small amount of protein in the center of the plate, covered with a delicious sauce and surrounded by an artistically arranged outer ring of vegetables, and a small side salad to cleanse the palate. Even though you could have gobbled down five meals at the all-you-can-eat pasta palace for less than you paid at the four-star French restaurant, the French restaurant is serving you a Zone meal: adequate amounts of protein, low glycemic vegetables, and perhaps a glass of wine. And the four-star Northern Italian restaurant? For the same fifty dollars you now get a glass of wine, a piece of fish in the center of the plate, surrounded by an outer ring of artistically prepared vegetables, and a small side dish of pasta.

Neither of these meals was more than 500 calories (a Zone Diet rule), and each had an appropriate balance of protein to carbohydrate (another Zone Diet rule). And no one can accuse you of not having a great meal.

But how do you play the game when you're going out to a typical restaurant where a satisfied customer is one who has to unbuckle his belt after the meal? Here are some simple rules to follow at any restaurant, four-star or family style.

Rule #1. Never eat the rolls. If you're going to eat unfavorable carbohydrates, save them for dessert.

Rule #2. Always choose your low-fat protein entree from the menu first. This sets the stage for selecting the rest of your meal.

Rule #3. Always ask the waiter to replace the rice, potatoes, or pasta with vegetables. You will be amazed how gracious the restaurant will be.

Rule #4. While you're waiting for dinner, have a glass of red wine or a glass of bottled water while everyone else is munching on rolls. Try conversation instead of eating to pass the time.

Rule #5. Once the dinner is served, use the eyeball method to survey the scene. Look at the size of the low-fat protein entree you ordered. If it is significantly greater in size than the palm of your hand, plan to take the excess home (it sure beats eating cottage cheese the next day). Then look at your plate and determine whether the carbohydrates are favorable or unfavorable.

Rule #6. The volume of the low-fat protein you plan to eat determines the volume of the carbohydrate you are going to eat. If you're eating favorable carbohydrates, then you can have double the volume of carbohydrates compared to your protein portion. If you are planning to eat unfavorable carbohydrates, then you can eat only the same volume of carbohydrates as in your protein portion.

Rule #7. If you really came to the restaurant to eat dessert, then don't eat any carbohydrates (favorable or unfavorable) at your meal. When the server comes back with a dessert menu, order whatever you want, but plan to eat only half of it (remember, you have saved up your carbohydrate allotment, so now it's time to cash in). The rest of the dessert? Offer it to your dinner companions. I'm sure they will be delighted to help out. And the best dessert? Try fresh fruit.

Now that wasn't too difficult. It's very easy to do in the four-star restaurant, where there isn't very much food to begin with. It's much more difficult to undertake at the typical American restaurant in which great masses of food are shoved in your direction. This is what has happened to American restaurants in the last generation. Because we have the cheapest food on earth, people expect to get their money's worth by consuming massive amounts of calories. Everything is oversized (the only exceptions are the above-mentioned four-star restaurants where presentation and quality count for more than sheer bulk). And since mass is in, restaurant owners make their money by making sure most of the mass comes in the form of carbohydrates (which are dirt cheap) as opposed to protein (which is relatively expensive).

But it can be easy to order hormonally correct meals, even in fast-food restaurants, if you keep in mind the rules from the last chapter. Let's take McDonald's, for example. Here's a very quick Zone meal. Buy two inexpensive, small hamburgers, then throw one of the buns away. Put the two patties together in the remaining bun, and enjoy. A little high on the saturated fat and all unfavorable carbohydrates, but if you're not doing it very often, it's not too bad hormonally. Now here's a far better choice at McDonald's: buy the grilled McChicken sandwich and a salad. Throw away three-quarters of the bun, add the grilled chicken and the rest of the bun (as croutons) to the salad, and, presto, you have a grilled chicken salad with a touch of bread. It's quick, it's easy, and it's hormonally correct.

Fast-food restaurants can be a great help to you when you don't have the time to cook or to sit down at a restaurant. A more comprehensive summary of many of those fast-food meals can be found in *The Zone,* but the best quick meals can be found in your supermarket at the salad bar. Simply grab a bunch of precut vegetables and fruits (especially the things you would never buy otherwise) and put them in the aluminum plate they provide along with some olives (your monounsaturated fat). Then walk over to the deli and buy a quarter pound of low-fat protein, like turkey, chicken, or tuna. Add the low-fat protein to the precut vegetables, fruits, and olives, and you've got a great hormonal meal. It may be a little expensive compared to a bagel and a cup of coffee, but isn't your health worth it?

What if you're constantly on the road? How do you stay in the Zone? Here are some easy tricks for the business-trip road warrior. If you are going to be staying a couple of days at a hotel that has a room refrigerator, go out and buy some fruit and sliced low-fat deli meat or low-fat cottage cheese. For every piece of fruit, plan to eat 1 ounce of low-fat meat or 2 ounces of cottage cheese. These can be quick snacks before you go out to eat (thereby making it easier to eat a Zone meal at the restaurant). And before you go to bed, remember to have a quick hormonal "touch-up" so that you get a good night's sleep in a strange bed.

Keep in mind that if you are a business person on the road, meals are your key to success because they are the main determinant of your mental alertness throughout the day. Here are three more hormonal winners you can always choose: For breakfast, have a three-egg omelette (try to have it made with egg substitutes or egg whites) and the fruit bowl, but don't eat the toast or the hash browns. For lunch, have a grilled chicken salad. And for dinner, eat fish with an extra serving of vegetables instead of the rice or potato. And, of course, never eat the rolls. Life is tough enough on the road without having to wander out of the Zone.

Eating out in the Zone is easy, if you know the rules. To quote Nancy Reagan, "just say no" to the overwhelming incoming tide of carbohydrates you're constantly exposed to when you eat. If you think it's difficult, then think of carbohydrates as a drug. The more you take of any drug, the more likely you are to get a drug overdose. In this case, an overdose of carbohydrates will generate an excess production of insulin, which can eventually kill you. That thought should make it easier to pass on the rolls the next time around.

12

YOUR ZONE REPORT CARD

The most important question a physician can ask a patient is "How do you feel?" That's the same question you want to ask yourself on the Zone Diet. My basic rule, whether it applies to a new diet, a vitamin, a mineral, an herb, etc., is to use as directed for two weeks. If you don't feel significantly better, then it's probably not going to happen.

The Zone Diet is no different. What results are you initially looking for? If you are like most people, you are after three simple things: thinking better, performing better, and looking better.

How do you think better? Once you begin to stabilize your blood sugar levels, you can expect your thinking to become much clearer and more focused. Think of what happens when you eat a big pasta meal at noon. By three o'clock you can barely keep your eyes open. The worst nightmare for a business executive is trying to negotiate a big business deal in the afternoon after eating a huge pasta lunch. If you want the world's greatest productivity tool, then think about following the Zone Diet.

Next, you should be performing better. When you're in the Zone, you essentially have a hormonal ATM card to tap into your body's stored fat, a virtually unlimited source of energy. So you should have more energy to spare for work, at home, and for play.

And finally, you will be looking better. You don't lose weight rapidly on a Zone Diet, but you do lose excess body fat at near a genetic maximum, which is 1 to 1½ pounds of fat per week. At the end of two weeks, your clothes, especially around your waist, will fit much better.

Even if you are having great success on the Zone Diet, every thirty days I strongly recommend that you eat a big carbohydrate-rich meal, like pasta. Why would you want to descend into carbo-hydrate hell? Just to let yourself know the difference between being in the Zone versus being out of it, even for one meal. What can you expect after eating that high-carbohydrate meal? An insulin hang-over with loss of mental focus after the meal, grogginess and trou-ble waking the next morning, puffiness in your hands and feet, etc. It's a very instructive lesson on the hormonal power of food. Consider it a form of dietary Anabuse (Anabuse is a drug used to treat alcoholics that makes them violently ill when they drink any alcohol). Don't worry, however; you're only one meal away from getting right back into the Zone.

And what about meals? How do you know if you're making a hormonally winning meal? Well, you could do a radioimmune assay on your blood insulin levels every two hours, but that's pretty unre-alistic. Or you could take blood sugar tests every two hours. Again, pretty unlikely. The easiest test is to just ask yourself how you feel during the next four to five hours after a meal. If you maintain a sharp mental focus and have no hunger for that four- to five-hour period, then you know the meal was a hormonal winner. Put that exact meal, with its ingredients and exact amounts, in your winner's cookbook so that you can come back to it at any time in the future. As with any drug, that meal will induce the same hormonal response.

Try to make your hormonal cookbook as large as possible. For most people that cookbook need consist of about only ten meals. Why? Well, most people really don't eat that many different meals at home. Of course, if you are like my wife and me, you probably have a million cookbooks as a result of joining some cookbook club years ago, but you still eat the same few meals you like to eat again and again. If each of those meals is a hormonal winner, eating any one of them will be the same as taking the most powerful drug known in order to think better, perform better, and look better. Most people would pay ungodly sums of money for such drugs, yet they exist right in your recipe file of hormonally winning meals.

Of course, feeling better, thinking better, performing better, and looking better are indicators that you're in the Zone, but in this age of technology most people want some hard numbers to confirm that they're feeling better. What can you do on your own to confirm that beneficial physiological changes are indeed happening? The first thing to track is the change in your percent body fat. You know your clothes are fitting better, but the weight on the scale isn't changing all that quickly. The reason you look at the scale at all is for a number that confirms the better fit of your clothes. Your weight, however, isn't nearly as important as your percent body fat in analyzing your overall health. So recalculate your percent body fat to confirm that your clothes are really fitting better. Using the tables in Appendix C allows you to make this measurement on a weekly basis.

And just how reliable are the tables found in the appendix? To answer that question, I did a study at the Medical Research Foundation in Houston, comparing the percent body fat of normal individuals determined by the tables in *The Zone* to the same number done by dual energy X-ray absorptiometry (DEXA) measurements (the new high-tech standard for measuring body fat). The variance of the results from the method in the appendix compared to the DEXA measurements was only about 1–2 percent in the body fat results. You might take a DEXA test once in your life, but you *can* measure yourself every day. Bear in mind that everything is relative to your starting point. And as you lower your percent body fat, know that you are lowering your insulin levels, too. As you lower your insulin levels, it is much more likely you are going to stay in the center of the Zone.

What if you still want more numbers? Well, this means getting a blood test. Most people (including me) hate seeing their blood leave their bodies. But when you know you're feeling better, you want every test in the book to confirm it. Most people dread going to a doctor's office to have a blood test, because they know they're there because they're sick, and they know the test is only going to confirm how sick they really are. Not surprisingly, when you're feeling great, you want to march in and demand as many tests as possible to congratulate yourself, if you only knew which tests.

One of the best is your blood pressure. No needles, no blood. It turns out that blood pressure is very sensitive to hyperinsulinemia. When you're done checking your blood pressure, have your physician take a blood sample (it's amazing how much braver you become in the Zone) and tell him or her you want the following tests:

- Fasting triglycerides
- HDL cholesterol
- Fasting-triglyceride-to-HDL-cholesterol ratio
- Fasting insulin
- Glycosylated hemoglobin (HgA$_1$C)

These are standard tests, but the last two are not routinely done, because they tend to be slightly more expensive. What results are you looking for? Your fasting triglycerides should be under 100 mg/dL, and your HDL cholesterol should be more than 50 mg/dL. This means your triglyceride-to-HDL-cholesterol ratio should be less than 2.0. Your fasting insulin should be less than 10 μ units/ml, and the HgA$_1$C should be less than 5 percent. The ratio of triglycerides to HDL cholesterol is indicative of your insulin levels. The higher the ratio, the higher your insulin. Likewise, your fasting insulin tells exactly how high your insulin levels are. Finally, the glycosylated hemoglobin tells you how well you have been keeping your blood sugar under control on a long-term basis. The lower your glycosylated hemoglobin, the better you have kept your insulin under control. The numbers of these clinical parameters give you very objective goals to mark your progress. In other words, your blood tells you whether you have been naughty or nice. These are your goals. It may take a little time to reach them, but if you are thinking better, performing better, and looking better as you progress toward them, you can afford the time.

Why are these numbers important? Because they indicate the extent of any hyperinsulinemia and therefore your likelihood of moving out of the Zone and toward chronic disease. If your triglycerides are greater than 200 mg/dL and your HDL cholesterol is less than 35 mg/dL, you're headed for big trouble, because you're hyperinsulinemic. Likewise, a fasting insulin greater than 15 μ units/ml means you're in danger, because you're hyperinsulinemic. And a glycosylated hemoglobin of greater than 9 percent means you're at high risk, because you're hyperinsulinemic.

Why do these numbers place you in such clinical trouble? It turns out that the primary risk factor that determines your likelihood to develop heart disease is not high cholesterol levels, or high blood pressure, but elevated insulin levels. If you're hyperinsulinemic, you'll be making more of a certain group of hormones (i.e., "bad" eicosanoids) that can actually make you ill. And if you have read *The Zone*, you know that represents very big trouble.

Why doesn't medical science just find some drug that lowers insulin? Actually, such a drug exists: It's called food. If you're hyper-insulinemic, then start using that drug. Your life depends on it.

13

LIVING IN THE ZONE

There's more to living in the Zone than simply eating. You really want to do everything you can to keep your insulin levels from rising.

What you eat and how you eat will have the greatest impact on getting you to the Zone, but there are two other ways you can enhance your diet to get to the Zone and stay there on a permanent basis. Not surprisingly, just like eating, you can do these things yourself. These extra magical hormonal elixirs are exercise and stress reduction. Before you go off to join some gym or find an appropriate guru in India, let me give you some very simple ways to integrate these two hormonal control strategies into your everyday life.

EXERCISE—JUST DO IT

The very word inspires dread for most people. Not because you don't think it's important, you just don't have the time to do it. There are two types of exercise you should do every day: aerobic and anaerobic.

Aerobic exercise simply means doing exercise that requires oxygen. As I pointed out in *The Zone,* the best exercise for most people is walking. Simply walk fifteen minutes in one direction, then turn around and walk back. You can do this in the morning, at lunch, after dinner. Just plan to do it once a day. You can even park your car a fifteen-minute walk from work, walk to your job, and then walk back to your car after work.

You don't need to join a health club, buy a designer Spandex exercise outfit, or invest in a pair of high-tech running shoes. That isn't to say there aren't benefits to more intensive aerobic exercise, but make this daily walking an integral part of your life before you decide to increase your level of activity. I have for one never yet figured out the logic of having valet parking at posh health clubs in California. Why not just park the car down the street and walk to the club?

What about anaerobic exercise, isn't that weightlifting? And doesn't this mean joining some dark and dingy gym surrounded by hulking figures that come out of central casting? No, in fact all the weight training you'll probably ever need can be done in your bedroom or for that matter any hotel room if you are on the road. All it takes is about five minutes a day.

The weight you're going to use is your own body, and you carry that piece of equipment with you wherever you go. You should work your upper and lower body muscles at every workout and you can do it with two simple exercises: pushups and squats.

Let's start with pushups. Many people, especially women, will have trouble doing a pushup at first, especially if they're out of shape. The key to all upper body exercises is to always keep your back straight. Correct form is always more important than the number of repetitions.

If you are really in bad shape, initially just lean toward a wall and push yourself away. These are really push-aways, not pushups. When you can easily do three sets of about ten to fifteen of these push-aways, then you're ready to progress to the next level, which is counter-pushes. Stand two to three feet away from a counter. With your hands on the counter, lower your body toward it and then push yourself away. After you can do three sets of ten to fifteen of these counter-pushes, you're ready for knee pushups (you're getting closer to that "dreaded" pushup all the time). Now simply kneel on the floor with your chest touching the floor. Place your hands on the floor at shoulder width and push your upper body up, keeping your knees touching the floor. After you can easily do three sets of knee pushups ten to fifteen times, you're finally ready for the traditional pushup. These are just like the knee pushups except now you lift your knees off the floor along with your upper body. All of your weight now rests upon your hands and your toes. Lower yourself until you are about one inch from the ground, and then raise yourself back up. Your goal is to do three sets of ten to fifteen of these traditional pushups on a daily basis.

Pushups are great for the upper body, but what about the lower body? For that you want to do squats (also described by your grandmother as deep knee bends). Squats are deceptive, because they require a lot of lower body strength. As with pushups, it's always best to start slowly, and always keep your back straight. Begin by using a chair with arms. Sit down and then stand up. If you initially have to use the arms of the chair for support, that's OK. Do three sets of this ten to fifteen times in each set. Your next progression is to do the same exercise without using the arms of the chair for support. The next step is to cross your arms across your chest and still be able to do three sets of ten to fifteen repetitions. Once you can do that, you're in position to begin to do a squat, which is essentially sitting down on a chair that isn't there. Don't let your knees bend more than 90 degrees, and at first do these squats with your arms extended. Once you reach that goal of three sets of ten to fifteen repetitions, then do the same exercise with your arms crossed on your chest.

So here's your daily exercise routine. Do one set of pushups (at whatever level you can), followed by one set of squats (at whatever level you can). Rest one minute, and then repeat both exercises again. Rest another minute and do both the pushups and squats a third time. When you can easily do fifteen repetitions on the third and last set, then go to the next level of difficulty the following day. The total time of your anaerobic exercise is five minutes a day in the privacy of your own home or in a hotel room if you're traveling. Just do it every day.

If you're walking thirty minutes a day and doing five minutes a day of strength training, you've got a pretty good exercise program. And you would be surprised how many people will still complain about the time it takes to do even this level of exercise. But if you really want to get into the Zone, this small expenditure of time and effort is certainly worth it.

Even if you have reached this level of exercise, before you join a health club, I would first recommend that you just buy a set of light barbells weighing between 1 and 15 pounds (or fill old plastic milk bottles that have handles partially with water, then grasp them by the handles) to do strength exercises in addition to your standard pushups and squats. Your pushups and squats now become great warm-ups for additional weight-bearing exercises. Any number of exercise books will describe more advanced barbell exercises for both the lower and upper body. The key point is that you should never let more than one minute go by between sets and should try not to go more than thirty minutes of exercise with weights. Beyond that point, hormonal levels begin to change significantly (i.e., testosterone drops and cortisol rises), and you can gain very little additional benefit with increased training. And if you want more aerobic activity? Walk one hour per day.

STRESS REDUCTION—STOP AND SMELL THE ROSES

Stress is a biochemical event that causes significant hormonal responses. The acute stress brought on by danger causes the release of hormones, such as adrenaline, which mobilize you for the typical "flight or fight" syndrome associated with acute stress. However, what is more common in our present society is chronic stress, which also has other hormonal consequences. During chronic stress, the hormone cortisol is being released at an elevated level. As cortisol levels rise, insulin resistance increases, which in turn causes insulin levels to rise. It's these rising insulin levels that drive you out of the Zone. The so-called Type A personality (aggressive, hard-charging, driven, etc.) is the type of individual with increased cortisol levels. And since cardiovascular disease is associated with such Type A personalities, it is not surprising that stress reduction can play an important role in reducing heart attack.

You don't have to find a guru or chant mantras all day long to reduce stress. Just carve out some personal time for the things you like to do (and I hope watching TV is not one of them). Probably the best stress reducer is walking. Not power walks where you are trying to pump up your heart rate, but the type of walks that let you stop and talk to neighbors, or enjoy the scenery, or even smell the roses. In each of these cases, there is a lot of stopping and starting, but since you have no particular agenda, it's a great stress reducer. Furthermore, walking is a two-in-one activity. Besides reducing stress, you're also reducing insulin by exercising aerobically. And insulin reduction is what it's all about.

So there you have it—diet, exercise, and stress reduction. Three low-tech ways to treat a high-tech problem: hyperinsulinemia. These are things you can begin tomorrow as you start your journey toward the Zone. Not only will these steps get you to the Zone, but they will allow you to live regularly there.

DRUGS THAT TAKE YOU OUT OF THE ZONE

You should be aware that a number of drugs can take you out of the Zone by raising insulin levels. Two of the most common are diuretics and beta-blockers, both commonly used in the treatment of high blood pressure. Newer hypertensive drugs such as angiotensin-converting enzyme (ACE) inhibitors have no effect on insulin levels. Corticosteroids, such as prednisone, also significantly raise insulin levels. Then there is another drug that only slightly elevates insulin levels. Unfortunately, that drug is ubiquitous in America. It's called caffeine. And one of the best ways to help yourself get to the Zone is to reduce the use of that drug.

14

FREQUENTLY ASKED QUESTIONS ABOUT THE ZONE

GENERAL

If I follow the Zone diet, does this mean I can never have rice, pasta, and bagels again?

Of course not. Following a Zone Diet only means that you should be using these sources of carbohydrates in moderation, like condiments. Simply make sure that most of your daily intake of carbohydrates comes from fruits and vegetables.

Do I have to be obsessive about the Zone Diet to be successful?

No. Obviously, the greater the precision, the greater the results, but if you only play by the rules of the Zone Game and use the eyeball method, you won't be too far away from the center of the Zone. Just remember to pay very close attention to your responses after a meal. Using the simple tools in this book, you will be able to adjust your hormonal carburetor with increasing precision without having to obsess about portion size, blocks, and calculations.

Should I be concerned about such a seemingly low daily caloric intake?

If you have excess body fat (greater than 15 percent for males and greater than 22 percent for females), then all the calories you need are already stored in your body. Remember that the typical male or female in this country carries about 100,000 calories of stored fat at all times. To put this in perspective, this represents approximately 1,700 pancakes, which is a pretty big breakfast. To access those 1,700 pancakes you simply need a "hormonal ATM card" to release these stored calories. The Zone Diet is that card. If you are using that ATM card correctly, you don't have to consume as many external calories to meet your body's energy requirements. On the Zone Diet, you are eating *as if* you are already at your ideal percentage of body fat because you are using a combination of your stored body fat and incoming calories to meet your total caloric requirements.

Doesn't any low-calorie diet cause fat loss?

Not necessarily. Research studies in the 1950s conducted by Kekwick and Pawan at the Middlesex Hospital in London examined diets consisting of 1,000 calories per day. All patients lost substantial weight on a high-protein (90 percent of calories) diet, high-fat (90 percent of calories) diet, and mixed (42 percent of calories as carbohydrate) diets, but most patients actually gained weight on a high-carbohydrate (90 percent of calories) diet. Cutting back on calories without gaining access to your hormonal ATM card is a surefire prescription for deprivation, constant hunger, and fatigue. Any time you reduce calories, you will lose some weight, but eventually you hit a hormonal plateau where the weight loss (and more importantly, fat loss) stops, but feelings of hunger, deprivation, and fatigue continue. The Zone Diet is not a diet; it's a hormonal control program that allows you to optimize your quality of life.

What is more important, the amount of carbohydrates you consume or the glycemic index of the carbohydrates you eat?

The total intake of carbohydrates is most important. However, you will get even greater results on the Zone Diet by making sure most of your carbohydrates come from low-glycemic carbohydrates. By eating low-glycemic foods, you are retarding their rates of entry into the bloodstream, thereby maintaining the best possible balance of your insulin levels. In addition, low-glycemic carbohydrates provide the maximum amounts of vitamins and minerals with the least amount of carbohydrate. Finally, by eating primarily low-glycemic carbohydrates, you will constantly be faced with a very hearty meal because low-glycemic carbohydrates are also usually low-density carbohydrates. It is simply very hard, if not impossible, to overconsume low-density carbohydrates such as fruits and vegetables.

How long before I can expect to see results on the Zone Diet?

Within two to three days you should see a noticeable reduction in your carbohydrate cravings and increased mental focus. Within five days you will notice a significant increase in your lack of hunger throughout the day, coupled with better physical performance. Within two weeks, although you will not have lost much weight, you will notice that your clothes are fitting much better. Keep in mind the maximum fat loss you can expect is 1 to 1½ pounds of fat per week. It is simply impossible to reduce excess body fat any faster.

Why doesn't the Zone Diet include the protein content of carbohydrate-rich sources like vegetables or grains?

Because people would get too bogged down in the calculations. A significant amount of the protein in these foods is not absorbed; therefore one has to impose correction factors to take into account the actual amount of protein that is absorbed and thus its effect on hormonal response. Since vegetable sources are not very protein-dense, it makes more sense to ignore their protein contribution. Vegetarians should make sure that they always include protein-rich vegetarian sources such as firm tofu, isolated protein powders, or soybean imitation meat products at every meal to ensure adequate protein intake.

What is the minimum amount of daily protein block intake?

Regardless of your protein calculations, we always recommend a minimum of eight protein blocks throughout the day for adults.

Won't a high-protein diet cause osteoporosis and kidney failure?

Not if you are eating a protein-adequate diet like the Zone Diet. No one should be eating more protein than his or her body requires, but, conversely, no one should be eating less, because to do so is to put yourself in a state of protein malnutrition. On the Zone Diet, not only are you eating adequate protein, but you are spreading it over three meals and two snacks. It's almost as if you are receiving an intravenous drip of protein. Excessive protein at any meal can't be stored by the body, and therefore has to be converted into fat. The first step in this conversion process is the removal of the amino group from the protein, which can put a strain on the kidneys if excessive protein is floating around in the bloodstream. Furthermore, the newest research indicates that even for patients with kidney failure, the earlier reports about the benefits of protein restriction may have been overstated. The calcium loss often associated with eating excessive amounts of protein is completely blocked if adequate dietary calcium is supplied with the protein. The one mineral many women don't get enough of is calcium. So if you are concerned, drink a glass of milk with each meal or take a calcium supplement.

Why don't the French have high rates of heart disease?

Nutritionists just hate the French. They smoke, they drink, they eat lots of fat, they don't exercise, they seem to have a very good time, and they have the lowest rates of heart disease in Europe. It's called the French Paradox. It's only a paradox if it is contrary to your expectations. Obviously, there are a number of reasons for these surprising statistics, but I believe the major factor is that their meals are moderate in calories, are rich in fruits and vegetables, always contain protein, and include fat. That's basically the Zone Diet. We also have the so-called Spanish Paradox. In the last twenty years, Spaniards have eaten more protein, more fat, and fewer grains than they used to as a population and their rates of cardiovascular disease are dropping. These are not paradoxes, simply adjustments in the hormonal responses of a population to a changing diet.

The Chinese eat a lot of rice; don't they have low rates of heart disease?

No, according to the American Heart Association. The rates of cardiovascular disease in urban Chinese males are nearly as great as the rates for Americans, and Chinese females, both rural and urban, actually have greater rates of cardiovascular disease than American females.

I'm concerned about pesticides on fruits and vegetables, and the hormones and antibiotics used in beef and chicken production. What should I do?

These are valid concerns. You should always try to eat organic fruits and vegetables and range-fed beef and chicken. However, be prepared to pay a significantly higher price and be willing to cope with reduced availability. Don't, however, make this an excuse for not eating the appropriate protein-to-carbohydrate ratio at every meal.

I'm not overweight. Why would I need to follow the Zone Diet?

The Zone Diet is not a diet. It's a lifelong hormonal control program. Loss of excess body fat is only a side effect (although a very beneficial side effect). The Zone Diet was originally developed for cardiovascular patients, and was tested on world-class athletes. Between those two extremes lies everyone else. If you are at your ideal percent body fat, and want to think better and perform better, then the Zone Diet is for you.

When was the Zone Diet developed?

The program has been undergoing constant testing and revision since 1984. The present program represents the seventh generation of my original concept to control hormonal responses using dietary intervention. *The Zone* provides a more detailed history of this development process. The Zone Diet has been used by thousands of individuals during this developmental period since 1984.

Can I still continue to use my vitamins and minerals?

Vitamins and minerals are an excellent low-cost insurance policy to ensure adequate levels of micronutrients. However, a Zone Diet—which is primarily composed of low-fat protein, fruits, and vegetables—provides an excellent base of vitamins and minerals, and requires much less supplementation. The only supplement that I strongly recommend is extra vitamin E, since the Zone Diet is still a low total fat diet, and most dietary vitamin E comes from fat.

What exactly do you mean by "use in moderation" when referring to unfavorable carbohydrates?

Try not to make unfavorable carbohydrates (grains, starches, breads, and pasta) more than 25 percent of the total carbohydrate blocks in a meal. Use them as condiments, not the primary source of your carbohydrate intake.

Should I be concerned about sodium?

Not if you are following a Zone Diet, because excess insulin activates another hormonal system that promotes sodium retention. However, it always makes sense not to use excessive amounts of sodium.

I'm a pure vegetarian. How can I make this diet work for me?

Simply add protein-rich vegetarian foods to your existing diet to maintain the correct protein-to-carbohydrate ratio. Ideal choices would be firm and extra-firm tofu and isolated soybean protein powder. The new generation of soybean-based imitation meat products (hot dogs, hamburgers, sausages, etc.) are another excellent way of getting protein-rich vegetarian foods into your existing meals. Traditional vegetarian protein sources, such as beans, have an exceptionally high amount of carbohydrate for the amount of protein they provide, which makes it impossible to achieve the desired protein-to-carbohydrate ratio needed to enter the Zone.

Which protein powders are best?

Excellent sources of isolated protein include egg and milk combinations and lactose-free whey powder. For vegetarians, isolated soy protein powders are excellent choices. Protein powders are available at most health food stores. These protein powders can be added to carbohydrate-rich meals, like oatmeal, to make them more hormonally favorable. They can also be added to flours and mixes (such as pancake, muffin, and cookie mixes) for cooking and baking to fortify the protein content.

What impact will various cooking methods have on the quality of the macronutrients or micronutrients?

Cooking has little effect on the macronutrients (except that excessive heat can damage and cross-link protein with carbohydrates). However, cooking can have a significant negative effect on micronutrients (vitamins and minerals). Vitamins are extraordinarily sensitive to heat. And minerals can be leached out of food when cooked with water. Therefore, steaming vegetables is an ideal preparation method to retain micronutrients and yet make the vegetables more digestible. Fruits are usually eaten raw, retaining all their micronutrients. The more carbohydrates are processed or cooked, the more rapid their rate of entry into the bloodstream. This is why instant forms of carbohydrate like instant rice or instant potatoes should be avoided.

Do I eat my meal or snack even if I'm not hungry?

Yes. This is the best time to eat in order to maintain hormonal equilibrium from one meal to the next.

Will this diet heal the damage done to my body over the years?

The body has a remarkable ability to repair itself, given the appropriate tools. The best of those tools is the diet, especially one that orchestrates the appropriate hormonal responses that accelerate the repair process.

Why don't I count all the protein, carbohydrate, and fat in everything I eat?

Because you would probably need a mini-computer to make all the calculations. This is why we devised the block method that takes into account fat content and protein digestibility, the fat content in low-fat protein, and the insulin-sensitive carbohydrate content of carbohydrates, making your calculations for preparing each meal exceptionally simple.

Will a liquid meal in the correct ratio get me to the Zone? If not, why not?

A liquid meal has a much greater surface area than a solid food. As a result, the digestion and entry rate of macronutrients into the bloodstream cannot be controlled as well, and there is a corresponding decrease in the desired hormonal control. Liquid meals are more convenient, but they are not as hormonally desirable as solid food. They can be used occasionally if you just don't have the time to cook.

Can children use the Zone Diet?

The diet is ideal for children because they need to be in the Zone even more than adults. For children, assume that they have 10 percent body fat when you make their lean body mass calculations. Then, whatever their activity factor actually is, increase it by two levels. This is to ensure more than adequate protein for growth spurts. The one protein source that virtually every child will eat is string cheese. Although a little high in saturated fat, string cheese is a good way to begin to introduce more protein in your child's diet. That leaves just the hard part for parents: getting your kids to eat fruits and vegetables instead of pasta and bread.

How do I know that two years from now the Zone Diet will not turn out to be like the other diets that initially produce great results?

The Zone Diet is not a diet, but a lifelong hormonal control program that allows you to maximize your full genetic potential. These hormonal systems have evolved over the last forty million years and are unlikely to change soon. Surprisingly, many diets are based on gluttony. Eat either all the carbohydrate you want (high-carbohydrate, low-fat diets) or all the protein and fat you want (high protein, low-carbohydrate diets). The Zone Diet is based on moderation. There are limits on the amount of protein, carbohydrate, and fat consumed at every meal.

I'm off the body fat calculation charts found in **The Zone.**
What should I do?

Assume that you have 50 percent body fat. With time you will lose
sufficient fat so that you can follow the percent body fat charts. If
you are off the weight charts, then also increase your physical activity level by one level, because with all the extra fat you have, you
are essentially doing light weight training twenty-four hours a day.

FAT FACTS

Why do I need extra fat? What does it do?

Paradoxically it takes fat to burn fat, if that fat is monounsaturated
fat. Remember, this is not an excuse for fat gluttony, but the need
to add back reasonable amounts of fat to each meal. First, fat acts
as a control rod to slow the rate of entry of carbohydrate into the
bloodstream, thereby reducing the insulin response. Second, it
releases a hormone (cholecystokinin, or CCK) from the stomach that
tells the brain to stop eating. Third, it supplies the building blocks
(i.e., essential fatty acids) for eicosanoids. Most of your fat intake
should be in the form of monounsaturated fat, and the amount of
fat you consume is dictated by the amount of protein you consume
at each meal.

Can I lose too much body fat?

Obviously it's possible to lose too much body fat. So once you reach
a percent of body fat that you are happy with and wish to stabilize
your weight at that point, simply add more monounsaturated fat to
your diet. This extra monounsaturated fat will act as a caloric ballast to provide the extra calories to maintain your percent body fat
without affecting insulin levels. Why? Monounsaturated fat has no
effect on insulin. It's hormonally neutral.

Why is the fat block only 1.5?

Every block of low-fat protein contains approximately 1.5 grams of
"hidden" fat. Therefore, by adding one extra fat block (which is
defined as 1.5 grams of fat) for each block of low-fat protein, you

are actually consuming 3 grams of fat or two fat blocks (one internal in the protein and one external) for each protein block. If you are using fat-free protein sources, such as isolated protein powders, then you should be adding two blocks of fat to achieve the same ratio. Obviously, if you are eating higher-fat protein choices, you would not be adding any extra fat blocks to your meal. Remember that every time you add additional fat blocks to a meal, they should be composed primarily of monounsaturated fat.

What's wrong with supplementing my diet with flaxseed oil?

A central theme in *The Zone* is the reduction of arachidonic acid levels by diet. Controlling insulin is your most powerful tool, but the addition of omega–3 fatty acids can also have a significant benefit. Flaxseed oil is rich in alpha linolenic acid (ALA), which is an omega–3 fatty acid and therefore has some use in controlling arachidonic acid production. But if you are going to supplement with an omega–3 oil, then I recommend fish oil, which is rich in the best omega–3 fatty acid, eicosapentaenoic acid (EPA). EPA has a tenfold greater impact on reducing the production of bad eicosanoids than does ALA on a gram-for-gram basis. Another reason I prefer fish oil over flaxseed oil is that the excess consumption of ALA in flaxseed oil tends to reduce the production of gamma linolenic acid (GLA), the building block of good eicosanoids. What's excess? Anything more than one tablespoon per day. Finally, the vast body of research data on the clinical benefits of EPA is overwhelming. Therefore, supplementation with EPA as opposed to ALA will have a far greater impact in getting you into the Zone. But before you add any omega–3 fatty acid supplements to your diet, try to get those fatty acids from food itself. The best source of EPA? Salmon. Of course, you could do what your grandmother did in her day to ensure adequate levels of EPA, and take cod liver oil.

Besides salmon, where can I get EPA, and how often should I eat fish each week?

Other sources that are rich in EPA include mackerel and sardines. Other marine sources that have a lower EPA content are common fish such as tuna, swordfish, scallops, shrimp, and lobster. Try to consume about 300 mg of EPA per week. This would translate into one serving of salmon or four servings of tuna or similar fish per week. One teaspoon of cod liver oil contains about 500 mg of EPA.

How can I tell if fish oil is safe?

The best indication that a fish oil capsule or cod liver oil containing EPA has been molecularly distilled, which removes harmful chemicals, is that it is cholesterol-free. This is a very expensive process that literally distills over chemicals, leaving the sensitive fish oil intact. This means that any residual PCBs, which contaminate virtually all fish and might be found in even refined fish oil, have been removed.

I'm a vegetarian and can't use fish oil. What should I do?

This is the one case I would suggest supplementation to your diet with flaxseed oil as a source of omega–3 fatty acids. But I would recommend no more than one tablespoon of refined flaxseed oil per day so that the natural production of GLA is not compromised.

FINE-TUNING

How do I adjust my hormonal carburetor?

Not everyone is genetically the same. Your hormonal carburetor is based on the protein-to-carbohydrate ratio that generates the best hormonal response for you. That hormonal response is easily measured by asking yourself, "How do I feel?" four to five hours after a meal. If you maintain excellent mental clarity and have no hunger, then the protein-to-carbohydrate ratio in the last meal you ate is correct for you. Your goal is to make every meal with that same ratio to generate the same hormonal response. For the vast majority of people, this ratio is 3 grams of protein for every 4 grams of effective carbohydrate. So the most efficient way to fine-tune your own carburetor is to start with this ratio and then experiment slightly on either side to determine your limits by using hunger and mental clarity as the parameters to optimize.

I'm still hungry on the Zone Diet. What should I do?

You need to make a slight adjustment to your hormonal carburetor. Always look back to your last meal. If you feel hungry within two to three hours after you eat, and experience a drop-off in mental focus (because of low blood sugar), it is because you consumed too much carbohydrate relative to the amount of protein. As a result, you're making too many bad eicosanoids because of an increase in insulin secretion that has taken you out of the Zone. Simply make that same meal in the future and keep the protein constant, but reduce the carbohydrate amount by one block. On the other hand, if you feel hungry before any four- to six-hour cycle ends, but maintain good mental focus, you're actually making too many good eicosanoids, which is pushing insulin levels too low. The brain has a sensing system that picks up low insulin levels in the bloodstream and tells you to eat to increase insulin levels, even though the brain is getting plenty of blood sugar (hence the good mental focus). Simply make that same meal in the future, and add one additional block of carbohydrate to the meal. In essence what you are doing is adjusting your personal hormonal carburetor to get to the center of the Zone. In either case, you should add more monounsaturated fat to either meal, as fat releases the hormone cholecystokinin (CCK), which promotes a feeling of fullness that is known as satiety.

I have developed some constipation. What should I do?

A Zone Diet will switch your body to a fat-burning metabolism instead of a carbohydrate-burning metabolism. The metabolism of fat requires greater amounts of water on a daily basis. So the first step is to increase your water intake by 50 percent. If this isn't sufficient to reduce the constipation, then it means that you are probably releasing stored arachidonic acid from your fat cells. For about 25 percent of the population, there will be a transitory release of stored arachidonic acid, the building block of bad eicosanoids, from stored body fat. The buildup of extra arachidonic acid in your stored fat is a result of your previous dietary patterns. This temporary increase in arachidonic acid can give rise to constipation by reducing water flow into the colon. Adding extra EPA to your diet will minimize this transitory effect. The best source of EPA is fish, but another good source is fish oil capsules. I would also recommend taking some crystalline vitamin C with each meal. Alternatively, you can slow down the access to your stored body fat by making a slight adjustment in your hormonal carburetor and adding one extra carbohydrate block to each meal.

As I drop weight, should I drop the number of protein blocks I eat?

No. The weight you are dropping is pure fat. The program is designed to maintain your lean body mass (LBM), which requires protein to maintain it. In essence, on the Zone Diet you are eating *as if* you are at your ideal body weight. The only time to change your protein block intake is when you change your physical activity level or see a significant change in your LBM, which you can measure using the tables found in *The Zone*. However, if you are overweight, you should recalculate your LBM after two weeks on the diet, since you may lose some retained water (which artificially inflates your real LBM, and therefore inflates your real protein requirements). This recalculation will provide you with your real LBM upon which to base your protein requirements.

Should I add protein if I'm trying to gain lean body mass? If so, how much?

The only way to build muscle mass is by exercise, primarily weight training. However, building one pound of new muscle mass per month is a noble goal. To do so, however, requires only one extra protein block per day in addition to the number of protein blocks required to maintain your existing lean body mass. One pound of new muscle equals 454 grams. But muscle is 70 percent water, which means that one pound of new muscle contains about 136 grams of protein. Divide 136 grams by 30 days, and you get 4.5 grams of extra protein per day required to build new muscle. Taking in one extra block of protein (7 grams) per day will be more than adequate in your quest to add one extra pound of muscle per month.

How should I alter this diet if I'm pregnant and/or nursing my child?

If you are pregnant or nursing, you should be using a Zone Diet to ensure adequate protein intake. For pregnant women, whatever your physical activity level actually is, increase it by two levels. For example, if you have a physical activity level of 0.7 grams of protein per pound of lean body mass, then increase it to 0.9 grams of protein per pound of lean body mass. For nursing mothers, increase your physical activity factor by one level over your actual physical activity level. However, if pregnant, always check with your physician before making any dietary change.

Can I cut back on fat blocks as long as I match my protein and carbohydrate requirements?

You can, but ironically you will not lose as much fat. The small amount of added fat acts as a control rod to reduce the rate of entry of carbohydrates into the bloodstream, thereby reducing insulin secretion. By reducing insulin, you can access your stored body fat more effectively. Also, the fat causes the release of the hormone cholecystokinin (CCK) that promotes satiety between meals. Of course, any added fat to your diet should be primarily monounsaturated fat, such as olive oil, guacamole, almonds, or macadamia nuts.

How do I get even more information?

Visit my site on the World Wide Web at http://www.Eicotech.com. This Web site is a virtual on-line Zone magazine, with weekly updates on new recipes, medical research news, and additional helpful tips to stay in the Zone. Consider this Web site your on-line Zone Community Center.

15

TALES FROM THE ZONE

Being in the Zone will help you think better, perform better, and look better. But the power of this dietary technology goes far beyond these benefits alone. It was developed to treat what I call "either/or" medical conditions: medical conditions that either have no treatment or those for which the treatments are less than desirable.

Hormonal control will be the key to twenty-first-century medicine, and much of this hormonal control comes from the food you eat: You take advantage of this fact when you enter the Zone. Once you are in the Zone, you are in position to control the most powerful hormones in your body, eicosanoids. You make over one hundred different types of these hormones, and they affect every cell in your body. They can keep you well or they can make you sick. You control them by controlling insulin levels. And you control insulin levels by your diet. The end result is that some very remarkable changes are possible if you treat food with the same respect that you treat a prescription drug.

While I can tell you this over and over, perhaps you would like to hear what other people have to say about the Zone Diet and how it has affected their life. These are their stories. They may begin like yours, or like the story of someone you know. Their endings, however, come straight from the Zone.

It's usually when you get bad news from your doctor that you begin to really appreciate health. And no news is worse than that your key organs are failing. Nothing can be more frightening than an organ transplant. The only time you undergo one is when you are literally days from death. Consider the story of Mary P., whose lung capacity was so compromised that she required a double lung transplant just to survive. Last year she began following the Zone Diet, and she won a gold medal in the 20-kilometer cycling event at the 1995 World Transplant Games. Nowadays, she routinely rides in 100-mile-plus events at the age of forty-nine. Does being in the Zone help? Mary likes to think so.

If organ transplants mean you're close to death, then having cancer is not far behind. Consider the tale of Willard H., a prostate cancer survivor who wrote,

> I just returned from the Mayo Clinic where I go for my annual physical. All of my tests came out well. My PSA [a marker for prostate cancer] is undetectable. My cholesterol has continued to decrease from 210 to 150. Thanks and congratulations go to you and The Zone. I spoke with my physicians about the Zone Diet. They were not experts on nutrition, but said they thought it was a good program. Neither their encouragement nor discouragement would have made a difference with me. I'm on your program for life. I give a lot of credit to your program for keeping my PSA at the bottom end of the scale.

Reaching the Zone is all about this improved quality of life. That's why I particularly like the letter that I got from Joan S., who wrote:

> This "incurable" multiple sclerosis is reversing after sixteen years. It feels like I'm living a miracle. I'm glad I've kept daily notes because it seems unbelievable. I keep pinching myself.

What is even more encouraging are letters from individuals who have been on medication for decades, like Louise P., who wrote the following:

> For 40 years I have been taking thyroid pills and drugs against depression. In addition, I had high blood pressure of 180/95 that was only controlled by medication. Since my understanding of your concept pertaining to the Zone and

applying its principles, I am a healthy person taking no more thyroid pills, no more anti-depressants, no more high blood pressure medications since my blood pressure is now 120/70. I thank you with the deepest gratitude for restoring my health through your dietary guidelines. And my husband and children feel the same way.

Reductions in blood pressure are common, as Steve W. wrote:

I tried your program and am very satisfied. My blood pressure was 132/103. Even after cutting out desserts and having my weight drop to 172, my blood pressure had not changed. After 45 days on the Zone Diet, my weight is in the low 160s but my blood pressure has dropped to 103/73. I guess you can say you probably saved my life. I am sorry I had to give up so many of my favorite things, such as bread, pizza, and rice. But I am developing new favorites such as cherries, peaches, blueberries, turkey breast and more. I guess it's a small price to pay to live longer.

I also received a letter from Pat G., who wrote:

I weighed 205 pounds and was a Type II diabetic. My brain was always foggy from the use of my medications. After 4 months on the Zone Diet, I have lost 41 pounds, I feel great. My body is still changing. My muscles are building and becoming more toned while I am losing fat. I take no medications. My blood sugar levels continue to remain in the normal range. I have very little, if any, pain now from my back and my leg. My doctor can't believe it.

Pat's experience in the Zone, with the resulting control of blood sugar, is no different from that of lots of other people, including Elisa L., who wrote:

During the month of September, I developed a strange taste of sawdust in my mouth and some needle pain in my liver, in addition to a small amount of foam in my urine. I decided to go to my doctor, and my blood tests of October 13 showed a fasting blood glucose level of 288, and inflammation of the liver. He prescribed a medication for diabetes, and then come back in 6 weeks for another test. I seriously pondered whether to try your Zone Diet and not the medication. I reported it to my doctor who, as expected, was not at all pleased. I bargained with him for four weeks of a trial. I confessed to him that I had abused my body for the last 40 years (I'm now 71), [and] therefore [wanted] to give my body a chance for recovery. Scared to death, I followed the Zone Diet to the letter. Four weeks later, my blood glucose test was 103, totally normal. Then, on purpose, I exited the Zone Diet a bit, and a week later my blood sugar had risen to 126. I am truly feeling that food must be perceived as a drug.

Relief from pain is crucial for quality of life. That's why I was happy to receive a letter from Belinda D. Belinda is a health care professional who was not only overweight, but also suffered from repetitive stress injuries that had required three separate surgeries. She was still taking eighteen aspirins per day to ease the pain. In her letter, Belinda wrote:

When I picked up your book in the bookstore, my first response was to put it back on the shelf and renew my promise not to try a diet program. What made me stop and buy the book was the section I read on chronic pain and arthritis. At that point, I was ready to try anything. Within a month of following the Zone Diet, my pain levels were reduced to a point where I stopped taking all medication, and I was actually returning to basically pain-free living. The weight loss I have experienced has been an added bonus to the way I feel. For the record I have lost 40 pounds in the last five months. I have a ways to go, but I feel no stress in getting to my ideal weight. My husband has been equally as successful in the Zone. He has returned to his ideal weight of 178 (from 220), and it is like having a new man around the house. The biggest improvement has come in his emotional well-being. Thank you again for your work and for publishing the information in such a clear and concise manner.

There are many more stories like these, but I feel the examples I have chosen are representative of my basic premise that food is a very powerful drug if used correctly.

But what about overweight individuals who use exercise to lose weight? Consider Steve G., who three years ago weighed 313 pounds. Determined to change his life Steve started biking and running 1.5 hours per day and sticking to a 1,000-calorie diet rich in carbohydrates and low in fat. Within a year, he had reached 250. For the next year and a half, he did the same exercise and low-calorie, high-carbohydrate diet, and nothing happened. His weight remained the same. As he wrote in a letter to me:

> I noticed your book this past summer one day in a bookstore, and could not believe what perfect sense you made. I actually cut back on some of my exercise and added more fat to my diet. I applied your technology and the weight has been dropping off. I'm down to 205 now, and headed toward my ultimate goal of 174. On top of it all, I feel energized, whereas on every other diet, I always felt very drained. The Zone simply works.

Probably the best summary letter came from Len D.:

> I don't usually write fan mail, but after reading about your research results in the *New York Times*, I was intrigued enough to buy your book. To say that it was the best health investment I have ever made would be an understatement. As I read your book, I found myself wondering if you wrote it specifically for me. Your book was an epiphany for me, and it made such incredible sense. The body fat that I could not lose began melting away after about three days on the Zone Diet. The cravings disappeared, yet I found I could eat just three ounces of ice cream and not crave the rest of the carton. I haven't had real ice cream in years. This was incredible. At the risk of sounding overly dramatic, you have

been instrumental in returning control back to me, and it is such a powerful feeling that I felt compelled to write you to thank you personally. I may sound like a TV infomercial, but my energy has tripled, my clothes had to be taken in so they would fit, I'm sleeping better than I have in years and I am experiencing a profound change in the way I view food. Food is no longer a reward for me; I still love to eat, but food has become a necessary fuel to be mixed properly for maximum energy output. Your comparison of food to medicine is brilliant, yet so simple. Why didn't I make that connection? I wish you continued success in your crusade and please add my name to the list of individuals who have seen the light.

Obviously, I am very gratified when I receive such letters, testimonials, and profound thanks from people who feel I have changed their lives. But I tell these people that I did not change their lives; they did. I only provided them with the rules and tools to make the changes. They are the ones who really deserve all the credit. After hearing their stories, something may have struck a resonant note in your life.

I hope that some of these stories illustrate the potential of the Zone Diet to influence your health and your performance. It's not that the Zone Diet is revolutionary (after all, it is similar to what your grandmother recommended), it's just that it requires you to look at food hormonally, and take responsibility when you eat.

A small price to pay for SuperHealth.

16

TALES FROM THE OLYMPIC ZONE

Although the Zone Diet was developed to treat disease, the same hormonal control technology can dramatically improve athletic performance. The crucible for testing that statement occurs every four years at the Olympic Games.

One of the most important events in the development of the Zone Diet was its introduction to the Stanford University Swim Team coaches, Skip Kenney and Richard Quick, many years ago. Their willingness to commit their highly successful programs to a radically new dietary approach was a testimony to their belief that this technology could take their athletes to a higher level. In 1992, their faith was rewarded when Stanford swimmers won eight gold medals in Barcelona.

Four years later, in 1996, Richard and Skip were the U.S. Olympic Men's and Women's head coaches for swimming. Not surprising, considering that they have won eight out of the last ten NCAA Swimming Championships since integrating the Zone Diet into the men's and women's programs in 1992.

The 1996 Olympics in Atlanta proved no different from the 1992 Olympics. Another eight gold medals in swimming, just as in 1992, and another gold medal in track and field, giving a total of nine.

In 1992 Jeff Rouse just missed Olympic gold in the 100-meter backstroke by a hundredth of a second. Vowing to return to the Olympics in 1996, for the next four years he remained the number one backstroker in the world. In Atlanta, he accomplished his goal and won the gold medal that had been just out of reach four years earlier. He also won another gold medal in the relays in Atlanta to go with a gold medal he won in relays in 1992, giving him a total of three gold medals and one silver medal for two Olympics.

Jenny Thompson completely dominated collegiate swimming during her four years at Stanford. In Atlanta, she won three gold medals to go with her two gold medals in Barcelona, making her the only U.S. woman ever to win that many Olympic gold medals in any sport. A Stanford teammate, Lisa Jacob, also won a gold medal in Atlanta.

Then there is Angel Martino, at age twenty-nine the oldest woman ever to make the U.S. Olympic Swim Team. She qualified not just in one event, but in four. Angel's husband, Dr. Mike Martino, is an exercise physiologist who contacted me several years ago after he read about the Zone Diet and the Stanford swimmers, and said it made perfect sense. Since that time, Angel has trained without the benefit of an organized program, just her own will and the Zone Diet. Her results in Atlanta: two gold medals and two bronze medals.

But winning medals is not the only goal of the Olympics; it is the opportunity for the best of the world to compete. Just the opportunity to participate in the Olympics is the dream of any athlete. And that's why some of the other stories from Stanford are illuminating.

Take the case of Kurt Grote, who came to Stanford in 1992. At that time, he wasn't good enough to get a swimming scholarship. But in 1996 he made the U.S. Olympic Team, just about the highest achievement any swimmer can reach. Or the case of Ray Carey, who so severely damaged the nerve in his arm that doctors at Stanford said he would never swim again, let alone compete in the butterfly. Ray not only won the national championship last year, but, like Kurt, was a member of the 1996 Olympic Team.

These swimmers were not the only Zoners in the 1996 Olympics. Others included Alvin Harrison in track and field, who the previous year was so disappointed in his progress that he had stopped running. Once he went on the Zone Diet, his training was elevated to a new level and he renewed his commitment to making the Olympic team. At the Olympic Trials in June, he dropped a full second off his 400-meter times to make the team. The ending to his story was a gold medal in the 4 x 400–meter relay. And there is Sinjin Smith, a legend in beach volleyball, who was competing in Atlanta at the age of thirty-nine.

Were the diets of these elite athletes radically different from the diets of the people you heard from in the previous chapter? No. In fact, as I have already shown you, the diets are remarkably similar to those recommended for the typical American, except that these athletes require more protein and much more fat than the average person. In essence, within everyone's body lies the potential to at least look like an Olympic athlete, even if you cannot perform like one.

17

WHAT THE CRITICS SAY

I have come to realize that two things are very visceral in life: religion and nutrition. Both are based on belief systems instead of hard science. Science is never going to explain religion, but it can explain nutrition if you think hormonally. Frankly, there is no good diet or bad diet, only a hormonally correct one based on the foods a person will eat. What is my definition of a hormonally correct diet? One that keeps insulin in a tight zone, not too high or too low.

Many critics have called the Zone Diet a high-protein diet, which simply isn't true. It's a protein-adequate diet. Calling the Zone Diet a low-carbohydrate diet isn't correct, either. You are actually consuming more carbohydrates than protein on the Zone Diet. It's a carbohydrate-moderate diet. Calling the Zone Diet a high-fat diet also doesn't hold water. The actual total fat consumed on the Zone Diet is similar to that consumed in a typical vegetarian diet. A protein-adequate, carbohydrate-moderate, low-fat diet rich in fruits and vegetables; that's the definition of a Zone Diet. What I tried to put forward in *The Zone* is the scientific foundation for this kind of hormonal diet.

If you try to define a hormonally correct diet, then first you have to articulate the clinical criteria required to judge its success. I outlined these criteria in Chapter 12, but let me repeat them again. A hormonally correct diet is one that results in:

1. Loss of excess body fat (not just weight).
2. Increased energy and well-being.
3. A decrease in ratio of triglycerides to HDL cholesterol.
4. A decrease in fasting insulin.
5. A decrease in glycosylated hemoglobin.

Every one of these criteria has to be met before a diet can be called hormonally correct, since they all relate to the reduction of insulin levels. This is not a multiple-choice test. You have to achieve all of these simultaneously to have a hormonally correct diet.

And when it comes to determining if these criteria have been met, the blood tells all. Your blood doesn't have a political agenda. Whatever diet you are following, your blood levels will indicate whether you're maintaining a tight control on insulin and are therefore in the Zone. If you're controlling insulin, then by definition your diet is hormonally correct.

Since the publication of *The Zone,* other important studies have been published that further reinforce my concepts about the relationship of elevated insulin to cardiovascular disease. The first, which appeared in the *New England Journal of Medicine,* in 1996, showed that very slight elevations in fasting insulin levels made a significant difference in predicting who did or did not develop heart disease. A second appeared in *Coronary Artery Disease,* and concluded that the existence and severity of existing cardiovascular disease is strongly related to very slight increases in serum insulin. These studies support the basic tenet of *The Zone:* that elevated insulin is exceptionally dangerous to your health.

The tenet is also strongly supported by recent research from Harvard Medical School, first presented at the 1995 American Heart Association meeting, where a research report demonstrated that the ratio of triglycerides to HDL cholesterol is a powerful predictor of heart disease. This conclusion should not be surprising since elevated triglycerides and decreased HDL cholesterol levels both correlated to insulin resistance and hyperinsulinemia. In fact, this study indicated that patients with the higher triglyceride-to-HDL-cholesterol ratios were seventeen times more likely to have a heart attack than those with lower triglyceride-to-HDL-cholesterol ratios. A seventeen-times greater risk seems like a very good reason to keep your triglyceride-to-HDL-cholesterol ratio under tight control.

The relationship of obesity, insulin, and heart disease is now emerging more clearly. For example, a Harvard Medical School study published in 1995 demonstrated that if a woman gains more than fifteen to twenty pounds after the age of eighteen, she greatly increases her risk of heart disease. Now since this study was based on 115,000 nurses, the large sample size should carry some validity. That paper published in the *Journal of the American Medical Association* also stated that the new "1990 weight guidelines are falsely reassuring to the large proportion of women who are within current guidelines but have potentially avoidable increased risks of cardiovascular heart disease because of their weight."

Likewise, studies done at Stanford University have investigated the relationship between carbohydrate and fat intake and their effects on insulin by comparing different diets using overweight Type II diabetic patients (defined as being hyperinsulinemic). These patients do much better on a higher-fat (if it is monounsaturated fat) and lower-carbohydrate diet in controlled clinical trials, compared to the standard high-carbohydrate diets recommended to such patients. If a higher-fat, lower-carbohydrate diet is better for overweight, hyperinsulinemic Type II diabetic patients, then isn't it also better for overweight, hyperinsulinemic (but not yet Type II diabetic) Americans? I would say so.

Many of my critics often rely on epidemiological studies to support their case for consuming high-carbohydrate diets, insisting that any study (like those at the Stanford University Medical School) of less than one year in duration isn't meaningful, since it takes a long time for heart disease to develop. However, when considering epidemiological data about heart disease, I feel the only statistic that really counts is mortality. Viewing the data from the American Heart Association shown in Figures 17–1 and 17–2, you will see that the mortality rates from cardiovascular disease of different populations give rise to interesting paradoxes.

It is clear from each of these figures that the Japanese have a low rate of cardiovascular mortality. But then so do the French. And the French diet is very dissimilar to the Japanese diet. Is one diet superior to the other? I have eaten both, and enjoy both. And what about the Chinese, who eat a lot of rice, but not nearly as much animal protein (like fish) as the Japanese? If you study the urban Chinese (the ones who are not doing heavy physical labor that will reduce insulin levels), and compare them to Americans, you see very little difference in mortality rate. Therefore, broad statements that eating copious amounts of low-fat rice will prevent heart disease may be true for urban Japanese, but not for urban Chinese.

CVD Mortality Rates
Ages 35–74

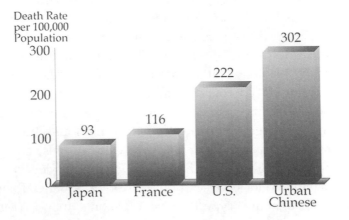

from American Heart Association *1996 Statistical Supplement*

Figure 17-1. Cardiovascular Mortality Figures (Female)

CVD Mortality Rates
Ages 35–74

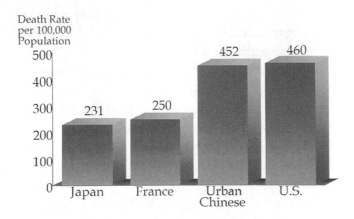

from American Heart Association *1996 Statistical Supplement*

Figure 17-2. Cardiovascular Mortality Figures (Male)

What this really demonstrates is that epidemiological studies can be misleading. As Charles Hennekens of Harvard Medical School has said, "Epidemiology is a crude and inexact science. Eighty percent of the cases are almost hypotheses." The power of epidemiology is to identify a potential hypothesis from large-scale population studies to set up controlled clinical experiments to prove or disprove the hypothesis.

Support for the claims that high-carbohydrate diets are truly superior should come from long-term clinical studies in which the diet has been tightly controlled. To my knowledge, only one such study has been published, and that was in 1995. In this particular study, cardiovascular patients were maintained on a high-carbohydrate, vegetarian diet coupled with exercise and stress reduction for a five-year period.

Although the patients had better blood flow, their triglyceride/HDL cholesterol ratio (an indicator of insulin levels), which was high to begin with, had risen another 25 percent during the five-year period that the patients were on the high-carbohydrate, low-fat diet. And if you want to believe preliminary work from Harvard Medical School, the increase in the triglyceride-to-HDL-cholesterol ratio of these patients is not a healthy long-term situation. In fact, the lead author of that study, Dr. K. Lance Gould, a highly respected cardiologist, said in a 1996 letter in the *Journal of the American Medical Association*: "Frequently, triglyceride levels increase and HDL cholesterol levels decrease for individuals on vegetarian, high-carbohydrate diets. Since low HDL cholesterol, particularly with high triglycerides, incurs substantial risk of coronary events, I do not recommend a high-carbohydrate strict vegetarian diet."

All the research cited indicates the tide is slowly shifting toward the realization that the high-carbohydrate diet may not be the panacea for our ills that we were led to believe. But none of the research directly confirms that the Zone Diet is the direction in which we should be headed. Therefore one question about *The Zone* is justified, and that is the following: Has any independent study verified the results of the Zone Diet in hyperinsulinemic patients? Science is based on the ability of any investigator to repeat a study and get basically the same results. Until that replication has been done, a study done by the single investigator remains only suggestive. In *The Zone,* I presented data on hyperinsulinemic subjects that demonstrated significant clinical improvements following the Zone Diet for eight weeks, and even further clinical improvement at sixteen weeks. But has anyone reproduced that data? Isn't that the real question?

Fortunately, in February 1996, such a study was done and the results were reported in the *American Journal of Clinical Nutrition.* This study controlled the diet of forty-three overweight, hyperinsulinemic patients by confining them to a hospital ward for six weeks. The composition of the diet used in this study was essentially equivalent to the Zone Diet. During this study, the patients lowered their blood glucose, triglycerides, and insulin.

How did the results compare to the data I presented in *The Zone* that resulted from my study conducted with overweight, hyperinsulinemic, Type II diabetic patients? For comparison purposes, I have outlined various diets used in the study published by the *American Journal of Clinical Nutrition* and the study I conducted comparing the Zone Diet and a diet recommended by the American Diabetes Association (ADA). The data is presented in terms of the various protein-to-carbohydrate ratios. This ratio of protein to carbohydrate (i.e., your hormonal carburetor), which the Zone Diet is based upon, ideally should be 0.75. The results are shown in Table 16–1.

Table 16-1
Comparison of Protein-to-Carbohydrate (P/C) Ratios
on Clinical Outcomes in Hyperinsulinemic Patients

P/C RATIO	GLUCOSE	INSULIN	TRIGLYCERIDES	TG/HDL
0.33 (ADA–8 weeks)*	–12%	+12%	+20%	+46%
0.64 (6 weeks)**	–7%	–8%	–18%	–12%
0.75 (Zone–8 weeks)*	–12%	–20%	–27%	–24%
0.75 (Zone–16 weeks)*	–15%	–30%	–35%	–30%

*From *The Zone* (1995), using Type II diabetic outpatients.
**From *American Journal of Clinical Nutrition* (1996), using metabolic ward patients.

As you can see from this table, changing the protein-to-carbo-hydrate ratio of a particular diet will alter insulin levels, and in turn lead to significant clinical improvement of blood glucose, triglyc-erides, and triglyceride-to-HDL-cholesterol ratio for the patients. And if you look at the clinical parameters, in particular the triglyc-eride-to-HDL-cholesterol ratio, the Zone Diet meets all the clinical criteria of a hormonally correct diet. And the longer the patients stayed on the Zone Diet, the better the clinical results.

If a growing body of research indicates something is wrong with our carbohydrate mania in treating overweight patients, why is it that the general population and vast majority of physicians still embrace the high-carbohydrate diet as the cure-all for our epidemic rise in obesity? One factor may be that the high-carbohydrate diet gives comfort if you're thinking calorically. After all, it's low in fat, and doesn't fat make you fat? And if fat is the enemy, then your bat-tle plan is to reduce all fat in the diet regardless of the type of fat.

On the other hand, if you are thinking hormonally, the high-car-bohydrate diet makes no sense whatsoever because it raises insulin levels in those who are genetically predisposed toward developing hyperinsulinemia or those who are already hyperinsulinemic. And it's increased insulin that not only makes you fat, but accelerates your progress toward heart disease. If insulin is the enemy, then your focus should be controlling the protein-to-carbohydrate ratio at every meal. There are two different potential enemies (fat versus insulin) and two different battle plans (a high-carbohydrate diet ver-sus a hormonally balanced diet). We have simply chosen the wrong enemy and the wrong battle plan for the past fifteen years.

The other factor that fuels this country's carbohydrate mania to keep Americans eating more and more carbohydrates is economics. One has to be realistic. There is a lot of money involved in pro-moting the high-carbohydrate diet. First, if you are a country pro-ducing millions of tons of wheat each year, what are you going to do with it? Animals won't eat it. The only thing wheat is good for is making bread, pasta, and bagels. And if you have a strong political lobby, you are going to do everything in your power to make sure the government encourages its citizens to buy as many wheat prod-ucts as possible. Maybe it's not so surprising that the base of the new U.S. food pyramid is composed primarily of wheat-based products. Also not surprisingly, consumption of pasta has increased by 115 percent in the past decade.

Second, if you're in the food manufacturing business, selling prepackaged carbohydrates makes excellent business sense. Protein is expensive, and fats go rancid. Given the opportunity to remove as much protein and fat as possible from packaged foods will improve shelf life and reduce costs. It makes good economic sense to do so. Furthermore, carbohydrates are dirt cheap, they last forever (remember pasta), they are politically correct, and they have the U.S. government seal of approval, plus billions of free advertising dollars to promote their consumption. It only makes sense to cater to this carbohydrate mania. And the sophistication of our food technology allows for virtually any product manufactured to consist primarily of carbohydrates.

Finally, the U.S. government, in an attempt to improve the health of the country, embraced a dietary concept (i.e., that eating more grain would decrease obesity) that was not well thought out in advance in terms of its hormonal consequences. It was a case of "shoot, ready, aim."

While there's no conspiracy to fatten Americans and make them less healthy, I do feel the convergence of these three trends (strong wheat lobby, profits in the food manufacturing sector, and government-driven "consensus") has been leading our country down a pathway toward a growing medical crisis.

And there is definite trouble lying ahead for the U.S. health care system. In early 1996, the American Heart Association announced that for the first time since 1980, deaths from cardiovascular disease are increasing. I'm afraid the hormonal chickens released during the last fifteen years of carbohydrate mania are coming home to roost.

Therefore, what is the best diet? It's one that you can stay on for the rest of your life and one that meets the clinical criteria I have outlined above. I believe that many of my critics will agree they are reasonable standards. Once we begin to treat nutrition as a science that can be judged by scientific standards, as opposed to some political or philosophical agenda, we as a country can get back to nutritional common sense.

What is desperately needed is a continuing dialog in this area as opposed to monolithic "consensus" based on belief systems.

Obviously, the belief system preached to Americans that carbohy-drates (and especially pasta and bagels) are the essence of good nutrition simply isn't working well. Rather than preaching more of the same, doesn't it make sense to try other directions, like the one your grandmother used? I hope my critics agree.

One last thing about your grandmother. A recent study in the *New England Journal of Medicine* revealed which nationalities had the greatest longevity once they had reached the age of eighty, start-ing in 1960 and beyond. By 1995 they had obtained enough data to come to their conclusions. This data would likely have included your grandmother. And who had the greatest longevity? Was it the Japanese? No. Was it the French? No. Was it the Swedes? No. The answer was the Americans.

18

WHERE YOU GO FROM HERE

Every American should wake up to the new realities about access to unlimited, low-cost medical care in the twenty-first century. It's not going to exist, especially with the growing crisis in entitlement programs like Medicare. So you had better start planning now. In other words, your best health insurance policy is to achieve SuperHealth as quickly as possible.

As I stated in the beginning, SuperHealth is a state beyond health (if health is defined as the absence of disease). SuperHealth is about doing everything in your power to control hormonal levels and reduce the likelihood of developing chronic disease. That is what this book is all about, giving you the strategies to master the Zone.

You have to eat, so you might as well eat smart. Americans have the greatest potential to do this because we have the cheapest food in the world. Nonetheless, virtually no one in this country eats adequate levels of fruits and vegetables. Instead, we can't get enough fat-free, prepackaged goods. And in the process we are moving rapidly toward a medical abyss.

And if you don't care about yourself, think about your kids. Childhood obesity has increased by 50 percent over the last decade. At least give them a chance to get the most out of their lives. You control their food choices, because you buy and prepare their food. If you don't like what has happened to your own body composition and energy levels in the last fifteen years of carbohydrate gluttony, you at least experienced what it was like to have less body fat and greater energy in your youth. Give your kids the same chance.

In this book I have tried to give you as many helpful hints as possible to allow you to reorganize your dietary life. In reality, the adjustments are very easy: Just begin thinking hormonally. This is the big leap—moving away from caloric thinking to embrace hormonal thinking.

And once you understand hormonal thinking, it becomes clear that in the last fifteen years, we have lost all common sense as to what constitutes a good diet. Your grandmother knew it intuitively, but we have forgotten how to listen to her common sense.

What I'm hoping is that after reading this book, you will end up like one of the characters from the film *Network*, yelling at the top of your lungs, "I'm mad as hell, and I'm not going to take it anymore." Why should you be mad? Because many of you could have had a far better quality of life in the past fifteen years if only you had been given the correct information. And this information has been in the scientific peer-reviewed literature for decades. It was conveniently ignored because it didn't fit into a preconceived notion of a "correct diet." *You* have the ultimate control of your diet. Just use the commonsense rules given to you by your grandmother, and retake the driver's seat of your destiny.

Although *The Zone* was written to show a better way to treat chronic disease, I'm the first to realize that disease prevention is a pretty low priority for people in today's world. People often think only of "What's in it for me today?" Well, the Zone has that element, too. If you want to think better, perform better, and look better, then use the tools found in this book, and the concepts found in *The Zone*. All I ask is that you follow the program for two weeks. At the end of two weeks, if you're thinking better, performing better, and looking better, then stick with the program for another two weeks. At the end of four weeks, if you're still feeling good, try another two weeks. That's not much of a sacrifice.

What I hope to accomplish is to show you how nutrition can dramatically alter your life, if nutrition is based on the combination of science and common sense.

The twenty-first century will be the century in which people will finally learn to harness the most powerful drugs known: hormones. And in the era of hormonal control, the most powerful drug of all will be called food.

Your grandmother knew this. I hope that, after reading this book, you do too.

APPENDIX A

FURTHER RESOURCES

CONTINUING TECHNICAL SUPPORT

Free technical support is available from our Web site at http://www.drsears.com. Consider this Web site your Zone Community Center containing our on-line magazine with constantly updated medical research news, new Zone recipes, new Zone Diet tips, and answers to selected questions received by e-mail. Our Web site will also contain my recommendations about products and services that will help you get to and maintain yourself in the Zone. If you don't have access to a computer, then call our toll-free number at 800-404-8171 to obtain further technical information.

FOOD PRODUCTS

Wild Game

Wild game or range-fed beef and chicken are excellent sources of low-fat protein. Range-fed protein sources can be found in most high-quality supermarkets. Wild game can be obtained from specialty suppliers listed here:

Denver Buffalo Company
1120 Lincoln Street
Denver, CO 80203-970
Telephone: 800-289-2833

Game Exchange/Polarica
105 Quint Street
San Francisco, CA 94124
Telephone: 800-426-3872
or

73 Hudson Street
New York, NY 10013
Telephone: 800-426-3487

Soybean Products
Soybean products are excellent sources of plant-based protein. Imitation soybean meat products provide an excellent source of high-density vegetable protein. Information about more specialized sources of soybean products can be obtained from the following:

Soya Bluebook
P.O. Box 84
Bar Harbor, ME 04609

RECOMMENDED READING

The Zone
Barry Sears
ReganBooks, 1995
The basic reference text on which this book is based. *The Zone* goes into far greater detail about the biochemistry of hormonal control mechanisms of food and their effects on disease conditions.

Protein Power
Michael and Mary Dan Eades
Bantam, 1996
An excellent book on hyperinsulinemia written by close personal friends and longtime colleagues of mine. Since the underlying science in their book is the same as that found in *The Zone*, I strongly recommend it as a companion book to the Zone series. Although their initial dietary approach to reduce insulin starts with a higher protein-to-carbohydrate ratio than I recommend in *The Zone*, they gradually reintroduce carbohydrates to their patients so that their maintenance plan is the same as found in *The Zone*. We both agree that an individual has to adjust the protein-to-carbohydrate ratio to control insulin on a permanent basis.

Beyond Prozac
Michael Norden
ReganBooks, 1995

Written by an early pioneer in Prozac research, this book shows how simple interventions, including the Zone Diet, can increase serotonin levels (the pharmacological action of Prozac). An excellent resource for anyone interested in the effects and implications of serotonin-modulating drugs.

The Complete Book of Food Counts
Corinne T. Netzer
Dell, 1991

This book provides a listing of virtually every food product in terms of macronutrient composition. Convert each item into appropriate blocks, multiply the protein content of vegetable sources by 75 percent to get the amount of absorbable protein, and subtract the fiber content from the total carbohydrates to get the amount of insulin-promoting carbohydrate.

COMPUTER PROGRAMS

A number of inexpensive, good nutritional computer programs are on the market. While many more will be appearing, I recommend the following:

General Programs

Personal Chef 2.0 for Windows
Parsons Technology
One Parsons Drive
Hiawatha, IA 52233-0100
319-395-9626

Key Home Gourmet
SoftKey International Corporation
One Athenaeon Street
Cambridge, MA 02142

Specific Zone Programs

These are specialty programs, especially designed for use with the Zone Diet.

The Zone Made Easy

Developed by Ted Wendler, this a useful program for determining body fat and block requirements, specifically based on *The Zone*. The program is available by calling 800-764-1019. Technical support for this program is available at 888-777-8839.

Zone Manager

A program developed by MetaMedix for automatically calculating Zone meals based on your protein requirements, using your favorite foods. The program contains over 5,000 foods to plan your meals, and you can add your own foods or recipes. This program is available by calling 800-455-4105. Technical support for this program is available at 800-684-3015.

FOOD BLOCKS

The concept of macronutrient food blocks gives a straightforward method to construct Zone meals. Listed below are the portion sizes of blocks of proteins, carbohydrates, and fats equal to one block. Note that the protein volumes are for uncooked portions. Each carbohydrate block represents the amount of insulin-promoting carbohydrate in that portion size. Although favorable carbohydrates are usually low-glycemic carbohydrates, there are exceptions (like ice cream and potato chips) that are also high in fat (see Glycemic Index in Appendix E).

I have rounded off the blocks to convenient sizes for easy memory. This list is by no means meant to be exhaustive. If you have a favorite food that is not listed, simply refer to Corinne Netzer's *Complete Book of Food Counts* (Dell, 1991) to expand the list. This list has been updated since the publication of *The Zone,* and as a result some block sizes have been altered from my original version.

When constructing a Zone meal, always remember the primary rule: Keep the protein and carbohydrate blocks in a 1:1 ratio.

PROTEIN BLOCKS (APPROXIMATELY 7 GRAMS PROTEIN PER BLOCK)

Meat and Poultry

Best Choices (low in saturated fat)

Beef (range-fed or game)	1 ounce
Chicken breast, skinless	1 ounce
Chicken breast, deli-style	1½ ounces
Turkey breast, skinless	1 ounce
Turkey breast, deli-style	1 ounce

Fair Choices (moderate in saturated fat)

Beef, lean cuts	1 ounce
Canadian bacon, lean	1 ounce
Chicken, dark meat, skinless	1 ounce
Corned beef, lean	1 ounce
Duck	1½ ounces
Ham, lean	1 ounce
Ham, deli-style	1½ ounces
Hamburger (less than 10 percent fat)	1½ ounces
Lamb, lean	1 ounce
Pork, lean	1 ounce
Pork chop	1 ounce
Turkey bacon	3 strips
Turkey, dark meat, skinless	1 ounce
Veal	1 ounce

Poor Choices (high in either saturated fat or arachidonic acid or both)

Bacon, pork	3 strips
Beef, fatty cuts*	1 ounce
Beef, ground (10 to 15 percent fat)	1½ ounces
Beef, ground (more than 15 percent fat)*	1½ ounces
Hot dog (pork or beef)	1 link
Hot dog (turkey or chicken)	1 link
Kielbasa	2 ounces
Liver, beef*	1 ounce
Liver, chicken*	1 ounce
Pepperoni	1 ounce
Salami	1 ounce

*Contains arachidonic acid.

Fish and Seafood

Bass	1 ounce
Bluefish	1 ounce
Calamari	2½ ounces

Catfish	1½ ounces
Clams	1½ ounces
Cod	1½ ounces
Crabmeat	1½ ounces
Haddock	1½ ounces
Halibut	1½ ounces
Lobster	1 ounce
Mackerel**	1½ ounces
Salmon**	1½ ounces
Sardines**	1 ounce
Scallops	1½ ounces
Shrimp	1½ ounces
Snapper	1½ ounces
Swordfish	1½ ounces
Trout	1 ounce
Tuna (steak)	1 ounce
Tuna, canned in water	1 ounce

**Rich in EPA.

Eggs

Best Choices

Egg whites	2
Egg substitute	¼ cup

Fair Choices

Cheese, non-fat	1 ounce
Whole egg*	1

*Contains arachidonic acid.

Protein-Rich Dairy

Best Choices

Cottage cheese, low-fat	¼ cup

Fair Choices

Cheese, reduced-fat	1 ounce
Mozzarella cheese, skim	1 ounce
Ricotta cheese, skim	2½ ounces

Poor Choice

Hard cheeses	1 ounce

Protein-Rich Vegetarian

Tofu, firm and extra-firm	3 ounces
Protein powder	⅓ ounce
Soy burgers	½ patty
Soy hot dog	1 link
Soy sausages	2 links
Soy sausage	1 patty

Mixed Protein/Carbohydrate (contains one block of protein and one block of carbohydrate)

Milk, low-fat (1 percent)	1 cup
Soy flour	⅓ cup
Tempeh	1½ ounces
Tofu, soft and regular	3 ounces
Yogurt, plain	½ cup

CARBOHYDRATE BLOCKS (APPROXIMATELY 9 GRAMS OF INSULIN-PROMOTING CARBOHYDRATE PER BLOCK)

Favorable Carbohydrates

Cooked Vegetables

Artichoke	1 medium
Asparagus	1 cup (12 spears)
Beans, green or wax	1 cup
Beans, black	¼ cup
Bok choy	3 cups

Broccoli	1¼ cups
Brussels sprouts	1½ cups
Cabbage, shredded	1⅓ cups
Cauliflower	2 cups
Chickpeas	¼ cup
Collard greens, chopped	2 cups
Eggplant	1½ cups
Kale	1¼ cups
Kidney beans	¼ cup
Leeks	1 cup
Lentils	¼ cup
Mushrooms (boiled)	1 cup
Okra, sliced	1 cup
Onions, chopped (boiled)	¾ cup
Sauerkraut	1 cup
Spinach, chopped	1¼ cups
Swiss chard, chopped	1½ cups
Turnip, mashed	1 cup
Turnip greens, chopped	1¾ cups
Yellow squash (summer), sliced	1¼ cups
Zucchini, sliced	1½ cups

Raw Vegetables

Alfalfa sprouts	11 cups
Bamboo shoots, cuts	1¼ cups
Broccoli	1½ cups
Cabbage, shredded	3 cups
Cauliflower, pieces	2 cups
Celery, sliced	2½ cups
Cucumber	1
Cucumber, sliced	4 cups
Endive, chopped	7½ cups
Escarole, chopped	7½ cups
Green or red peppers	3
Green pepper, chopped	2¼ cups
Hummus	¼ cup
Lettuce, iceberg (six-inch diameter)	1 head

Lettuce, romaine, chopped	4 cups
Mushrooms, chopped	3 cups
Onion, chopped	1 cup
Radishes, sliced	2½ cups
Salsa	½ cup
Snow peas	1 cup
Spinach, chopped	6 cups
Spinach salad (3 cups raw spinach, ¼ raw onion, ¼ cup raw mushrooms, and ¼ raw tomato)	1
Tomato	2
Tomato, chopped	1¼ cups
Tossed salad (2 cups shredded lettuce, ¼ raw green bell pepper, ¼ raw cucumber, and ¼ raw tomato)	1
Water chestnuts	⅓ cup

Fruits (fresh, frozen, or canned light)

Apple	½
Applesauce	⅓ cup
Apricots	3
Blackberries	¾ cup
Blueberries	½ cup
Boysenberries	¾ cup
Cantaloupe	¼ melon
Cantaloupe, cubed	¾ cup
Cherries	¾ cup
Fruit cocktail	½ cup
Grapefruit	½
Grapes	½ cup
Honeydew melon, cubed	½ cup
Kiwi fruit	1
Lemon	1
Lime	1
Nectarine, medium	½

Orange	½
Orange, mandarin, canned	⅓ cup
Peach	1
Peaches, canned	½ cup
Pear	½
Pineapple, cubed	½ cup
Plum	1
Raspberries	1 cup
Strawberries	1 cup
Tangerine	1
Watermelon, cubed	¾ cup

Grains

Barley (dry)	½ tablespoon
Oatmeal (slow-cooking)***	⅓ cup (cooked)
Oatmeal (slow-cooking)***	½ ounce dry

***Contains GLA.

Unfavorable Carbohydrates (use in moderation)

Cooked Vegetables

Acorn squash	½ cup
Baked beans	⅛ cup
Beets, sliced	½ cup
Butternut squash	½ cup
Carrot	1
Carrot, shredded	1 cup
Carrot, sliced	½ cup
Corn	¼ cup
French fries	5
Lima beans	¼ cup
Parsnip	⅓ cup
Peas	⅓ cup
Pinto beans	¼ cup
Potato, baked	⅓
Potato, boiled	⅓ cup
Potato, mashed	⅕ cup

Refried beans	¼ cup
Sweet potato, baked	⅓
Sweet potato, mashed	⅕ cup

Fruits

Banana	⅓
Cranberries, chopped	¾ cup
Cranberry sauce	3 teaspoons
Dates	2 pieces
Fig	1 piece
Guava	½ cup
Kumquat	3
Mango, sliced	⅓ cup
Papaya, cubed	¾ cup
Prunes (dried)	2
Raisins	1 tablespoon

Fruit Juices

Apple	⅓ cup
Apple cider	⅓ cup
Cranberry	¼ cup
Fruit punch	¼ cup
Grape	¼ cup
Grapefruit	⅓ cup
Lemon	⅓ cup
Lemonade	⅓ cup
Orange	⅓ cup
Pineapple	¼ cup
Tomato	1 cup
V–8	¾ cup

Grains, Cereals, and Breads

Bagel (small)	¼
Biscuit	½
Bread crumbs	½ ounce

Bread, whole grain	½ slice
Bread, white	½ slice
Breadstick, soft	½
Breadstick, hard	1
Buckwheat, dry	½ ounce
Bulgur wheat, dry	½ ounce
Cereal, dry	½ ounce
Cornbread	one-inch square
Cornstarch	1 teaspoon
Couscous, dry	1 ounce
Cracker, saltine	4
Cracker, Triscuit	3
Croissant, plain	½
Crouton	½ ounce
Doughnut, plain	¾
English muffin	¼
Granola	½ ounce
Grits, cooked	⅓ cup
Melba toast	½ ounce
Millet	½ ounce
Muffin, blueberry	½
Noodles, egg (cooked)	¼ cup
Pancake (four-inch)	½
Pasta, cooked	¼ cup
Pita bread	¼ pocket
Pita bread, mini	½ pocket
Popcorn, popped	2 cups
Rice, brown (cooked)	⅕ cup
Rice, white (cooked)	⅕ cup
Rice cake	1
Roll, bulkie	¼
Roll, dinner	½ small
Roll, hamburger	½
Taco shell	1 small
Tortilla, corn (six-inch)	1
Tortilla, flour (eight-inch)	½
Waffle	½

Alcohol

Beer	6 ounces
Distilled spirits	1 ounce
Wine	4 ounces

Others

Barbecue sauce	2 tablespoons
Candy bar	¼
Cake	⅓ slice
Cocktail sauce	2 tablespoons
Cookie (small)	1
Crackers (saltine)	4
Crackers (graham)	1½ pieces
Honey	½ tablespoon
Ice cream, regular	¼ cup
Ice cream, premium	⅙ cup
Jam or jelly	2 tablespoons
Ketchup	2 tablespoons
Molasses, light	1½ teaspoons
Plum sauce	1½ tablespoons
Potato chips	½ ounce
Pretzels	½ ounce
Relish, pickle	4 teaspoons
Sugar, brown	2 teaspoons
Sugar, granulated	2 teaspoons
Sugar, confectionery	1 tablespoon
Syrup, maple	2 teaspoons
Syrup, pancake	2 teaspoons
Teriyaki sauce	1 tablespoon
Tortilla chips	½ ounce

FAT BLOCKS (APPROXIMATELY 1.5 GRAMS OF FAT PER BLOCK)

Best Choices (rich in monounsaturated fat)

Almond butter	⅓ teaspoon
Almonds (slivered)	1½ teaspoons

Almonds (whole)	3
Avocado	1 tablespoon
Canola oil	⅓ teaspoon
Guacamole	1 tablespoon
Macadamia Nut	1
Olive oil	⅓ teaspoon
Olive oil and vinegar dressing (⅓ teaspoon olive oil and ⅔ teaspoons vinegar)	1 teaspoon
Olives	3
Peanut butter, natural	½ teaspoon
Peanut oil	⅓ teaspoon
Peanuts	6
Tahini	½ teaspoon

Fair Choices (low in saturated fat)

Mayonnaise, regular	⅓ teaspoon
Mayonnaise, light	1 teaspoon
Sesame oil	½ teaspoon
Soybean oil	⅓ teaspoon
Walnuts, shelled and chopped	1 teaspoon

Poor Choices (rich in saturated fat)

Bacon bits (imitation)	1½ teaspoons
Butter	⅓ teaspoon
Cream (half-and-half)	1 tablespoon
Cream cheese	1 teaspoon
Cream cheese, light	2 teaspoons
Lard	⅓ teaspoon
Sour cream	½ tablespoon
Sour cream, light	1 tablespoon
Vegetable shortening	⅓ teaspoon

APPENDIX C

CALCULATION OF LEAN BODY MASS

A rapid way to determine your lean body mass is simply to use a tape measure and scale. You should make all measurements on bare skin (not through clothing), and make sure that the tape fits snugly but does not compress the skin and underlying tissue. Take all measurements three times and calculate the average. All measurements should be in inches. The tables used to calculate the percentage of body fat were used with the permission of Dr. Michael Eades from his book *Thin So Fast.*

Calculating Body-Fat Percentages for Females

There are five steps you must take to calculate your percentage of body fat:

1. While keeping the tape level, measure your hips at their widest point, and your waist at the umbilicus (i.e., belly button). It is critical that you measure at the belly button and not at the narrowest point of your waist. Take each of these measurements three times and compute the average.
2. Measure your height in inches without shoes.
3. Record your height, waist, and hip measurements on the accompanying worksheet.
4. Find each of these measurements in the appropriate column in the accompanying tables and record the constants on the worksheet.
5. Add Constants A and B, then subtract Constant C for this sum and round to the nearest whole number. That figure is your percentage of body fat.

Worksheet for Women to Calculate Their Percentage of Body Fat

Average hip measurement _____ (used for Constant A)

Average abdomen measurement _____ (used for Constant B)

Height _____ (used for Constant C)

Using Table 1, look up each of the average measurements and your height in the appropriate column.

Constant A = _____

Constant B = _____

Constant C = _____

To determine your approximate percentage of body fat, then add Constant A and B. From that total, subtract Constant C. The result is your percentage of body fat.

Calculating Body-Fat Percentages for Men

There are four steps you must take to determine your body-fat percentage:

1. While keeping the tape level, measure the circumference of your waist at the umbilicus (i.e., belly button). Measure three times and compute the average.
2. Measure your wrist at the space between your dominant hand and your wrist bone, at the location where your wrist bends.
3. Record these measurements on the worksheet for males.
4. Subtract your wrist measurement from your waist measurement and find the resulting value listed in the table. On the left-hand side of this table, find your weight. Proceed to right from your weight and down from your waist-minus-wrist measurement. Where these two points intersect, read your body fat percentage.

Worksheet for Men to Calculate Their Percentage of Body Fat

Average waist measurement _____ (inches)

Average wrist measurement _____ (inches)

Subtract the wrist measurement from the waist measurement. Use Table 2 to find your weight. Then find your "waist minus wrist" number. Where the two columns intersect is your approximate percentage of body fat.

Calculating Lean Body Mass for Both Females and Males

Now that you know your body-fat percentage, the next step is to use this figure to calculate the weight in pounds of the fat portion of your total body weight. This is done by multiplying your weight by your percentage of body fat. (Remember to use a decimal point—15 percent is 0.15 for example.)

(Weight) × (% of body fat) = total body-fat weight

Once you know the weight of your total body fat, you subtract that total fat weight from your total weight, which results in your lean body mass. Lean body mass is the total weight of all nonfat body tissue.

        _____ Your total weight

− _____ Your total of body fat

= _____ Your lean body mass

Lean body mass = total weight − total body-fat weight

TABLE 1

CONVERSION CONSTANTS FOR PREDICTION OF PERCENTAGE OF BODY FAT IN FEMALES

Hips		Abdomen		Height	
Inches	Constant A	Inches	Constant B	Inches	Constant C
30	33.48	20	14.22	55	33.52
30.5	33.83	20.5	14.40	55.5	33.67
31	34.87	21.0	14.93	56	34.13
31.5	35.22	21.5	15.11	56.5	34.28
32	36.27	22	15.64	57	34.74
32.5	36.62	22.5	15.82	57.5	34.89
33	37.67	23	16.35	58	35.35
33.5	38.02	23.5	16.53	58.5	35.50
34	39.06	24	17.06	59	35.96
34.5	39.41	24.5	17.24	59.5	36.11
35	40.46	25	17.78	60	36.57
35.5	40.81	25.5	17.96	60.5	36.72
36	41.86	26	18.49	61	37.18
36.5	42.21	26.5	18.67	61.5	37.33
37	43.25	27	19.20	62	37.79
37.5	43.60	27.5	19.38	62.5	37.94
38	44.65	28	19.91	63	38.40
38.5	45.32	28.5	20.27	63.5	38.70
39	46.05	29	20.62	64	39.01
39.5	46.40	29.5	20.80	64.5	39.16
40	47.44	30	21.33	65	39.62
40.5	47.79	30.5	21.51	65.5	39.77
41	48.84	31	22.04	66	40.23
41.5	49.19	31.5	22.22	66.5	40.38
42	50.24	32	22.75	67	40.84
42.5	50.59	32.5	22.93	67.5	40.99
43	51.64	33	23.46	68	41.45
43.5	51.99	33.5	23.64	68.5	41.60
44	53.03	34	24.18	69	42.06
44.5	53.41	34.5	24.36	69.5	42.21
45	54.53	35	24.89	70	42.67

| Hips | | Abdomen | | Height | |
Inches	Constant A	Inches	Constant B	Inches	Constant C
45.5	54.86	35.5	25.07	70.5	42.82
46	55.83	36	25.60	71	43.28
46.5	56.18	36.5	25.78	71.5	43.43
47	57.22	37	26.31	72	43.89
47.5	57.57	37.5	26.49	72.5	44.04
48	58.62	38	27.02	73	44.50
48.5	58.97	38.5	27.20	73.5	44.65
49	60.02	39	27.73	74	45.11
49.5	60.37	39.5	27.91	74.5	45.26
50	61.42	40	28.44	75	45.72
50.5	61.77	40.5	28.62	75.5	45.87
51	62.81	41	29.15	76	46.32
51.5	63.16	41.5	29.33		
52	64.21	42	29.87		
52.5	64.56	42.5	30.05		
53	65.61	43	30.58		
53.5	65.96	43.5	30.76		
54	67.00	44	31.29		
54.5	67.35	44.5	31.47		
55	68.40	45	32.00		
55.5	68.75	45.5	32.18		
56	69.80	46	32.71		
56.5	70.15	46.5	32.89		
57	71.19	47	33.42		
57.5	71.54	47.5	33.60		
58	72.59	48	34.13		
58.5	72.94	48.5	34.31		
59	73.99	49	34.84		
59.5	74.34	49.5	35.02		
60	75.39	50	35.56		

TABLE 2
MALE PERCENTAGE BODY FAT CALCULATIONS

Waist-Wrist (in inches)	22	22.5	23	23.5	24
Weight (in lbs.)					
120	4	6	8	10	12
125	4	6	7	9	11
130	3	5	7	9	11
135	3	5	7	8	10
140	3	5	6	8	10
145		4	6	7	9
150		4	6	7	9
155		4	5	6	8
160		4	5	6	8
165		3	5	6	8
170		3	4	6	7
175			4	6	7
180			4	5	7
185			4	5	6
190			4	5	6
195			3	5	6
200			3	4	6
205				4	5
210				4	5
215				4	5
220				4	5
225				3	4
230				3	4
235				3	4
240					4
245					4
250					4
255					3
260					3
265					
270					
275					
280					
285					
290					
295					
300					

24.5	25	25.5	26	26.5	27	27.5
14	16	18	20	21	23	25
13	15	17	19	20	22	24
12	14	16	18	20	21	23
12	13	15	17	19	20	22
11	13	15	16	18	19	21
11	12	14	15	17	19	20
10	12	13	15	16	18	19
10	11	13	14	16	17	19
9	11	12	14	15	17	18
9	10	12	13	15	16	17
9	10	11	13	14	15	17
8	10	11	12	13	15	16
8	9	10	12	13	14	16
8	9	10	11	13	14	15
7	8	10	11	12	13	15
7	8	9	11	12	13	14
7	8	9	10	11	12	14
6	8	9	10	11	12	13
6	7	8	9	11	12	13
6	7	8	9	10	11	12
6	7	8	9	10	11	12
6	7	8	9	10	11	12
5	6	7	8	9	10	11
5	6	7	8	9	10	11
5	6	7	8	9	10	11
5	6	7	8	9	9	10
5	6	6	7	8	9	10
4	5	6	7	8	9	10
4	5	6	7	8	9	10
4	5	6	7	8	8	9
4	5	6	7	7	8	9
4	5	5	6	7	8	9
4	4	5	6	7	8	9
4	4	5	6	7	8	8
3	4	5	6	7	7	8
3	4	5	6	6	7	8
3	4	5	5	6	7	8

Waist-Wrist (in inches)	28	28.5	29	29.5	30	30.5	31
Weight (in lbs.)							
120	27	29	31	33	35	37	39
125	26	28	30	32	33	35	37
130	25	27	28	30	32	34	36
135	24	26	27	29	31	32	34
140	23	24	26	28	29	31	33
145	22	23	25	27	28	30	31
150	21	23	24	26	27	29	30
155	20	22	23	25	26	28	29
160	19	21	22	24	25	27	28
165	19	20	22	23	24	26	27
170	18	19	21	22	24	25	26
175	17	19	20	21	23	24	25
180	17	18	19	21	22	23	25
185	16	18	19	20	21	23	24
190	16	17	18	19	21	22	23
195	15	16	18	19	20	21	22
200	15	16	17	18	19	21	22
205	14	15	17	18	19	20	21
210	14	15	16	17	18	19	21
215	13	15	16	17	18	19	20
220	13	14	15	16	17	18	19
225	13	14	15	16	17	18	19
230	12	13	14	15	16	17	18
235	12	13	14	15	16	17	18
240	12	13	14	15	16	17	17
245	11	12	13	14	15	16	17
250	11	12	13	14	15	16	17
255	11	12	13	14	14	15	16
260	10	11	12	13	14	15	16
265	10	11	12	13	14	15	15
270	10	11	12	13	13	14	15
275	10	11	11	12	13	14	15
280	9	10	11	12	13	14	14
285	9	10	11	12	12	13	14
290	9	10	11	11	12	13	14
295	9	10	10	11	12	13	14
300	9	9	10	11	12	12	13

31.5	32	32.5	33	33.5	34	34.5
41	43	45	47	49	50	52
39	41	43	45	46	48	50
37	39	41	43	44	46	48
36	38	39	41	43	44	46
34	36	38	39	41	43	44
33	35	36	38	39	41	43
32	33	35	36	38	40	41
31	32	34	35	37	38	40
30	31	33	34	35	37	38
29	30	31	33	34	36	37
28	29	30	32	33	34	36
27	28	29	31	32	33	35
26	27	28	30	31	32	34
25	26	28	29	30	31	33
24	26	27	28	29	30	32
24	25	26	27	28	30	31
23	24	25	26	28	29	30
22	23	25	26	27	28	29
22	23	24	25	26	27	28
21	22	23	24	25	26	28
20	22	23	24	25	26	27
20	21	22	23	24	25	26
19	20	21	22	23	24	25
19	20	21	22	23	24	25
18	19	20	21	22	23	24
18	19	20	21	22	23	24
18	18	19	20	21	22	23
17	18	19	20	21	22	23
17	18	19	19	20	21	22
16	17	18	19	20	21	22
16	17	18	19	19	20	21
16	16	17	18	19	20	21
15	16	17	18	19	19	20
15	16	17	17	18	19	20
15	15	16	17	18	19	19
14	15	16	17	17	18	19
14	15	16	16	17	18	19

Waist-Wrist (in inches)	35	35.5	36	36.5	37
Weight (in lbs.)					
120	54				
125	52	54			
130	50	52	53	55	
135	48	50	51	53	55
140	46	48	49	51	53
145	44	46	47	49	51
150	43	44	46	47	49
155	41	43	44	46	47
160	40	41	43	44	46
165	38	40	41	43	44
170	37	39	40	41	43
175	36	37	39	40	41
180	35	36	37	39	40
185	34	35	36	38	39
190	33	34	35	37	38
195	32	33	34	35	37
200	31	32	33	35	36
205	30	31	32	34	35
210	29	30	32	33	34
215	29	30	31	32	33
220	28	29	30	31	32
225	27	28	29	30	31
230	26	27	28	30	31
235	26	27	28	29	30
240	25	26	27	28	29
245	25	26	27	27	28
250	24	25	26	27	28
255	24	24	25	26	27
260	23	24	25	26	27
265	22	23	24	25	26
270	22	23	24	25	25
275	22	22	23	24	25
280	21	22	23	24	24
285	21	21	22	23	24
290	20	21	22	23	23
295	20	21	21	22	23
300	19	20	21	22	22

37.5	38	38.5	39	39.5	40	40.5
54						
52	54	55				
50	52	53	55			
49	50	52	53	55		
47	48	50	51	53	54	
45	47	48	50	51	52	54
44	45	47	48	49	51	52
43	44	45	47	48	49	51
41	43	44	45	47	48	49
40	41	43	44	45	46	48
39	40	41	43	44	45	46
38	39	40	41	43	44	45
37	38	39	40	41	43	44
36	37	38	39	40	41	43
35	36	37	38	39	40	42
34	35	36	37	38	39	40
33	34	35	36	37	38	39
32	33	34	35	36	37	38
32	33	34	35	36	37	38
31	32	33	34	35	36	37
30	31	32	33	34	35	36
29	30	31	32	33	34	35
29	30	31	31	32	33	34
28	29	30	31	32	33	34
27	28	29	30	31	32	33
27	28	29	29	30	31	32
26	27	28	29	30	31	31
26	27	27	28	29	30	31
25	26	27	28	29	29	30
25	26	26	27	28	29	30
24	25	26	27	27	28	29
24	25	25	26	27	28	28
23	24	25	26	26	27	28

Waist-Wrist (in inches)	41	41.5	42	42.5	43	43.5
Weight (in lbs.)						
120						
125						
130						
135						
140						
145						
150						
155						
160						
165	55					
170	54	55				
175	52	53	55			
180	50	52	53	54		
185	49	50	51	53	54	55
190	48	49	50	51	52	54
195	46	47	49	50	51	52
200	45	46	47	48	50	51
205	44	45	46	47	48	49
210	43	44	45	46	47	48
215	42	43	44	45	46	47
220	41	42	43	44	45	46
225	40	41	42	43	44	45
230	39	40	41	42	44	44
235	38	39	40	41	42	43
240	37	38	39	40	41	42
245	36	37	38	39	40	41
250	35	36	37	38	39	40
255	34	35	36	37	38	39
260	34	35	35	36	37	38
265	33	34	35	36	36	37
270	32	33	34	35	36	37
275	32	32	33	34	35	36
280	31	32	33	33	34	35
285	30	31	32	33	34	34
290	30	31	31	32	33	34
295	29	30	31	32	32	33
300	29	29	30	31	32	33

44	44.5	45	45.5	46	46.5	47
55						
53	55					
52	53	54	55			
51	52	53	54	55		
49	50	51	53	54	55	
48	49	50	51	52	53	54
47	48	49	50	51	52	53
46	47	48	49	50	51	52
45	46	47	48	49	50	51
44	45	46	47	48	49	50
43	44	45	46	46	47	48
42	43	44	44	45	46	47
41	42	43	44	44	45	46
40	41	42	43	44	44	45
39	40	41	42	43	43	44
38	39	40	41	42	43	43
37	38	39	40	41	42	43
37	38	38	39	40	41	42
36	37	38	38	39	40	41
35	36	37	38	39	39	40
35	35	36	37	38	39	39
34	35	36	36	37	38	39
33	34	35	36	36	37	38

Waist-Wrist (in inches)	47.5	48	48.5	49	49.5	50
Weight (in lbs.)						
120						
125						
130						
135						
140						
145						
150						
155						
160						
165						
170						
175						
180						
185						
190						
195						
200						
205						
210						
215	55					
220	54	55				
225	53	54	55			
230	52	53	54	55		
235	51	51	52	53	54	55
240	49	50	51	52	53	54
245	48	49	50	51	52	53
250	47	48	49	50	51	52
255	46	47	48	49	50	51
260	45	46	47	48	49	50
265	44	45	46	47	48	49
270	43	44	45	46	47	48
275	43	43	44	45	46	47
280	42	43	43	44	45	46
285	41	42	43	43	44	45
290	40	41	42	43	43	44
295	39	40	41	42	43	43
300	39	39	40	41	42	43

Day in the Zone Meal Construction Template

Breakfast

	Protein	Carbohydrate	Added Fat
Protein Course			
Main Carb. Course			
Total			

Lunch

	Protein	Carbohydrate	Added Fat
Salad			
Protein Course			
Main Carb. Course			
Dessert			
Alcohol			
Total			

Dinner

	Protein	Carbohydrate	Added Fat
Salad			
Protein Course			
Main Carb. Course			
Dessert			
Alcohol			
Total			

APPENDIX E

GLYCEMIC INDEX

Terms such as "simple" and "complex" carbohydrates are meaningless when it comes to reaching the Zone. What really matters to the body is the amount and the rate at which a carbohydrate enters into the bloodstream (which in turn determines the extent of insulin secretion). The body is extremely efficient in absorbing carbohydrates so that all the carbohydrate that you consume will eventually enter the bloodstream. This is why controlling the overall amount of carbohydrate in a meal is critical. However, the rate at which the carbohydrate component of a particular food is converted to glucose and enters the blood can be variable. This rate of carbohydrate entry into the bloodstream is known as the glycemic index. Foods that contain no carbohydrate will not have a glycemic index.

To determine a glycemic index of a food, usually 50 grams of insulin-promoting carbohydrate (subtracting the fiber content from the total carbohydrate content) is given to a test subject. Blood sugar levels are carefully and periodically monitored over the next three hours, and the response curve is plotted. The response to the reference food is tested at least three times and the results are averaged.

From these time points, the area under the response curve for the test food is expressed as a percent of the mean value for the reference food (e.g., white bread) for the same subject. The percentages from several subjects are then averaged together to obtain the glycemic index for any particular food. The higher the glycemic index for a food, the faster it will raise blood sugar levels, and therefore increase insulin secretion.

The actual glycemic index of a food is a number relative to the standard of white bread, which is given a glycemic index of 100. Although the glycemic index of a food is fairly standard, the insulin response of an individual to a defined amount of carbohydrate entering the bloodstream can be highly variable.

The glycemic index is also affected by the way a food is prepared. Greater processing of the food results in a breakdown of the cell walls, allowing the carbohydrates in a food to be broken down faster into simple sugars for absorption. This is why refried beans have a much higher glycemic index than kidney beans. In addition, fat will always decrease the glycemic index of a given carbohydrate because the fat content will decrease the rate of carbohydrate absorption into the blood. This is why potato chips have a lower glycemic index than potatoes, even though they have been highly processed.

The glycemic index is a valuable tool to help determine which carbohydrates will most likely get you to the Zone. Regardless of the glycemic index of a food, never consume more carbohydrate blocks from that food in a meal than protein blocks. It is the ratio of the protein to carbohydrate that is the primary determining factor to get you to the Zone. The glycemic index should be viewed as a broad guide to help you choose more favorable carbohydrates in constructing your Zone meals. Within a particular grouping, each food is ranked in order of its measured glycemic index.

GLYCEMIC INDEX OF FOODS BASED ON THE RATE OF ENTRY INTO THE BLOODSTREAM

Extremely high (greater than 100)

Grain-based foods
Puffed rice
Cornflakes
Millet
Rice, instant
Potato, instant
Bread, French

Vegetables

Parsnips, cooked
Potato, russet, baked
Potato, instant
Carrots, cooked
Broad beans (Fava beans)

Simple sugars

Maltose
Glucose
Honey

Glycemic Standard=100 percent

Bread, white

High (80–100)

Grain-based foods

Bread, wheat, whole meal
Grapenuts
Tortilla, corn
Shredded wheat
Muesli
Bread, rye, crispbread
Bread, rye, whole meal
Rice, brown
Porridge oats
Corn, sweet
Rice, white

Vegetables

Potato, mashed
Potato, new, boiled

Simple sugars

Sucrose

Fruits

Apricots
Raisins
Banana

Papaya
Mango

Snacks
Corn chips
Mars Bar
Crackers
Cookies
Pastry
Ice cream, low-fat

Moderately high (60–80)

Grain-based foods
Buckwheat
All Bran
Bread, rye, pumpernickel
Bulgur
Macaroni, white
Spaghetti, white
Spaghetti, brown

Vegetables
Yam
Potato, sweet
Green peas, marrowfat
Green peas, frozen
Baked beans (canned)
Kidney beans (canned)

Fruits
Fruit cocktail
Grapefruit juice
Orange juice
Pineapple juice
Pears, canned
Grapes

Snacks
Cookies, oatmeal
Potato chips
Sponge cake

Moderate (40–60)

Vegetables
Haricot (white) beans
Tomato soup
Brown beans
Lima beans
Green peas, dried
Chickpeas (garbanzo)
Butter beans
Black-eyed peas
Kidney beans
Black beans

Fruits
Orange
Apple juice
Pears
Apple

Dairy
Yogurt
Ice cream, high-fat
Whole milk
2 percent milk
Skim milk

Low (less than 40)

Grain-based food
Barley

Vegetables
Red lentils
Soybeans, canned
Soybeans, dried

Fruits
   Peaches
   Plums

Simple sugars
   Fructose

Snacks
   Peanuts

APPENDIX F

REFERENCES

American Heart Association. "Heart and Stroke Facts: 1996 Statistical Supplement."

_____. "Heart Disease and Strokes Deaths Rising." January 24, 1996, press release.

Anderson, G.H. "Metabolic Regulation of Food Intake." In *Modern Nutrition in Health and Disease*, edited by M.E. Shils and V.R. Young, 557–569. Philadelphia: Lea and Febiger, 1988.

Bao, W., S.R. Srinivasan, and G.S. Berenson. "Persistent Elevation of Plasma Insulin Levels Is Associated with Increased Cardiovascular Risk in Children and Young Adults." *Circulation* 93 (1996): 54–59.

Bidoli, E., S. Franceschi, R. Talamini, S. Barra, and C. La Vecchia. "Food Consumption and Cancer of the Colon and Rectum in North-Eastern Italy." *International Journal of Cancer* 50 (1992): 223–229.

Blum, M., M. Auerbuch, V. Wolman, and A. Aviram. "Protein Intake and Kidney Function in Humans: Its Effect on Normal Aging." *Archives Internal Medicine* 149 (1989): 211–212.

Blundell, J.E., and V.J. Burley. "Evaluation of the Satiating Power of Dietary Fat in Man." In *Progress in Obesity Research*, edited by Y. Onumura, 453–457. New York: John Libbey, 1990.

Brothwell, D., and A.T. Sandison, eds. *Diseases in Antiquity: A Survey of the Disease.* Springfield, Ill.: C.C. Thomas, 1967.

Brunning, P.F., J.M.G. Bonfrer, P.A.H. van Noord, A.A.M. Hart, M. de Jong-Bakker, and W.J. Nooijen. "Insulin Resistance and Breast Cancer Risk." *International Journal of Cancer* 52 (1992): 511–516.

Chen, Y.I., A.M. Coulston, M. Zhou, C.B. Hollenbeck, and G.M. Reaven. "Why Do Low-Fat High-Carbohydrate Diets Accentuate Postprandial Lipemia in Patients with NIDDM?" *Diabetes Care* 18 (1995): 10–16.

Cockburn, A., and E. Cockburn, eds. *Mummies, Disease, and Ancient Cultures.* Cambridge, England: Cambridge University Press, 1980.

Corti, M-C., J.M. Guraink, M.E. Saliva, T. Harris, T.S. Field, R.B. Wallace, L.F. Berkman, T.E. Seeman, R.J. Glynn, C.H. Hennekens, and R.J. Havlik. "HDL Cholesterol Predicts Coronary Heart Disease Mortality in

Older Persons." *Journal of the American Medical Association* 274 (1995): 539–544.

Crawford, M., and D. Marsh. *The Driving Force: Food, Evolution and the Future.* New York: Harper and Row, 1989.

Despres, J.P., B. Lamarche, P. Mauriege, B. Cantin, G.R. Dagenais, S. Moorjani, and P.J. Lupen. "Hyperinsulinemia as an Independent Risk Factor for Ischemic Heart Disease." *New England Journal of Medicine* 334 (1996): 952–957.

Drexel, H., F.W. Amann, J. Beran, K. Rentsch, R. Candinas, J. Muntwyler, A. Leuthy, T. Gasser, and F. Follath. "Plasma Triglycerides and Three Lipoprotein Cholesterol Fractions Are Independent Predictors of the Extent of Coronary Atherosclerosis." *Circulation* 90 (1994): 2230–2235.

Eades, M., and M.D. Eades. *Protein Power.* New York: Bantam, 1996.

Eaton, S.B. "Humans, Lipids, and Evolution." *Lipids* 27 (1992): 814–820.

Eaton, S.B., and M.J. Konner. "Paleolithic Nutrition." *New England Journal of Medicine* 312 (1985): 283–289.

Eaton, S.B., M. Konner, and M. Shostalle. "Stone Agers in the Fast Lane: Chronic Degenerative Diseases in Evolutionary Implications." *American Journal of Medicine* 84 (1988): 739–749.

Eaton, S.B., M. Shostalle, and M. Konner. *The Paleolithic Prescription.* New York: Harper and Row, 1988.

Flatt, J-P. "Use and Storage of Carbohydrate and Fat." *American Journal of Clinical Nutrition* 61 (1995): 952S–959S.

Fontbonne, A., G. Tchobroutsky, E. Eshwege, J.L. Richard, J.R. Claude, and G.E. Rosselin. "Coronary Heart Disease Mortality Risk; Plasma Insulin Level Is a More Sensitive Marker Than Hypertension or Abnormal Glucose Tolerance in Overweight Males." *International Journal of Obesity* 12 (1988): 557–565.

Franceschi, S., A. Favero, A. Decarli, E. Negri, C. La Vecchia, M. Ferranroni, A. Russo, S. Salvini, D. Amadori, E. Conti, M. Montella, and A. Giacosa. "Intake of Macronutrients and Risk of Breast Cancer." *Lancet* 347 (1996): 1351–1356.

Garg, A., J.P. Bantle, R.R. Henry, A.M. Coulston, and G.M. Reaven. "Effects of Varying Carbohydrate Content of Diet in Patients with Non-Insulin Dependent Diabetes Mellitus." *Journal of the American Medical Association* 271 (1994): 1421–1428.

Gaziano, M., and C. Hennekens. "Triglycerides, HDL, and Risk of Myocardial Infarction in a Case-Control Study." Abstract presented at the annual meeting of the American Heart Association, Anaheim, CA, November 1995.

Golay, A., A.F. Allaz, Y. Morel, N. de Tonnac, S. Tankova, and G. Reaven. "Similar Weight Loss with Low- or High-Carbohydrate Diets." *American Journal of Clinical Nutrition* 63 (1996): 174–178.

Gould, K.L. "Very Low-Fat Diets for Coronary Heart Disease: Perhaps, but Which One?" *Journal of the American Medical Association* (1996) 275: 1402–1403.

Gould, K.L., D. Ornish, L. Scherwitz, S. Brown, R.P. Edens, M.J. Hess, N. Mullani, L. Bolomey, F. Dobbs, W.T. Armstrong, T. Merritt, T. Ports, S. Sparier, and J. Billings. "Changes In Myocardial Perfusion Abnormalities by Positron Emission Tomography After Long-Term, Intense Risk Factor Modification." *Journal of the American Medical Association* 274 (1995): 894–901.

Hollenbeck, C., and G.M. Reaven. "Variations in Insulin-Stimulated Glucose Uptake in Healthy Individuals with Normal Glucose Tolerance." *Journal of Clinical Endocrinology and Metabolism* 64 (1987): 1169–1173.

Holt, S., J. Brand, C. Soveny, and J. Hansky. "Relationship of Satiety to Postprandial Glycemic, Insulin, and Cholecystokinin Responses." *Appetite* 18 (1992): 129–141.

Hunt, J.R., S.K. Gallagher, L.K. Johnson, and G.I. Lykken. "High versus Low-Meat Diets: Effects on Zinc Absorption, Iron Status, and Calcium, Copper, Iron, Magnesium, Manganese, Nitrogen, Phosphorous, and Zinc Balance in Postmenopausal Women." *American Journal of Clinical Nutrition* 62 (1995): 621–632.

Jiang, W., M. Babyak, D.S. Krantz, R.A. Waugh, E. Coleman, M.M. Hanson, D.J. Frid, S. McNulty, J.J. Morris, C.M. O'Connor, and J.A. Blumenthal. "Mental Stress-Induced Myocardial Ischemia and Cardiac Events." *Journal of the American Medical Association* (1996) 275: 1651–1656.

Job, F.P., J. Wolfertz, R. Meyer, A. Hubinger, F.A. Gries, and H. Kuhn. "Hyperinsulinism in Patients with Coronary Artery Disease." *Coronary Artery Disease* 5 (1994): 487–492.

Karhapaa, P., M. Malkki, and M. Laakso. "Isolated Low HDL Cholesterol: An Insulin-Resistant State." *Diabetes* 43 (1994): 411–417.

Kekwick, A., and G.L.S. Pawan. "Calorie Intake in Relation to Body-Weight Changes in the Obese." *Lancet* 2 (1956): 155–161.

_____. "Metabolic Study in Human Obesity with Isocaloric Diets High in Fat, Protein or Carbohydrate." *Metabolism* 6 (1957): 447–460.

Klarhr, S., A.S. Levey, G.J. Beck, A.W. Caggiula, L. Hunsicker, J.W. Kusek, and G. Striker. "The Effects of Dietary Protein Restriction and Blood-Pressure Control on the Progression of Chronic Renal Disease." *New England Journal of Medicine* 330: (1994) 877–884.

La Vecchia, C., E. Negri, A. Decarli, B. D'Avanzo, and S. Franceschi. "A Case-Control Study of Diet and Gastric Cancer in Northern Italy." *International Journal of Cancer* 40 (1992): 484–489.

Laws, A., A.C. King, W.L. Haskell, and G.M. Reaven. "Relation of Fasting Plasma Insulin Concentration to High-Density Lipoprotein Cholesterol and Triglyceride Concentrations in Men." *Arteriosclerosis and Thrombosis* 11 (1991): 1636–1642.

Leek, F.F. "Dental Health and Disease in Ancient Egypt with Special Reference to the Manchester Mummies." In *Science in Egyptology*, edited by R.A. Davis, 35–42. Manchester, England: Manchester University Press, 1986.

Mallick, N.P. "Dietary Protein and Progression of Chronic Renal Disease: Large Randomized Controlled Trial Suggests No Benefit from Restriction." *British Medical Journal* 309 (1994): 1101–1102.

Manton, K.G., and J.W. Vaupel. "Survival After Age of 80 in the United States, Sweden, France, England, and Japan." *New England Journal of Medicine* 333 (1995): 1232–1235.

Miller, M., A. Seidler, P.O. Kwiterovich, and T.A. Pearson. "Long-Term Predictors of Subsequent Cardiovascular Events with Coronary Artery Disease and 'Desirable' Levels of Plasma Total Cholesterol." *Circulation* 86 (1992): 1165–1170.

Modan, M., H. Halkin, J. Or, A. Karasik, Y. Drory, Z. Fuchs, A. Lusky, and A. Chetrit. "Hyperinsulinemia, Gender and Risk of Atherosclerotic Cardiovascular Disease." *Circulation* 84 (1991): 1165–1175.

Norman, A.W., and G. Litwack. *Hormones.* New York: Academic Press, 1987.

Oates, J.A., G.A. FitzGerald, R.A. Branch, E.K. Jackson, H.R. Knapp, and L.J. Roberts. "Clinical Implications of Prostaglandin and Thromboxane A_2 Formation. Part 1." *New England Journal of Medicine* 319 (1988): 689–698.

———. "Clinical Implications of Prostaglandin and Thromboxane A_2 Formation. Part 2." *New England Journal of Medicine* 319 (1988): 761–767.

Paffenbarger, R.S., and W.E. Hale. "Physical Activity as an Index of Heart Attack Risk in College Alumni." *American Journal of Epidemiology* 108 (1978): 161–175.

Paffenbarger, R.S., R.T. Hyde, A.L. Wing, and C. Hsieh. "Physical Activity, All-Cause Mortality, and Longevity of College Alumni." *New England Journal of Medicine* 314 (1986): 613–615.

Parillo, M., A.A. Rivellese, A.V. Ciardul, B. Capaldo, A. Giacco, S. Genovese, and G. Riccardi. "A High Monounsaturated-Fat/Low-

Carbohydrate Diet Improves Peripheral Insulin Sensitivity in Non-Insulin-Dependent Diabetic Patients." *Metabolism* 41 (1992): 1373–1378.

Patch, J.R., G. Miesenbock, T. Hopferwieser, V. Muhlberger, E. Knapp, J.K. Dunn, A.M. Gotto, and W. Patsch. "Relation of Triglyceride Metabolism and Coronary Artery Disease." *Arteriosclerosis and Thrombosis* 12 (1992): 1336–1345.

Phinney, S.D., P.G. Davis, S.B. Johnson, and R.T. Holman. "Obesity and Weight Loss Alter Polyunsaturated Metabolism in Humans." *American Journal of Clinical Nutrition* 52 (1991): 831–838.

Phinney, S.D., R.S. Odin, S.B. Johnson, and R.T. Holman. "Reduced Aracidonate in Serum Phospholipids and Cholesteryl Esters Associated with Vegetarian Diets in Humans." *American Journal of Clinical Nutrition* 51 (1991): 385–392.

Puech, P.F., and F.F. Leek. "Dental Microwear As an Indication of Plant Food in Early Man." In *Science in Egyptology*, edited by R.A. Davis, 239–242. Manchester, England: Manchester University Press, 1986.

Pyorala, K., E. Savolainen, S. Kaukula, and J. Haapakoski. "Plasma Insulin As Coronary Heart Disease Risk Factor." *Acta Med Scandinavia* 701 (1985): 38–52.

Reaven, G.M. "Role of Insulin Resistance in Human Disease." *Diabetes* 37 (1988): 1595–1607.

_____. "The Role of Insulin Resistance and Hyperinsulinemia in Coronary Heart Disease." *Metabolism* 41 (1992): 16–19.

Remer, T., and F. Manz. "Dietary Protein As a Modulator of the Renal Net Acid Excretion Capacity: Evidence That an Increased Protein Intake Improves the Capability of the Kidney to Excrete Ammonium." *Nutritional Biochemistry* 6 (1995): 431–437.

Renauld, S., and M. De Lorgeril. "Wine, Alcohol, Platelets and the French Paradox for Coronary Heart Disease." *Lancet* 339 (1992): 1523–1528.

Schapira, D.V., N.B. Kumar, G.H. Lyman, and C.E. Cox. "Abdominal Obesity and Breast Cancer Risk." *Ann Int Medicine* 112 (1990): 182–186.

Schwartz, M.W., D.P. Figlewicz, D.G. Baskin, S.C. Woods, and D. Porte. "Insulin in the Brain: A Hormonal Regulator of Energy Balance." *Endocrine Review* 13 (1992): 387–414.

Sears, B. *The Zone*. New York: HarperCollins, 1995.

Serra-Majem, L., L. Ribas, R. Tresserras, and L. Salleras. "How Could Changes in Diet Explain Changes in Coronary Heart Disease Mortality in Spain? The Spanish Paradox." *American Journal of Clinical Nutrition* 61 (1995): 1351S–1359S.

Silver, M.J., W. Hoch, J.J. Kocsis, C.M. Ingerman, and J.B. Smith.

"Arachidonic Acid Causes Sudden Death in Rabbits." *Science* 183 (1974): 1085–1087.

Smith, N.J.D. "Dental Pathology in an Ancient Egyptian Population." In *Science in Egyptology*, edited by R.A. Davis, 43–48. Manchester, England: Manchester University Press, 1986.

Spencer, H., L. Kramer, M. DeBartolo, C. Morris, and D. Osis. "Further Studies of the Effect of a High Protein Diet As Meat on Calcium Metabolism." *American Journal of Clinical Nutrition* 37 (1983): 924–929.

Spencer, H., L. Kramer, and D. Osis. "Do Protein and Phosphorus Cause Calcium Loss?" *Journal of Nutrition* 118 (1988): 657–660.

United States Department of Agriculture. *Research News.* January 16, 1996.

Wellborn, T.A., and K. Wearne. "Coronary Heart Disease Incidence and Cardiovascular Mortality in Busselton with Reference to Glucose and Insulin Concentrations." *Diabetes Care* 2 (1979): 154–160.

Willett, W.C., J.E. Manson, M.J. Stampfer, G.A. Colditz, B. Rosner, F.E. Speizer, and C.H. Hennekens. "Weight, Weight Change, and Coronary Heart Disease in Women." *Journal of the American Medical Association* 273 (1995): 461–465.

Wolever, T.M.S., D.J.A. Jenkins, A.L. Jenkins, and R.G. Josse. "The Glycemic Index: Methodology and Clinical Implications." *American Journal of Clinical Nutrition* 54 (1991): 846–854.

Wu, D., S.N. Meydani, M. Meydani, M.G. Hayek, P. Huth, and R.J. Nicolosi. "Immunologic Effects of Marine- and Plant-Derived N–3 Polyunsaturated Fatty Acids in Nonhuman Primates." *American Journal of Clinical Nutrition* 63 (1996): 273–280.

Young, V.R., and P.L. Pellett. "Plant Proteins in Relation to Human Protein and Amino Acid Nutrition." *American Journal of Clinical Nutrition* 59 (1994): 1203–1212S.

ZONE PERFECT MEALS IN MINUTES

Other books by Barry Sears, Ph.D.

The Zone
Mastering the Zone

ZONE
PERFECT
MEALS
IN MINUTES

150 Fast and Simple
Healthy Recipes
from the Bestselling Author of
THE ZONE and
MASTERING THE ZONE

BARRY SEARS, Ph.D.

ReganBooks
An Imprint of HarperCollins*Publishers*

HarperCollins books may be purchased for educational, business, or sales promotional use. For information please write: Special Markets Department, HarperCollins Publishers, Inc., 10 East 53rd Street, New York, NY 10022.

FIRST EDITION

Designed by Nancy Singer Olaguera

Library of Congress Cataloging-in-Publication Data
Sears, Barry, 1947–
    Zone-perfect meals in minutes / by Barry Sears.
      p. cm.
    Includes index.
    ISBN 0-06-039241-X
    1. Reducing diets—Recipes. I. Title.
  RM222.2.S393   1997
  613.2'5—dc21   97-31133

97 98 99 00 01 ❖/RRD 10 9 8 7 6 5 4 3 2 1

CONTENTS

Appendixes:

ACKNOWLEDGMENTS

Rarely is any work done alone, and this book is no exception. As usual, primary thanks must be given to my wife, Lynn Sears, and my brother, Doug Sears, not only for their editorial comments, but also for their valuable feedback on how to better communicate Zone concepts to the general public.

Other important contributions have resulted from the thousands of responses from readers of the Zone books. Also, many thanks must go to Todd Silverstein for his exceptionally insightful editing of the manuscript and his constant support.

Much of the early part of this book is inspired by the educational materials developed for teaching Type II diabetics how to use the Zone Diet as part of their treatment programs. But all this would be for naught without the recipes skillfully created and tested by Scott C. Lane, who also crafted the recipes for *Mastering the Zone*. Scott combines the rare talent of being a gourmet chef with a background in food technology. His contributions have been invaluable. The results of his work are recipes that are not only great-tasting, but have powerful hormonal benefits that can be considered the cutting edge of food technology for the twenty-first century.

I also want to thank my friends Dr. Michael Eades and Dr. Michael Norder for their unique insights into the role of diet and hormonal response. Furthermore, much credit must also go to the medical staff at Eicotech consisting of Dr. Paul Kahl and Dr. Eric Freeland for their extremely valuable contributions.

Finally, and most important, my deepest thanks must be given to Judith Regan, who had the courage to publish the first of the Zone books, and who has given invaluable insight into how to best communicate these concepts to the general public. Without her continuing support, the concept of the Zone might never have come to light.

WOULD YOU BUY
THIS DRUG?

What if you could buy a drug that keeps you mentally focused throughout the day? What if the same drug could increase your physical stamina, leaving you with excess energy when you get home? What if it would eliminate hunger between meals? What if it could reduce the likelihood of developing chronic diseases that rob life of its dignity? Would you buy such a drug? Of course.

Would you be startled to learn that such a drug already exists? That the side effects of taking this drug are the loss of excess body fat at the maximum rate possible, and a slowing of the aging process? Best of all, this wonder drug won't cost you a thing. Why? Because you are already taking it every day.

This magical elixir I am describing is food. The food you eat is probably the most powerful drug you will ever encounter. But to use this drug correctly you have to apply the hormonal rules about food that haven't changed in the past 40 million years, and are unlikely to change any time soon. Beware, the door swings both ways on the application of these hormonal rules. Used correctly, food becomes the exceptionally powerful drug that mankind has searched millenniums for. Used incorrectly, on the other hand, food can become your worst nightmare, as tens of millions of Americans have already discovered.

How does this drug work? Simply stated, you must learn how to administer food in the appropriate combination, at the right time, and in the correct dosage to keep the hormone insulin in a tight zone—not too high, not too low. That's the definition of the Zone. The Zone is about maintaining a steady range of insulin in your bloodstream, and food is the only drug known to medical science that you can use to reach that goal. The Zone Diet is the prescription you need to use that drug (i.e., food) correctly.

In my first book, *The Zone,* I outlined the science behind my approach of using food as a drug to control insulin. My second book, *Mastering the Zone,* was a how-to book to apply the principles of the Zone to daily living. This third book addresses the greatest enemy to reaching the Zone—time. The biggest complaint about the Zone Diet is that it takes too much time. No longer. If you follow a few simple rules and use the recipes provided in this book, it will now take you only minutes to enter the Zone.

Why has the Zone Diet become the rage of Hollywood? Why is the Zone Diet followed by world-class athletes? Why is the Zone Diet used by millions of average Americans like yourself? Because it works. That's also why the Zone Diet has become the scourge of the nutritional establishment, which has told you for the past fifteen years that eating bagels and pasta is a surefire way to reach nutritional nirvana. Yet, no one can say with a straight face that Americans are healthier now than they were fifteen years ago.

So if you are one of the millions of Americans who are not happy with what has happened to your body and your health in the past fifteen years, this book will be your primer on using a powerful drug, food, to get into the Zone, quickly and effortlessly. Consider this book a lifelong prescription for a better quality of life.

You can, if you wish, jump directly to the recipes in Chapter 6 to start your Zone prescription. But if you want a little more background on the Zone, then read the next few short chapters.

HORMONAL THINKING VERSUS CALORIC THINKING

This chapter will give you a capsule summary of the concepts that are the foundation of the Zone, as detailed in both *The Zone* (1995) and *Mastering the Zone* (1997).

I have come to realize that two things in life are visceral: our beliefs about nutrition and religion. Both generate passionate feelings, and neither responds well to challenge. Both have also been responsible for the deaths of more people than all the wars mankind has waged thus far. Diet and religion are fightin' words.

As part of our war on obesity, Americans have been told for the past fifteen years that fat is the enemy, and we have lined up as very willing soldiers to wage war against fat. If fat is the enemy, we should have won the war by now. Today we are eating less fat than at any other time in our history, yet we have become the fattest people on the face of the earth.

This is why health authorities like Dr. C. Everett Koop have called obesity the greatest public health crisis currently facing the nation. Why? As readers of *The Zone* already know, this epidemic explosion in obesity may be just the tip of the iceberg, a precursor to an unprecedented increase in chronic disease in the next decade.

What went wrong with our noble war against fat? Doesn't fat cause you to become fat? No. Unfortunately it never has, and it never will. The real cause of increased accumulation of body fat (and our inability to shed it) is the excess production of the hormone insulin. This same excess of insulin also accelerates the likelihood of heart disease, diabetes, and possibly cancer.

We're losing the war against obesity because nutritionists continue to think calorically, instead of looking at food from a hormonal perspective.

You can sum up caloric thinking in a single phrase: "If no fat touches my lips, then no fat will reach my hips." Seductive thinking, but alas, it's not true. Hormonal thinking, on the other hand, says: "It's excess insulin that makes you fat and keeps you fat." Since fat has no effect on insulin, our perceived enemy, fat, is really a neutral bystander in the war on obesity. And this is one war that we are rapidly losing on every front.

Hormonal thinking, which is the foundation of the Zone Diet, can be summarized by the following points. Each of these points may challenge the very core of what you think you know about nutrition.

1. **It is impossible for dietary fat alone to make you fat.** It is the hormone insulin that makes you fat and keeps you fat. How do you increase insulin levels? By eating too many fat-free carbohydrates or too many calories at any one meal. Americans have done both in the past fifteen years. People tend to forget that the best way to fatten cattle and pigs is to raise their insulin levels by feeding them lots and lots of low-fat grain. The best way to fatten humans is to raise their insulin levels by feeding them lots and lots of low-fat grain, but now in the form of pasta and bagels.

2. **Your stomach is politically incorrect.** The stomach is basically a vat of acid that breaks all food into its basic components. From that perspective, one Snickers bar has the same amount of carbohydrate as two ounces of pasta. Most people would not eat four Snickers bars at one sitting, but they would have no problem eat-

ing eight ounces of pasta. Your stomach can't tell the difference. And the more carbohydrates you eat, the more insulin you produce. And the more insulin you produce, the fatter you become.

3. **Not everyone is genetically the same**. About 25 percent of the U.S. population is genetically lucky because they have a low insulin response to carbohydrates. These people will never become fat, and they will always do well on any high-carbohydrate diet whether it's pasta, Snickers, or Twinkies. Unfortunately, the other 75 percent of the U.S. population isn't so lucky. As they increase the amount of fat-free carbohydrates in their diet, they increase the production of insulin.

   Next time you look at that breakfast bagel, ask the question: "Do I feel lucky?" You have a 25 percent chance that you might be. On the other hand, you have a 75 percent chance that your morning bagel will be your worst hormonal nightmare.

4. **Ten thousand years ago there were no grains on the face of the earth.** During mankind's evolution, our ancestors were exposed to two food groups only: low-fat protein and low-density carbohydrates (fruits and vegetables). As a result, this is what we are genetically designed to eat. When grains were first introduced into the human diet 10,000 years ago, the archaeological record clearly reflects three immediate and dramatic changes in grain-eating societies:
   a. Mankind shrank in height from lack of adequate protein.
   b. Diseases of "modern civilization," such as heart attacks, first appeared.
   c. Obesity first became apparent.

   Nowhere is this clearer than in the comparison of Egyptian mummies to the skeletons of Neo-Paleolithic man. Ancient Egyptians were shorter by about six inches than Neo-Paleolithic man, probably because the Egyptians' protein consumption had dropped so dramatically.

More ominously for us, ancient Egyptian medical textbooks dating back as far as 3,500 years ago describe heart disease in frightening detail. Their medical descriptions of heart disease are confirmed when one examines those mummies with preserved visceral tissue that show extensive atherosclerotic lesions, even though the average Egyptian lifespan was only twenty years.

Finally, it is estimated that the extent of obesity in ancient Egypt was similar to the extent of obesity currently found in the United States. We can determine this from the excess amount of skin folds found around the midsections of preserved Egyptian mummies. (Keep in mind that the diet eaten by the ancient Egyptians was very similar to the diet now recommended by the U.S. government for every American. Talk about history repeating itself.)

5. **It takes fat to burn fat.** This statement makes no sense if you are thinking calorically, but it makes perfect sense if you are thinking hormonally. Fat acts like a control rod in a nuclear reactor, slowing down the entry rate of carbohydrates into the bloodstream, and thereby decreasing the production of insulin. Fat also sends a hormonal signal to the brain, telling you to stop eating, which is another way it reduces insulin production.

   Since it's excess insulin that makes you fat, having more fat in the diet becomes an important tool for reducing insulin. The best type of fat to add to your meals? Monounsaturated fat, like olive oil, guacamole, almonds, and macadamia nuts.

6. **You can use food as a hormonal ATM card.** The average American male or female carries a minimum of 100,000 calories of stored body fat on their bodies at any one time. To put this in perspective, this amount of stored body fat is equivalent to eating 1,700 pancakes for breakfast. That's a pretty big breakfast. In fact, the calories you need for your daily energy are already stored in your body. What you need is a hormonal ATM card to release this stored fat for energy. The Zone Diet is that hormonal ATM card,

allowing you to access this massive amount of energy already stored in your body.

7. **The number-one predictor of heart disease is not high cholesterol, not high blood pressure, but elevated levels of insulin.** How can you tell if you have elevated levels of insulin? Look in the mirror. If you're fat and shaped like an apple, you have elevated insulin levels, and you are probably fast-tracking to an early heart attack. But you can still be thin and have elevated insulin. How can you tell? You have high triglycerides and low HDL cholesterol. This is why high-carbohydrate, low-fat diets can be extremely dangerous to cardiovascular patients even if they lose weight, because they often also see an increase in triglycerides and a decrease in HDL cholesterol levels.

8. **Carbohydrates are a drug.** Make no mistake about it. Your body needs some carbohydrate at every meal for optimal brain function. But like any drug, too much will give rise to toxic side effects. The toxic side effect of consuming too much carbohydrate at any meal is an overproduction of insulin, and that can be very dangerous to your health.

The central theme of the Zone Diet is to understand the importance of thinking of food hormonally, rather than calorically. Once you do so, you begin to understand why virtually every dietary recommendation of the U.S. government and leading nutritionists is hormonally wrong (and maybe dead wrong) for millions of Americans.

All that remains for you is to get into the Zone as easily and as quickly as possible. That's what this book is all about. But before we begin getting into the Zone, a little background on nutrition is needed to explain how and why the Zone Diet works.

3

WHAT IS FOOD?

Food can be divided into three groups: protein, carbohydrate, and fat. What these food groups are and how they affect the Zone Diet are the keys to understanding what and how you must eat to get and stay in the Zone.

PROTEIN

Protein comes primarily from animal sources because animals are very efficient concentrators of protein compared to plants. Protein levels in plants, on the other hand, are usually very low and, unfortunately, often require you to eat massive and unrealistic amounts of vegetable sources to obtain adequate protein intake (while also consuming massive amounts of carbohydrates that take you out of the Zone). Eating adequate protein is essential to health, because eating less than adequate protein is equivalent to protein malnutrition. But while virtually no one in America suffers from caloric malnutrition, a surprising number of people today suffer from protein malnutrition because they have eliminated protein from the diet and replaced it with increasing amounts of grains and pasta in their relentless effort to reduce dietary fat.

Why do you have to have adequate protein? Your body's immune system, the integrity of all your tissues, each of the body's cells, the enzymes (the engines of life) contained in each cell, and the amount of your muscle mass all depend on having adequate levels of new incoming protein, since you are losing protein every day through normal metabolism. If you don't have at least an equal amount of protein coming into the body to balance the amount that is being constantly lost from the body, you have protein malnutrition. Protein malnutrition can be insidious, leading to a decrease in the ability of your immune system to fight infection. You will also lose muscle mass as your body cannibalizes existing muscle in a losing effort to keep up with the demand for new protein building blocks for your immune system and new enzyme formation.

The key to the Zone Diet is to ensure that adequate amounts of protein are being supplied to your body like an intravenous drug that is delivered throughout the day in relatively controlled amounts based on your own unique protein requirements.

Notice, too, that you need *adequate*, not excessive protein. The Zone Diet is *not* a high-protein diet, but rather a protein-adequate diet. In fact, the Zone Diet has absolutely no relationship to the high-protein diets of the 1970s (this is explained in far greater detail in Chapter 13). Simply stated, no one should ever eat more protein than his or her body requires, but no one should ever eat less.

To make the picture a little more complex, not all protein is the same. On the Zone Diet, you want to keep the amount of saturated fat to a minimum. Therefore your primary source of protein will consist of low-fat choices such as chicken, fish, turkey, egg whites, low-fat cottage cheese, tofu, soybean imitation meat products, and isolated protein powders as opposed to bacon, steaks, and sausages.

Besides meeting the needs I have described above, protein also plays another critical hormonal role—it stimulates the release of the hormone called glucagon. Glucagon is a mobilization hormone that allows your body to use stored energy, both fat and carbohydrate, as energy sources.

CARBOHYDRATES

Carbohydrates come from plants and trees. Examples are grains (the basis of all pastas, breads, and cereals), or vegetables, or fruits.

In human nutrition, there is no such thing as an essential carbo-hydrate! You don't need to eat carbohydrates to live. This was demon-strated in 1927 when a noted Arctic explorer, Vihajalmur Stefansson and a colleague, confined themselves in a hospital ward for a year, eat-ing only protein and fat, and no carbohydrates whatsoever. After one year on this diet, they were both perfectly normal.

Although you can live without carbohydrate, this is not true for protein or fat, as the human body cannot make essential protein (i.e., essential amino acids) and essential fat (i.e., essential fatty acids), and therefore these must be obtained in the diet if you are to survive. On the other hand, the body can make carbohydrate (necessary for brain function) from both protein and fat.

A complex carbohydrate is simply a large quantity of simple sug-ars strung together and looks something like this:

—glucose—O—glucose—O—glucose—O—glucose—O—glucose—

This is the configuration of pasta, starches, bagels, or cereals at the molecular level. Notice that a typical complex carbohydrate is simply a simple sugar (glucose) held together by an oxygen bond. These oxy-gen bonds are broken down in the stomach, thus allowing a complex carbohydrate to be absorbed.

How quickly this breakdown occurs determines how fast your blood sugar level rises. This is very important because it's the combi-nation of the amount of carbohydrates you eat and the speed with which they enter into the bloodstream that dictate how much of insulin is produced.

The average American currently consumes the carbohydrate equivalent of more than two cups of sugar per day. This is because all carbohydrates, no matter how complex they might be when they enter your mouth, must be broken down to simple sugars to be absorbed.

Your stomach is politically incorrect because it can't tell the difference between a bagel, pasta, or cotton candy. And the more carbohydrates you consume, the more insulin you make.

Insulin (unlike glucagon) is a storage hormone. One of its functions is to push incoming calories into cells. And any excess carbohydrates or protein that can't be stored immediately are converted to fat. Insulin will then drive this newly converted fat into your fat cells for storage.

The Zone Diet is based on keeping glucagon and insulin balanced at every meal. This means maintaining the appropriate balance of protein and carbohydrate at every meal.

FATS

Finally, what about fat? Fats come from both animal and plant sources. There are three types of fat: saturated fat, which is solid at room temperature; monounsaturated fat, which is liquid at room temperature but solid in the freezer; and polyunsaturated fat, which remains a liquid even when frozen. An example of saturated fat is butter, a monounsaturated fat is olive oil, and a polyunsaturated fat is soybean oil. Since all your cells are composed of fat, the ratio of these types of fat in your diet will determine how effectively your body's cell membranes function. There is a fluidity zone (not too viscous, but not too fluid) that allows membranes to operate at optimal efficiency. This is the reason why the Zone Diet recommends the use of primarily monounsaturated fat.

Hormonally, fat has no direct effect on insulin or glucagon, but it does affect their balance by slowing down the absorption rate of any carbohydrate into the bloodstream, thereby decreasing insulin production. Furthermore, fat plays a critical role, because it provides the building blocks (essential fatty acids) for the production of the most important hormones in your body, called eicosanoids.

As explained in greater detail in *The Zone,* there are both "good" and "bad" eicosanoids, and their balance will determine whether your body works at peak efficiency or suffers from disease. As with insulin and glucagon, it's a matter of balance. And what controls this balance? The ratio of insulin and glucagon in your bloodstream determines whether your body makes "good" or "bad" eicosanoids.

The Zone Diet keeps all three hormonal systems (insulin, glucagon, and eicosanoids) working smoothly by treating food with the same respect that you would treat a prescription drug.

Preparing meals based on hormonal thinking may seem like a radical new approach to eating. So radical, in fact, that you might think no one has ever done it before in human history. As you read the next chapter, you will be surprised to learn just who has been eating in the Zone for a long time.

WHO ACTUALLY EATS IN THE ZONE?

Balancing your protein and carbohydrate to maintain insulin in a tight zone might sound almost impossible at first. Yet your grandmother had no problem doing it. Remember what your grandmother told you (or should have told you) about food? Probably these four simple rules.

1. **Eat small meals throughout the day.** One of the best ways to maintain insulin levels in the Zone is not to eat too much carbohydrate or protein at any one meal. Although carbohydrate has a powerful effect on stimulating insulin, protein can also stimulate its release. By not eating too much of either at any one meal, you are well on your way to the Zone. One of the frightening consequences of having the cheapest food on the face of the earth is that Americans have come to expect massive portions of food at every meal. And in the last fifteen years they have gotten their wish, but with a correspondingly massive increase in insulin production.

2. **Have some protein at every meal**. Protein's primary hormonal role is to stimulate the release of glucagon, which is a mobilization hormone. Glucagon also does a real bang-up job on control-

575

ling insulin output. Therefore, if you really want to get to the Zone, protein is your passport. But be careful about eating too much protein and remember the palm-of-your-hand rule discussed in *Mastering the Zone:* At any one meal, never consume any more protein than can fit on the palm of your hand (and no thicker than the palm of your hand). Your body simply can't handle any more at a meal, and any excess protein at a meal is converted to fat.

3. **Always eat your fruits and vegetables.** Any one can eat one cup of pasta, but it's hard work to eat six cups of steamed broccoli. Yet both contain the same amount of carbohydrates (due to the large amounts of fiber and water they contain which dilute out the carbohydrate). Why? Because fruits and vegetables are low-density carbohydrates. By eating primarily low-density carbohydrates, such as fruits and vegetables, you set up a natural control system that helps control the total amount of carbohydrates being consumed at any one meal. In addition, the fiber (especially if it's soluble fiber) in low-density carbohydrates helps slow down the rate of entry of carbohydrates into the bloodstream, thus lowering insulin secretion. On the other hand, grains, starches, pasta, and bagels are very high-density carbohydrates (which means it's very easy to overconsume them). This is why I recommend using high-density carbohydrates in moderation, as condiments, if you want to control insulin.

    Remember when your grandmother told you that you couldn't leave the table until you finished all your vegetables? She was simply being a good Zone coach.

4. **Take your cod liver oil.** Nothing is more disgusting than cod liver oil. However, it contains a special fatty acid called eicosapentaenoic acid, or EPA, that does a very good job of keeping insulin under control by affecting eicosanoids. You can still take cod liver oil like your grandmother did, but a better choice today is eating salmon, which is rich in that same fatty acid, but tastes a lot better.

Now, look at your grandmother's four Zone rules and compare them to what nutrition "experts" are advocating today. According to the U.S. Department of Agriculture Food Pyramid you are supposed to get most of your calories from breads, grains, starches, and pasta. A typical recommended daily menu might include a bagel for breakfast, pasta for lunch, and probably more pasta for dinner. By eating bountiful amounts of these recommended "healthy" foods, you may find it very easy to have large meals (at least in carbohydrate content) throughout the day: the first violation of your grandmother's rules.

Remember that famous commercial in which Clara demanded to know, "Where's the beef?" We could paraphrase her now and ask, "Where's the protein?" Because protein contains fat, it almost never appears at most breakfasts, rarely appears at lunch, and finally may make an almost apologetic appearance at dinner. Another violation of your grandmother's rules to have some protein at *every* meal.

Why eat lots of fruits and vegetables? Where do you think you get your vitamins and minerals from? They are found primarily in fruits and vegetables, not breads, starches, and pasta. In the land of plenty, we suffer from a massive underconsumption of fruits and vegetables, and a gross overconsumption of pasta and bagels. No wonder vitamin sales are booming.

Finally, what about cod liver oil? Your grandmother didn't know how or why it worked. It just seemed to work. We now know the fatty acids in cod liver oil favorably change the levels of eicosanoids.

OK, so the Zone Diet was fine for your grandmother, but that was nearly two generations ago. Is there anyone who eats in the Zone today? Actually, the French do. No one has ever accused the French of not eating well, yet they don't have the rampant obesity we have in this country, and their rate of heart disease is half of what it is in America. This is why our nutritional "experts" hate the French. They smoke, they drink, they don't exercise, they eat lots of fat, and their worst sin is that they seem to have a good time when they eat.

In reality, the French are Zoners. They eat a balance of protein to carbohydrate at every meal. They eat primarily fruits and vegetables, they eat in moderation, and they are not afraid of fat, especially in the form of sauces. And therein lies one of the secrets of French cooking—the sauces. And their drinking? Well, every time they drink wine (which the body treats like a carbohydrate), they always have a protein chaser (like cheese). If you ate gourmet French meals three times a day with slight adaptations, I guarantee you would be in the Zone.

The bottom line is that (1) you are genetically designed to eat a Zone Diet, (2) your grandmother told you to eat a Zone Diet, and (3) the French have demonstrated that the Zone Diet is really the pinnacle of gourmet cooking.

Now that you have had a basic primer on nutrition, all that remains is to teach you some very simple Zone rules. Once you know these easy rules, you will be well on your way to reaching the Zone.

5

ZONE RULES

Any drug use comes with certain rules and instructions to follow. The Zone Diet is no different. Does this mean Zone rules are hard to understand? Not at all. Just follow your grandmother's four simple dietary rules as I outlined in the previous chapter. To make it even easier for yourself, for the first two weeks you're on the Zone Diet, simply put starch, pasta, cereals, bread, and bagels out of sight. During these two weeks, you will get your carbohydrates the old-fashioned way, from fruits and vegetables.

Now each time you sit down for a meal simply divide your plate into three equal sections. In one section you will put a portion of low-fat protein (chicken, turkey, fish, etc.) that is no larger than the palm of your hand (and no thicker than the palm). Fill the other two-thirds of the plate with fruits and vegetables. Then add a dash of monounsaturated fat (olive oil, slivered almonds, guacamole, etc.).

You're probably telling yourself, "It can't be this easy." Well, it is. Just do it at every meal and snack and you'll be pretty close to the center of the Zone throughout the day.

What if you want even greater precision? Can you achieve it? Yes, it's called the Zone food block method and its use is explained in greater detail in *Mastering the Zone*. Since different foods have different densities of protein, carbohydrate, and fat, what the Zone food block method does is put them on an equal footing by standardizing the amount of protein, carbohydrate, and fat in each block. If you don't want to bother to calculate your individual block requirements, keep in mind that the average American male requires four blocks of each (protein, carbohydrate, and fat) at every meal, whereas the average American female will require three blocks of each at every meal. (In fact, my latest clinical trials with Type II diabetics have led me to conclude that no adult should consume fewer than three blocks per meal.) No minicomputer required.

I have taken most of the foods you will ever eat and broken them down into Zone food blocks, and these are listed in Appendix B. Just remember to look up the amounts of your favorite foods that constitute one Zone food block, and as you reconstruct your Zone meal, just make the number of protein blocks equal the number of carbohydrate blocks, and then add an equal number of fat blocks.

If you are going to err in making a Zone-Perfect meal, then do so in the fat blocks, since fat has no effect on insulin. Furthermore, always pay close attention to the amount of carbohydrates you're adding to a meal, as you can use up your carbohydrate block allotment very quickly, especially if you are using high-density carbohydrates.

Another important Zone rule on meal timing. Never let more than five hours go by without eating a Zone meal or snack. Remember, the best time to eat is when you are not hungry.

Finally, there's exercise. Exercise will lower insulin levels, so it should be part of your Zone lifestyle. However, I like to apply the 80/20 rule to exercise. Most (more than 80 percent) of your insulin control will come from the diet, and a much smaller part (less than 20 percent) will come from exercise. The best exercise? Try walking 30 minutes every day. Just like the Zone Diet, exercise works only if you do it consistently.

To show you how easy and delicious Zone meals can be, the next chapter features 150 balanced Zone-Perfect meals, many of which can be prepared in minutes.

6

150 ZONE-PERFECT MEALS

This chapter is probably the reason you bought this book. These Zone-Perfect meals were designed by Scott C. Lane, an exceptionally talented culinary expert who is also trained in the most advanced food technology. Each meal not only looks great and tastes delicious, but it is also designed to control insulin levels for the next four to six hours. This is the definition of a Zone-Perfect meal. Each meal has been crafted with the same kind of precision that pharmaceuticals use in manufacturing their drugs.

Furthermore, these meals have been constructed so that you can reduce their cooking times by nearly 50 percent by substituting frozen vegetables in place of fresh vegetables. (Birds Eye frozen vegetables are a good commercial source since they often contain combinations of several Zone-favorable vegetables.) Each Zone-Perfect meal is designed to provide four blocks of protein, carbohydrate, and fat. This is the typical size for an American male, whereas the typical American female would require the slightly smaller meal using only three blocks.

As I explained in *Mastering the Zone,* Zone meals are incredibly flexible. Each recipe is organized into Zone food blocks, so that with a quick turn to the Appendix, you can modify any Zone-Perfect meal. Think of this chapter not as 150 Zone-Perfect meals, but as literally thousands of Zone-Perfect meals.

BREAKFAST

TEXAS-STYLE OMELETTE

Servings: 1 Breakfast Entrée (4 blocks)

Block Size:	Ingredients:
2 Protein	3 ounces lean ground turkey
2 Protein	½ cup egg substitute
1 Carbohydrate	¼ cup canned kidney beans, rinsed and diced*
1 Carbohydrate	½ cup salsa**
1 Carbohydrate	1 cup Zoned Country-Style Chicken Gravy (see page 709)
½ Carbohydrate	1½ cups bean sprouts
½ Carbohydrate	¾ cup red and green bell peppers
4 Fat	1⅓ teaspoons olive oil

Spices:

¼ teaspoon hot sauce

Method:

In a nonstick sauté pan, add the oil, and heat over medium-high heat. In a medium bowl, blend the ground turkey, egg substitute, kidney beans, salsa, and hot sauce. Add egg mixture to heated pan. Let cook until set, then (flip) turn over egg mixture. While omelette is cooking, heat a second nonstick sauté pan. In a small bowl, mix the chicken gravy, bean sprouts, and mixed peppers. Pour into second pan. Cook over medium heat, to blend flavors. When omelette is browned on both sides, place it on a serving dish and top it with the gravy.

*Note: When using canned beans, always rinse them before using.

**Note: Salsa comes with different levels of heat. Choose one that best fits your family's tastes.

SCRAMBLED EGG POCKET WITH MIXED FRUIT SALAD

Servings: 1 Breakfast Entrée (4 blocks)

Block Size:	Ingredients:
3 Protein	¾ cup egg substitute
1 Protein	1 ounce low-fat cheddar cheese, shredded
1 Carbohydrate	½ mini pita pocket
1 Carbohydrate	½ apple, chopped*
1 Carbohydrate	½ pear, chopped
1 Carbohydrate	¾ cup cantaloupe**
4 Fat	4 teaspoons almonds, slivered

Spices:

1 teaspoon chives, chopped
⅛ teaspoon dill
Dash chili powder
Dash celery salt
Black pepper to taste
1 teaspoon lemon juice

Method:
Combine egg substitute, chives, dill, chili powder, celery salt, and pepper. Pour mixture into a microwave-safe 10-ounce dish. Cook in microwave on high (100 percent) setting for 1 to 2½ minutes, until almost set. Push cooked egg portions to center of the dish and continue cooking in 30-second intervals on high setting. When the egg is set, sprinkle with cheese and let stand 2 minutes. Scoop egg mixture into pita pocket. In a medium bowl combine fruit and almonds. Place pita pocket and fruit on a breakfast plate and serve.

*Note: To stop apples from turning brown, dip cut apples in a little lemon juice and water mixture.

**Note:* Depending on the size of the cantaloupe, you may not need all the flesh—store the excess for use in another recipe.*

HERBED OMELETTE

Servings: 1 Breakfast Entrée (4 blocks)

Block Size:	Ingredients:
4 Protein	1 cup egg substitute
½ Carbohydrate	5½ cups alfalfa sprouts
½ Carbohydrate	½ cup onion, chopped
½ Carbohydrate	¾ cup red and green bell peppers
½ Carbohydrate	1½ cups mushrooms, sliced
1 Carbohydrate	½ cup salsa*
1 Carbohydrate	⅓ cup mandarin orange sections
4 Fat	1⅓ teaspoons olive oil

Spices:

¼ teaspoon garlic, minced
⅛ teaspoon dried oregano
⅛ teaspoon dill
⅛ teaspoon chili powder
⅛ teaspoon dried parsley
⅛ teaspoon Worcestershire sauce
⅛ teaspoon cilantro
Dash lemon herb seasoning

Method:

In a nonstick sauté pan, heat oil over medium-high heat. In a medium bowl, combine the onion, bell peppers, and mushrooms. Add garlic, oregano, dill, chili powder, parsley, Worcestershire sauce, cilantro, and lemon herb seasoning. Spoon vegetable/herb mixture into pan and sauté for 3 minutes, until vegetables soften and herbs are heated. Pour egg substitute into pan, stir to distribute vegetables, and cook until almost set.

Sprinkle sprouts onto half of omelette and fold over. Remove to serving plate. Decorate with orange sections and top omelette with salsa.

Note: Salsa comes with different levels of heat. Choose one that best fits your family's tastes.

YOGURT-TOPPED APPLE

Servings: 1 Breakfast Entrée (4 blocks)

Block Size:	Ingredients:
3 Protein	¾ cup low-fat cottage cheese
1 Protein	½ cup plain low-fat yogurt
1 Carbohydrate	
2 Carbohydrate	1 apple, cored and halved lengthwise*
1 Carbohydrate	1 teaspoon raisins, diced
4 Fat	4 teaspoons almonds, slivered

Spices:

⅛ teaspoon nutmeg
⅛ teaspoon orange zest
⅛ teaspoon cinnamon

Method:
Place apple cut side up in a small microwaveable dish. Spoon raisins into core of apple. Cook the apple in microwave set on high (100 percent) for 4 to 5 minutes. In a small mixing bowl combine yogurt, nutmeg, orange zest, and cinnamon. Place cottage cheese in a serving dish, sprinkled with almonds. When the apple is cooked (slightly soft) place apple on top of cottage cheese, top with yogurt, and serve.

Note: To stop apples from turning brown, dip cut apples in a little lemon juice and water mixture.

COTTAGE CHEESE FRUIT SALAD

Servings: 1 Breakfast Entrée (4 blocks)

Block Size:	Ingredients:
4 Protein	1 cup low-fat cottage cheese
2 Carbohydrate	1 apple, cored and chopped*
1 Carbohydrate	1 teaspoon raisins, chopped
1 Carbohydrate	½ cup pineapple, chopped
4 Fat	4 teaspoons almonds, chopped

Spices:

⅛ teaspoon cinnamon
⅛ teaspoon cilantro
⅛ teaspoon nutmeg

Method:

In a medium serving bowl combine cottage cheese, apple, raisins, pineapple, and almonds. Sprinkle with cinnamon, cilantro, and nutmeg. Serve immediately.

*Note: To stop apples from turning brown, dip cut apples in a little lemon juice and water mixture.

POACHED FRUIT WITH CHEESE

Servings: 1 Breakfast Entrée (4 blocks)

Block Size:	Ingredients:
4 Protein	1 cup low-fat cottage cheese
2 Carbohydrate	1 apple, cored and cut in 8 wedges*
1 Carbohydrate	⅓ cup Mandarin orange sections
1 Carbohydrate	½ pear, cut in 3 wedges
4 Fat	4 teaspoons almonds, chopped

Spices:

1 cup water
1-inch piece cinnamon stick
⅛ teaspoon nutmeg

Method:

In medium saucepan bring water, cinnamon, and nutmeg to a boil. Add apple and pear, return to a boil, and cover. Reduce heat to a simmer and cook 5 to 6 minutes. Add orange sections and simmer 1 minute more. Place cottage cheese sprinkled with almonds in a serving bowl. Remove apple and pear with slotted spoon to serving bowl, and place on top of cottage cheese. Serve immediately.

*Note: To stop apples from turning brown, dip cut apples in a little lemon juice and water mixture.

CURRIED ASPARAGUS OMELETTE

Servings: 1 Breakfast Entrée (4 blocks)

Block Size:	Ingredients:
4 Protein	1 cup egg substitute
1 Carbohydrate	½ cup tomato, seeded and chopped
½ Carbohydrate	1½ cups mushrooms, chopped
2 Carbohydrate	2 cups steamed asparagus, 1-inch pieces
½ Carbohydrate	½ cup onion, chopped
4 Fat	1⅓ teaspoons olive oil, divided

Spices:

½ teaspoon garlic, minced
½ to 1 teaspoon curry powder
⅛ teaspoon Worcestershire sauce
1 teaspoon parsley, chopped
⅛ teaspoon turmeric
Salt and pepper to taste

Method:

In a medium nonstick sauté pan, heat half of the oil. Add garlic and cook until lightly browned. Stir in curry powder, Worcestershire sauce, turmeric, and salt and pepper. Cook 1 minute to heat through. Add tomato and mushrooms, asparagus and onion. Cook until softened, about 5 minutes. Cover and remove from heat. In a second nonstick sauté pan, heat remaining oil. Pour egg substitute into second sauté pan and cook until set. Place omelette on serving plate and spoon asparagus mixture onto half of omelette and fold other half over. Sprinkle with parsley and serve immediately.

ORIENTAL VEGETABLE OMELETTE

Servings: 1 Breakfast Entrée (4 blocks)

Block Size:	Ingredients:
4 Protein	1 cup egg substitute
½ Carbohydrate	½ cup scallions, thinly sliced diagonally
1 Carbohydrate	1 cup canned mushrooms, sliced
½ Carbohydrate	2¼ cups red and green bell peppers
1 Carbohydrate	¼ cup chickpeas
1 Carbohydrate	3 cups bean sprouts
4 Fat	1⅓ teaspoons olive oil, divided

Spices:

½ teaspoon garlic, minced
3 tablespoons cider vinegar
½ teaspoon gingerroot, grated*
1 tablespoon soy sauce
⅛ teaspoon Worcestershire sauce

Method:

In large nonstick sauté pan, heat half of the oil. Stir-fry scallions for 1 minute over medium-high heat. Add mushrooms and cook another 2 minutes, then add peppers, chickpeas, sprouts, garlic, vinegar, ginger, soy sauce, and Worcestershire sauce. Cook 3 to 5 minutes or until bean sprouts are tender. In a second large nonstick sauté pan, heat remaining oil on medium-high heat. Pour in egg substitute. As it cooks, push cooked portions toward center of pan with a spatula. When eggs are set, remove omelette to warmed serving plate and place filling from first pan into one side of omelette and fold other side and serve.

*Note: When a recipe calls for fresh gingerroot (available in most grocery stores or Asian markets), it is not advisable to substitute ground ginger. The flavors are very different.

OMELETTE ROCKEFELLER

Servings: 1 Breakfast Entrée (4 blocks)

Block Size:	Ingredients:
4 Protein	1 cup egg substitute
½ Carbohydrate	2 cups watercress, chopped
½ Carbohydrate	½ cup onion, chopped
½ Carbohydrate	3 cups raw spinach*
1 Carbohydrate	1 cup canned mushrooms, chopped
½ Carbohydrate	1½ cups bean sprouts
1 Carbohydrate	½ cup salsa**
3 Fat	1 teaspoon olive oil, divided
1 Fat	1 teaspoon almonds, finely chopped

Spices:

½ teaspoon garlic, minced, divided
⅛ teaspoon cayenne pepper
⅛ teaspoon nutmeg
⅛ teaspoon celery salt
1 tablespoon balsamic vinegar
Salt and pepper to taste

Method:
In a medium nonstick sauté pan, heat oil. Mix egg substitute, ¼ teaspoon garlic, salt and pepper. Pour into sauté pan and cook until set. In a small nonstick saucepan heat onion, salsa, ¼ teaspoon garlic, cayenne, nutmeg, celery salt, vinegar, and salt and pepper. Bring to boil, reduce heat, cover and gently simmer 2 to 3 minutes. On half of serving plate combine watercress, spinach, mushrooms, and sprouts. Place omelette on the other side, top all with sauce, sprinkle with almonds, and serve.

*Note: Fresh spinach needs to be cleaned very well, because of its tendency

to have sand on it, so be sure to soak spinach in water to remove any sand or dirt before using.

Note: *Salsa comes with different levels of heat. Choose one that best fits your taste.*

FLORENTINE FILLED CREPES

Servings: 1 Breakfast Entrée (4 blocks)

Block Size:	Ingredients:
4 Protein	1 cup egg substitute
1 Carbohydrate	3 cups mushrooms, sliced
½ Carbohydrate	½ cup onion, chopped
½ Carbohydrate	3 cups fresh spinach, torn*
1 Carbohydrate	2 cups alfalfa sprouts
1 Carbohydrate	1 kiwi fruit, peeled and sliced
4 Fat	1⅓ teaspoons olive oil, divided

Spices:

⅛ teaspoon celery salt
⅛ teaspoon nutmeg
⅛ teaspoon cinnamon
4 tablespoons balsamic vinegar
Salt and pepper to taste

Method:

In a large nonstick sauté pan, heat ⅔ teaspoon oil. Combine egg substitute, celery salt, nutmeg, and cinnamon. Pour into sauté pan. When browned on one side flip over with spatula and brown the other side. Heat remaining oil in a second nonstick sauté pan, over a medium-high heat. When heated, add mushrooms and onion. Cook for 3 to 5 minutes, then add balsamic vinegar, spinach, and sprouts. Continue cooking until spinach is just wilted. Place omelette onto serving plate. Spoon vegetable mixture onto omelette and fold over. Decorate with kiwi fruit and serve.

Note: Fresh spinach needs to be cleaned very well, because of its tendency to have sand on it, so be sure to soak spinach in water to remove any sand or dirt before using.

SPICY SHRIMP AND MUSHROOM OMELETTE

Servings: 1 Breakfast Entrée (4 blocks)

Block Size:	Ingredients:
1 Protein	1½ ounces shrimp, chopped
3 Protein	¾ cup egg substitute
1 Carbohydrate	1 cup onion, chopped
1 Carbohydrate	3 cups mushrooms, chopped
1 Carbohydrate	1 kiwi fruit, peeled and sliced
1 Carbohydrate	1 cup asparagus spears
4 Fat	1⅓ teaspoons olive oil

Spices:

⅛ teaspoon garlic, minced
¼ teaspoon dried parsley, chopped
⅛ teaspoon dry mustard
⅛ teaspoon dried basil
⅛ teaspoon cayenne pepper
⅛ teaspoon turmeric
Salt and pepper to taste

Method:

In a medium nonstick sauté pan, heat oil. Add asparagus and spices to sauté pan and cook for 1 minute, then add onion and mushrooms. Cook for 3 to 5 minutes or until vegetables are tender. Remove vegetables and keep warm. Place shrimp in sauté pan and cook for 1 minute. Pour egg substitute into sauté pan. Stir to make sure shrimp is distributed throughout the egg. Cook on medium-high heat until omelette is almost set. Remove omelette to serving plate. Spoon onion/mushroom mixture onto omelette and fold over. Decorate omelette with kiwi slices and serve.

FRUITY-NUT COTTAGE CHEESE WITH RASPBERRY SAUCE

Servings: 1 Breakfast Entrée (4 blocks)

Block Size:	Ingredients:
4 Protein	1 cup low-fat cottage cheese
½ Carbohydrate	¼ cup fresh blueberries
1 Carbohydrate	½ cup peaches, diced
½ Carbohydrate	¾ cup cantaloupe, diced
½ Carbohydrate	¼ cup grapes
1½ Carbohydrate	1½ cups raspberries
4 Fat	4 macadamia nuts, chopped

Method:
This recipe requires a blender or food processor. Mound cottage cheese in center of serving plate. Arrange blueberries, peaches, cantaloupe, and grapes around cottage cheese. Place raspberries in blender and puree. Pour pureed raspberries over cottage cheese and fruit, then sprinkle with nuts and serve.

JAPANESE-STYLE CHICKEN AND SPINACH OMELETTE

Servings: 1 Breakfast Entrée (4 blocks)

Block Size:	Ingredients:
2 Protein	½ cup egg substitute
2 Protein	2 ounces chicken tenderloins, diced
1 Carbohydrate	6 cups spinach*
1 Carbohydrate	3 cups mushrooms, sliced
1 Carbohydrate	3 cups bean sprouts
1 Carbohydrate	1 cup onion, diced
4 Fat	1⅓ teaspoons olive oil, divided

Spices:

1 tablespoon soy sauce
¼ teaspoon Worcestershire sauce
2 tablespoons balsamic vinegar
⅛ teaspoon chili powder
⅛ teaspoon cayenne pepper
⅛ teaspoon celery salt

Method:

Heat 1 teaspoon oil in a medium nonstick sauté pan. Sauté chicken and onion until lightly browned. Add spinach, mushrooms, and bean sprouts. Cook 3 to 5 minutes. Add remaining oil to another sauté pan. In a small bowl stir soy sauce, Worcestershire sauce, balsamic vinegar, and seasonings into egg substitute, then pour into sauté pan. Cook until almost set. Spoon vegetables onto half of omelette. Fold over and cook 1 additional minute. Place omelette on serving plate and serve.

*Note: Fresh spinach needs to be cleaned very well, because of its tendency to have sand on it, so be sure to soak spinach in water to remove any sand or dirt before using.

TOMATO OMELETTE WITH SAUTÉED PEPPER AND CHEESE

Servings: 1 Breakfast Entrée (4 blocks)

Block Size:	Ingredients:
3 Protein	¾ cup egg substitute
1 Protein	1 ounce shredded low-fat cheddar cheese
¾ Carbohydrate	¾ cup canned mushrooms, chopped
1 Carbohydrate	2¼ cups bell peppers, chopped
½ Carbohydrate	½ cup pearl onions, frozen
1 Carbohydrate	1¼ cups tomato, seeded and diced
½ Carbohydrate	¼ cup salsa*
¼ Carbohydrate	1 teaspoon cornstarch
4 Fat	1⅓ teaspoons olive oil, divided

Spices:

½ teaspoon garlic, minced
⅛ teaspoon celery salt
¼ teaspoon Worcestershire sauce
1 tablespoon cider vinegar
Salt and pepper to taste

Method:
In a medium nonstick sauté pan heat ⅔ teaspoon oil. Add mushrooms and sauté for 3 minutes. Stir in peppers and cook an additional 3 minutes. Add onions, tomatoes, salsa, and cornstarch to form a sauce. (Mix cornstarch with a little water to dissolve it before adding to pan.) Heat remaining oil in a second sauté pan. In a small bowl combine egg substitute, garlic, celery salt, Worcestershire sauce, cider vinegar, and salt and pepper. Pour into second sauté pan. Cook until almost set. Spoon mushroom mixture onto half of omelette. Fold over and cook for an additional 3 to 5 minutes. Lift with spatula onto serving dish. Top with shredded cheese and serve.

Note: Salsa comes with different levels of heat. Choose one that best fits your family's tastes.

SOUTHWESTERN HAM OMELETTE WITH TACO CHEESE

Servings: 1 Breakfast Entrée (4 blocks)

Block Size:	Ingredients:
2 Protein	½ cup egg substitute
1 Protein	1 ounce low-fat taco-style cheese, shredded
1 Protein	1½ ounces deli-style ham, diced
½ Carbohydrate	½ cup onion, diced
1 Carbohydrate	2¼ cups peppers, chopped
1 Carbohydrate	1¼ cups tomatoes, chopped
½ Carbohydrate	¼ cup salsa*
½ Carbohydrate	¼ cup cooked kidney beans, rinsed
½ Carbohydrate	2 teaspoons cornstarch
4 Fat	1⅓ teaspoons olive oil, divided

Spices:

½ teaspoon garlic, minced
⅛ teaspoon chili powder
1 tablespoon apple cider
½ teaspoon cilantro, chopped
⅛ teaspoon celery salt
Salt and pepper to taste

Method:

In a medium nonstick sauté pan, heat ⅔ teaspoon of oil. Combine onion, peppers, tomato, salsa, kidney beans, cornstarch, and seasonings. (Mix cornstarch with a little water to dissolve it before adding to pan.) Cook for 5 to 8 minutes, stirring occasionally. In a second sauté pan, heat remaining oil. Using a medium bowl, blend egg substitute, ham, and salt and pepper. Pour into pan and stir to distribute ham evenly. Cook until set. Flip omelette over with spatula and cook another 2 minutes. Place omelette on serving plate and spoon pepper mixture onto half of omelette. Fold omelette over and sprinkle with cheese and serve.

Note: Salsa comes with different levels of heat. Choose one that best fits your taste. We used a medium salsa here.

ASPARAGUS OMELETTE WITH CHEESE

Servings: 1 Breakfast Entrée (4 blocks)

Block Size:	Ingredients:
3 Protein	¾ cup egg substitute
1 Protein	1 ounce shredded low-fat cheese
1 Carbohydrate	1 cup pearl onions, frozen
1 Carbohydrate	1¼ cups tomatoes, chopped
1 Carbohydrate	¼ cup cooked kidney beans, rinsed and chopped
1 Carbohydrate	1 cup asparagus spears, chopped
4 Fat	1⅓ teaspoons olive oil, divided

Spices:

1 teaspoon garlic, minced
⅛ teaspoon celery salt
⅛ teaspoon lemon herb seasoning
⅛ teaspoon chili powder
½ teaspoon balsamic vinegar
⅛ teaspoon Worcestershire sauce
Salt and pepper to taste

Method:

In a medium nonstick sauté pan heat ⅔ teaspoon oil. Sauté onion, tomato, beans, asparagus, and seasonings for 5 to 7 minutes. Heat remaining oil in second sauté pan. Pour in egg substitute, spread around pan, and lightly season with salt and pepper. When set, spoon mixture onto half of omelette. Fold over and remove to serving plate. Top with cheese and serve.

BLUEBERRY COTTAGE CHEESE

Servings: 1 Breakfast Entrée (4 blocks)

Block Size:	Ingredients:
3 Protein	¾ cup low-fat cottage cheese
1 Protein and 1 Carbohydrate	½ cup plain low-fat yogurt
1 Carbohydrate	⅓ cup unsweetened applesauce
2 Carbohydrate	1 cup blueberries, fresh or frozen
4 Fat	4 teaspoons slivered almonds

Spices:

¼ teaspoon cinnamon
¼ teaspoon nutmeg

Method:

This recipe requires a blender or food processor. Place blueberries and applesauce, nutmeg and cinnamon in a blender and pulse 2 or 3 times. In a medium bowl, combine blueberry mixture, yogurt, and cottage cheese. Sprinkle with almonds and serve.

STEAK WITH MORNING VEGETABLE MEDLEY

Servings: 1 Breakfast Entrée (4 blocks)

Block Size:	Ingredients:
4 Protein	4 ounces sirloin steak, ¾ inch thick
1 Carbohydrate	1¼ cups tomatoes, chopped
1 Carbohydrate	1 cup pearl onions, frozen
1 Carbohydrate	1 cup green beans
½ Carbohydrate	3 cups fresh spinach*
½ Carbohydrate	¼ cup cooked kidney beans
4 Fat	1⅓ teaspoons olive oil, divided

Spices:

2 teaspoons garlic, minced
¼ teaspoon Worcestershire sauce
⅛ teaspoon celery salt
1 tablespoon cider vinegar
1 teaspoon parsley, chopped
Salt and pepper to taste

Method:

In a medium nonstick sauté pan, heat ⅔ teaspoon oil. Combine all vegetables and seasonings and sauté 5 to 7 minutes until crisp-tender. In a second sauté pan, heat remaining oil and sauté steak until cooked to the desired degree. Place steak on one side of serving dish and vegetables on the other.

*Note: Fresh spinach needs to be cleaned very well, because of its tendency to have sand on it, so be sure to soak spinach in water to remove any sand or dirt before using.

WINTER FRUIT COMPOTE

Servings: 1 Breakfast Entrée (4 blocks)

Block Size:	Ingredients:
4 Protein	1 cup low-fat cottage cheese
1 Carbohydrate	½ grapefruit, in sections
1 Carbohydrate	⅓ cup mandarin orange sections
2 Carbohydrate	1 Granny Smith apple, cored and chopped
4 Fat	4 teaspoons almonds, slivered and toasted

Spices:
⅛ teaspoon cinnamon
⅛ teaspoon nutmeg
Paprika to taste

Method:
In small mixing bowl combine cottage cheese with cinnamon and nutmeg. Mound onto serving dish. Arrange grapefruit and orange sections around cheese. Combine almonds and apple pieces and spoon over cheese. Sprinkle paprika over cheese and serve.

CHICKEN AND CHICKPEA HASH

Servings: 1 Breakfast Entrée (4 blocks)

Block Size:	Ingredients:
4 Protein	6 ounces ground chicken
½ Carbohydrate	1½ cups mushrooms, diced
½ Carbohydrate	½ cup onion, diced
1 Carbohydrate	⅓ cup boiled potato, mashed (without butter or milk)
2 Carbohydrate	½ cup cooked chickpeas, mashed
4 Fat	1⅓ teaspoons olive oil

Spices:

⅛ teaspoon Worcestershire sauce
⅛ teaspoon lemon herb seasoning
⅛ teaspoon chili powder
Paprika for garnish
Parsley for garnish

Method:

In a medium nonstick sauté pan, heat oil. Sauté chicken, onion, and mushrooms until chicken is cooked. Add remaining ingredients (except paprika and parsley) and cook on medium-high heat until browned, about 3 to 5 minutes. Place on a heated serving dish. Garnish with parsley and paprika.

MANDARIN ORANGE COTTAGE CHEESE SCRAMBLE

Servings: 1 Breakfast Entrée (4 blocks)

Block Size:	Ingredients:
1 Protein	¼ cup low-fat cottage cheese
3 Protein	¾ cup egg substitute
½ Carbohydrate	1½ cups mushrooms, sliced
½ Carbohydrate	½ cup onion, chopped
1 Carbohydrate	2¼ cups mixed peppers, cut in half and sliced*
1 Carbohydrate	1 cup snow peas, julienned
1 Carbohydrate	⅓ cup mandarin orange sections
4 Fat	1⅓ teaspoons olive oil

Spices:

1 tablespoon balsamic vinegar
¼ teaspoon Worcestershire sauce
⅛ teaspoon celery salt
¼ teaspoon dried dill
¼ teaspoon lemon herb seasoning

Method:

Heat oil in a medium nonstick sauté pan. Sauté mushrooms, onion, peppers, vinegar, Worcestershire sauce, celery salt, and dill. Cook until the vegetables are crisp-tender, about 5 to 7 minutes. Then pour in the egg substitute and snow peas. Cook, stirring, until set. Remove from heat and stir in cottage cheese and mandarin orange sections. Sprinkle on lemon herb seasoning and serve.

*Note: Equal portions of red, yellow, and green peppers.

ITALIAN SAUSAGE AND APPLE COMPOTE

Servings: 1 Breakfast Entrée (4 blocks)

Block Size:	Ingredients:
4 Protein	8 links Italian soy sausages, chopped
2 Carbohydrate	1 Granny Smith apple, cored and chopped
2 Carbohydrate	⅔ cup unsweetened applesauce
4 Fat	1⅓ teaspoons olive oil

Spices:

1 tablespoon balsamic vinegar
2 tablespoons cider vinegar
⅛ teaspoon celery salt
⅓ cup water
⅛ teaspoon cinnamon

Method:

Heat oil in a medium nonstick sauté pan. Sauté sausage with celery salt and vinegars. Cook until sausage is browned. Add apple and cook until it begins to soften but is still crunchy. Add applesauce, cinnamon, and water; reduce heat, and simmer 2 to 3 minutes. Spoon into bowl and serve.

BERRY OMELETTE

Servings: 1 Breakfast Entrée (4 blocks)

Block Size:	Ingredients:
4 Protein	1 cup egg substitute
1 Carbohydrate	½ nectarine, pitted and chopped
1 Carbohydrate	½ cup blueberries
½ Carbohydrate	½ cup raspberries
½ Carbohydrate	¼ cup seedless grapes
1 Carbohydrate	⅓ cup applesauce
4 Fat	1⅓ teaspoons olive oil

Spices:

⅛ teaspoon celery salt
⅓ cup water
⅛ teaspoon cinnamon
Salt and pepper to taste

Method:

Heat oil in medium nonstick sauté pan. Season egg substitute and pour into pan. Cook until set and flip over with a spatula. Cook an additional minute. Fold omelette onto serving dish and keep warm. Combine fruits, water, and cinnamon in a saucepan, heat until hot, then spoon over omelette and serve.

CILANTRO EGG SALAD

Servings: 1 Breakfast Entrée (4 blocks)

Block Size:

4 Protein

¼ Carbohydrate
½ Carbohydrate
¼ Carbohydrate
1 Carbohydrate
½ Carbohydrate
½ Carbohydrate
1 Carbohydrate

4 Fat

Ingredients:

1 cup egg substitute

¼ cup celery, minced
½ cup canned mushrooms, diced
¼ cup onion, chopped
¼ cup kidney beans
2 cups lettuce
2 cups cucumber, peeled and sliced
1¼ cups tomatoes, diced

4 teaspoons reduced-fat mayonnaise

Spices:

⅛ teaspoon dry mustard
½ teaspoon garlic, minced
⅛ teaspoon cilantro
Salt and pepper to taste

Method:
Pour egg substitute into a 10-ounce microwave-safe dish and cook on high (100 percent) setting for 1 to 2½ minutes, or until set, push cooked egg portions to center of the dish and continue cooking in 30-second intervals on high setting. When done, cool and dice cooked egg substitute. In a small bowl, blend mayonnaise and seasonings. Combine cooked egg substitute with the other ingredients in a medium bowl and toss to coat with mayonnaise and serve.

LUNCH

MEDITERRANEAN BEEF SALAD

Servings: 1 Lunch Entrée (4 blocks)

Block Size:	Ingredients:
4 Protein	4 ounces beef eye of round, ⅛-inch slices, cut in ½-inch pieces
1 Carbohydrate	2¼ cups red and green pepper strips
1 Carbohydrate	1 cup onion, chopped
1 Carbohydrate	1 cup Zoned Mushroom Sauce (see page 708)
1 Carbohydrate	3 cups garden salad mix (lettuce and shredded red cabbage)
4 Fat	1⅓ teaspoons olive oil

Spices:

⅛ teaspoon Worcestershire sauce
⅛ teaspoon red wine
Salt and pepper to taste

Method:

In a nonstick sauté pan, add oil, beef, peppers, onion, Worcestershire sauce, and red wine. Cook until beef is browned and pepper and onions are tender, then add Zoned Mushroom Sauce. Cover and simmer for 5 minutes until mixture is hot, stirring occasionally to blend flavors. On a large oval plate, arrange garden salad mix. Spoon beef and vegetable mixture into the center of plate, on top of garden salad. Sprinkle with salt and pepper and serve immediately.

GERMAN TURKEY SALAD

Servings: 1 Lunch Entrée (4 blocks)

Block Size:	Ingredients:
4 Protein	6 ounces ground turkey
½ Carbohydrate	¾ cup broccoli florets
½ Carbohydrate	1 cup cauliflower florets
1 Carbohydrate	2¼ cups bell pepper strips*
1 Carbohydrate	3 cups shredded cabbage (or coleslaw mix)
1 Carbohydrate	½ cup Zoned French Dressing (see page 717)
4 Fat	1⅓ teaspoons olive oil

Spices:

⅛ teaspoon balsamic vinegar
⅛ teaspoon Worcestershire sauce
1 teaspoon minced garlic
Salt and pepper to taste

Method:

In a nonstick sauté pan, add oil, ground turkey, broccoli, cauliflower, bell pepper strips, balsamic vinegar, Worcestershire sauce, and garlic. Cook until ground turkey is browned and vegetables are tender, then add Zoned French Dressing. Cover and simmer for 5 minutes until mixture is hot, stirring occasionally to blend flavors. On a large oval plate arrange shredded cabbage. Spoon ground turkey and vegetable mixture into the center of plate, on top of the shredded cabbage. Sprinkle with salt and pepper and serve immediately.

Note: Equal portions of red, yellow, and green peppers.

BARBECUE CHICKEN SALAD

Servings: 1 Lunch Entrée (4 blocks)

Block Size:	Ingredients:
4 Protein	4 ounces chicken tenderloin, diced (or skinless chicken breast)
1 Carbohydrate	2¼ cups bell pepper strips
1 Carbohydrate	1 cup onions, diced
1 Carbohydrate	½ cup Zoned Barbecue Sauce (see page 714)
½ Carbohydrate	1½ cups garden salad mix (lettuce and shredded red cabbage)
½ Carbohydrate	1½ cups shredded cabbage (or coleslaw mix)
4 Fat	1⅓ teaspoons olive oil

Spices:

⅛ teaspoon cider vinegar
⅛ teaspoon Worcestershire sauce
1 teaspoon minced garlic
Salt and pepper to taste

Method:

In a nonstick sauté pan, add oil, chicken tenderloins, pepper, onion, vinegar, Worcestershire sauce, and garlic. Cook until chicken is browned and vegetables are tender, then add Zoned Barbecue Sauce. Cover and simmer for 5 minutes until mixture is hot, stirring occasionally to blend flavors. Blend together garden salad mix and shredded cabbage, then place blended salad-cabbage mixture on a large oval plate. Spoon chicken and vegetable mixture into the center of plate on top of salad-cabbage mixture. Sprinkle with salt and pepper and serve immediately.

HERBED SEAFOOD SALAD

Servings: 1 Lunch Entrée (4 blocks)

Block Size:	Ingredients:
2 Protein	3 ounces clams
2 Protein	3 ounces bay scallops
1 Carbohydrate	½ cup Zoned Herb Dressing (see page 706)
½ Carbohydrate	1½ cups shredded cabbage
½ Carbohydrate	1½ cups garden salad mix (lettuce and shredded red cabbage)
½ Carbohydrate	2 cups cucumber, peeled, seeded, and roughly chopped
1 Carbohydrate	2¼ cups bell pepper strips
½ Carbohydrate	½ cup onion, chopped
4 Fat	1⅓ teaspoons olive oil

Spices:

⅛ teaspoon Worcestershire sauce
1 teaspoon dry mustard
⅛ teaspoon white wine

Method:

Heat oil in medium nonstick sauté pan. Add clams, scallops, pepper strips, onion, Worcestershire sauce, mustard, and wine. Sauté until cooked through; add Zoned Herb Dressing. Simmer for 3 to 5 minutes. Combine vegetables in medium bowl. Pour seafood mixture over vegetables.

DILLED CHICKEN GARDEN SALAD

Servings: 1 Lunch Entrée (4 blocks)

Block Size:	Ingredients:
4 Protein	4 ounces chicken tenderloin
1 Carbohydrate	½ cup Zoned Herb Dressing (see page 716)
1 Carbohydrate	1 cup onion, chopped
½ Carbohydrate	2 cups romaine lettuce, torn
½ Carbohydrate	1½ cups garden salad mix (lettuce and shredded red cabbage)
1 Carbohydrate	3 cups mushrooms, sliced
4 Fat	1⅓ teaspoons olive oil

Spices:

⅛ teaspoon Worcestershire sauce
¼ teaspoon lemon herb seasoning
1 tablespoon cider vinegar
1 teaspoon dried dill weed
Salt and pepper to taste

Method:
Heat oil in medium nonstick sauté pan. Add chicken, mushrooms, onion, Worcestershire sauce, lemon and herb seasoning, cider vinegar, dill, and salt and pepper. Sauté until cooked through. Drain off excess liquid. Stir in Zoned Herb Dressing and simmer 3 to 5 minutes. Combine romaine and salad mix in a medium bowl. Top with chicken mixture and serve.

FLORENTINE CRAB SALAD

Servings: 1 Lunch Entrée (4 blocks)

Block Size:	Ingredients:
4 Protein	6 ounces canned crabmeat
½ Carbohydrate	½ cup scallions, sliced (white and green parts)
½ Carbohydrate	1½ cups mushrooms, sliced
1 Carbohydrate	¼ cup cooked kidney beans, rinsed
½ Carbohydrate	2 cups raw spinach, stems removed
½ Carbohydrate	1½ cups shredded cabbage (or coleslaw mix)
1 Carbohydrate	½ cup Zoned Herb Dressing (see page 716)
4 Fat	1⅓ teaspoons olive oil

Spices:

1 tablespoon balsamic vinegar
⅛ teaspoon Worcestershire sauce
⅛ teaspoon celery salt
½ teaspoon garlic, minced
2 teaspoons white Zinfandel wine
⅛ teaspoon chili powder
Pepper to taste

Method:
Heat oil in a medium nonstick sauté pan. Add crab, scallions, mushrooms, kidney beans, vinegar, Worcestershire sauce, celery salt, garlic, wine, chili powder, and pepper. Sauté until cooked through. Stir in Zoned Herb Dressing. Simmer 3 to 5 minutes. In a medium bowl combine spinach and cabbage. Top with crab mixture and serve.

TUNA SALAD WITH CABBAGE

Servings: 1 Lunch Entrée (4 blocks)

Block Size:	**Ingredients:**
4 Protein	4 ounces albacore tuna in water
1 Carbohydrate	½ cup Zoned French Dressing (see page 717)
½ Carbohydrate	1½ cups shredded cabbage (or coleslaw mix)
½ Carbohydrate	1½ cups garden salad mix (lettuce and shredded red cabbage)
1 Carbohydrate	1¼ cups tomato, diced
½ Carbohydrate	1¼ cups celery, chopped
¼ Carbohydrate	¼ cup asparagus, chopped
¼ Carbohydrate	¼ cup scallion, chopped (white and green parts)
2 Fat	6 olives, chopped coarsely
2 Fat	⅔ teaspoon olive oil

Spices:

⅛ teaspoon lemon herb seasoning
⅛ teaspoon chili powder
1 tablespoon cider vinegar

Method:
Combine tuna, tomato, celery, asparagus, scallion, olives, oil, Zoned French Dressing, lemon herb seasoning, chili powder, and vinegar. Arrange garden salad mix and shredded cabbage on a serving plate. Place tuna mixture on top of greens and serve.

HERBED STIR-FRY SCALLOPS WITH MIXED VEGETABLES

Servings: 1 Lunch Entrée (4 blocks)

Block Size:	Ingredients:
4 Protein	6 ounces baby bay scallops
½ Carbohydrate	¾ cup broccoli florets
¾ Carbohydrate	¾ cup green beans
¾ Carbohydrate	¾ cup pearl onions, frozen
½ Carbohydrate	1⅛ cups red pepper strips
½ Carbohydrate	1½ cups mushrooms, sliced
1 Carbohydrate	½ cup Zoned Herb Dressing* (see page 716)
4 Fat	1⅓ teaspoons olive oil, divided

Spices:

2 tablespoons lemon- or lime-flavored spring water

Method:

In a nonstick sauté pan, place ⅔ teaspoon oil, flavored water, and scallops. Cook until scallops are done. While the scallops are cooking over medium heat, in another sauté pan, place vegetables, ⅔ teaspoon oil, and Zoned Herb Dressing. Heat vegetables until entire mixture is hot, then add scallops. Cook for 3 to 4 minutes until entire stir-fry is hot and vegetables and dressing have coated scallops. Spoon onto a lunch dish and serve immediately.

*Note: All the seasonings you need for this dish are in the Zoned Herb Dressing.

SAUTÉED SCALLOPS WITH ARTICHOKE HEARTS

Servings: 1 Lunch Entrée (4 blocks)

Block Size:

4 Protein

2 Carbohydrate
1 Carbohydrate
1 Carbohydrate

4 Fat

Ingredients:

6 ounces baby bay scallops

6 small artichoke hearts, canned*
½ cup salsa**
1 cup Zoned Mushroom Sauce (see page 708)

1⅓ teaspoons olive oil

Spices:

⅛ teaspoon Worcestershire sauce

Method:
Cut artichoke hearts into pieces. Combine with oil and Worcestershire sauce in heated nonstick sauté pan. Heat for 2 to 3 minutes. Add scallops and remaining ingredients and cook on high until the scallops are cooked through.

*Note: 3 small artichoke hearts equal 1 medium artichoke.

**Note: We used a medium-heat salsa, but you can adjust the strength to your family's taste.

SAUTÉED SCALLOPS WITH SPICED PEPPERS AND MUSHROOMS

Servings: 1 Lunch Entrée (4 blocks)

Block Size:	Ingredients:
4 Protein	6 ounces bay scallops
1 Carbohydrate	2¼ cups red and green pepper strips
1 Carbohydrate	¼ cup canned kidney beans, rinsed
1 Carbohydrate	½ cup salsa*
½ Carbohydrate	1½ cups mushrooms, sliced
½ Carbohydrate	2 teaspoons cornstarch
4 Fat	1⅓ teaspoons olive oil

Spices:

1 tablespoon balsamic vinegar
⅛ teaspoon chili powder
⅛ teaspoon hot pepper sauce
⅛ teaspoon ground red pepper

Method:
Heat oil in a nonstick sauté pan and add peppers and salsa. Stir-fry 2 to 3 minutes. Add mushrooms, scallops, kidney beans, spices, and cornstarch. (Mix cornstarch with a little water to dissolve it before adding to pan.) Stir-fry until scallops are cooked through. Just before dish is cooked, add vinegar. Stir and serve.

*Note: We used a medium-heat salsa, but you can adjust the strength to your family's tastes.

FLORENTINE TURKEY SALAD

Servings: 1 Lunch Entrée (4 blocks)

Block Size:	Ingredients:
4 Protein	6 ounces lean ground turkey
½ Carbohydrate	3 cups spinach, chopped*
1 Carbohydrate	½ cup Zoned French Dressing (see page 717)
1½ Carbohydrate	¾ cup salsa**
½ Carbohydrate	1½ cups cabbage, shredded (or coleslaw mix)
½ Carbohydrate	½ cup onion, chopped
4 Fat	1⅓ teaspoons olive oil

Spices:

1 tablespoon cider vinegar
⅛ teaspoon Worcestershire sauce
⅛ teaspoon celery salt
⅛ teaspoon chili powder

Method:
Heat oil in a medium nonstick sauté pan. Add turkey, salsa, onion, vinegar, Worcestershire sauce, celery salt, and chili powder. When turkey is cooked, add Zoned French Dressing. Sauté 3 to 5 minutes. In a medium bowl combine spinach and cabbage. Top with turkey mixture and serve.

*Note: Fresh spinach needs to be cleaned very well, because of sand, so be sure to soak spinach in water to remove any sand or dirt before using.

**Note: We used a medium-heat salsa, but you can adjust the strength to your family's tastes.

CALIFORNIA-STYLE TACOBURGER

Servings: 1 Lunch Entrée (4 blocks)

Block Size:	Ingredients:
4 Protein	6 ounces lean ground turkey
½ Carbohydrate	5½ cups bean sprouts
½ Carbohydrate	1 cup red and green pepper strips
1 Carbohydrate	½ cup salsa*
1 Carbohydrate	½ mini pita pocket (6-inch)
1 Carbohydrate	¼ cup canned kidney beans, rinsed
2 Fat	2 teaspoons almonds, slivered
2 Fat	6 olives, sliced

Spices:

½ teaspoon garlic, minced
¼ teaspoon chili powder, divided
⅛ teaspoon Worcestershire sauce
⅛ teaspoon celery salt
⅛ teaspoon cider vinegar

Method:

Combine the turkey, ⅛ teaspoon chili powder, Worcestershire sauce and 1 cup sprouts and form into patty and bake in a 425-degree Fahrenheit oven for 15 minutes. Mix peppers, salsa, kidney beans, 4½ cups sprouts, and remaining spices. Cook for several minutes, then add vinegar. Add olives and almonds. Stir to blend and heat through. When heated, stuff mini pita with burger and place vegetable mixture on plate and serve.

*Note: We used a medium-heat salsa, but you can adjust the strength to your family's tastes.

ORIENTAL TURKEY WITH SNOW PEAS

Servings: 1 Lunch Entrée (4 blocks)

Block Size:	Ingredients:
4 Protein	6 ounces lean ground turkey
1 Carbohydrate	¾ cup Zoned Espagnol (Brown) Sauce (see page 715)
½ Carbohydrate	5½ cups alfalfa sprouts
1 Carbohydrate	2¼ cups bell pepper strips
½ Carbohydrate	½ cup snow peas
½ Carbohydrate	½ cup pearl onions, frozen
½ Carbohydrate	¾ cup broccoli florets
4 Fat	1⅓ teaspoons olive oil, divided

Spices:

1 teaspoon soy sauce
1 teaspoon Worcestershire sauce
1 tablespoons balsamic vinegar

Method:

In nonstick sauté pan heat ⅔ teaspoon of the olive oil and cook the turkey (breaking it up as it cooks) and alfalfa sprouts. In second non-stick sauté pan, heat remaining olive oil. Sauté peppers, snow peas, onions, broccoli, soy sauce, Worcestershire sauce, and vinegar. Cook until tender, then add Zoned Espagnol Sauce. Blend turkey mixture with vegetables and serve.

STIR-FRY BEEF WITH GREEN BEANS

Servings: 1 Lunch Entrée (4 blocks)

Block Size:	Ingredients:
4 Protein	4 ounces lean beef, small cubes
3 Carbohydrate	3 cups green beans
1 Carbohydrate	½ cup Zoned Tarragon Mustard Sauce (see page 720)
4 Fat	1⅓ teaspoons olive oil, divided

Spices:

¼ teaspoon Worcestershire sauce
½ teaspoon cider vinegar
⅛ teaspoon chili powder
⅛ teaspoon celery salt
⅛ teaspoon tarragon

Method:

Heat ⅔ teaspoon oil in a medium nonstick sauté pan. Add beef and sauté until cooked through. Stir in Zoned Tarragon Mustard Sauce and simmer for 3 to 5 minutes. In second sauté pan, heat remaining oil and sauté green beans, Worcestershire sauce, vinegar, chili powder, celery salt, and tarragon. Cook until beans are crisp-tender, about 5 minutes. Place beans on serving dish and either top with beef mixture or spoon it beside beans.

BEEF ITALIANO

Servings: 1 Lunch Entrée (4 blocks)

Block Size:	Ingredients:
4 Protein	4 ounces lean beef, small cubes
1 Carbohydrate	½ cup Zoned Italian Sauce (see page 710)
1 Carbohydrate	1 cup Italian-style green beans
1 Carbohydrate	2¼ cups red and green pepper strips
½ Carbohydrate	½ cup onion, diced
½ Carbohydrate	¼ cup salsa*
4 Fat	1⅓ teaspoons olive oil, divided

Spices:

½ teaspoon parsley flakes
½ teaspoon Worcestershire sauce
⅛ teaspoon celery salt
⅛ teaspoon lemon herb seasoning
⅛ teaspoon dried oregano

Method:
Heat ⅔ teaspoon oil in a medium nonstick sauté pan. Add beef and sauté until cooked. Add Zoned Italian Sauce and simmer for 3 to 5 minutes. In second nonstick sauté pan, heat remaining oil. Sauté the green beans, pepper strips, onion, salsa, parsley, Worcestershire sauce, celery salt, lemon herb seasoning, and oregano. Cook until crisp-tender, about 5 minutes. Spoon vegetables onto serving dish and top with beef mixture.

*Note: We used a medium-heat salsa. Use whatever strength you prefer.

SCALLOPS ROMA

Servings: 1 Lunch Entrée (4 blocks)

Block Size:	Ingredients:
4 Protein	6 ounces bay scallops
1 Carbohydrate	3 cups mushrooms, sliced
1½ Carbohydrate	1½ cups asparagus, cuts and tips
½ Carbohydrate	½ cup onion, chopped
1 Carbohydrate	½ cup Zoned Italian Sauce (see page 710)
4 Fat	1⅓ teaspoons olive oil, divided

Spices:

½ teaspoon dried dill
⅛ teaspoon lemon herb seasoning
⅛ teaspoon celery salt
⅛ teaspoon dried oregano
Pepper to taste

Method:

Heat ⅔ teaspoon oil in a medium nonstick sauté pan. Sauté scallops until cooked through. Stir in Zoned Italian Sauce and simmer 3 to 5 minutes. In second nonstick sauté pan, heat remaining oil and add mushrooms, asparagus, onion, dill, lemon herb seasoning, pepper, celery salt, and oregano. Cook until crisp-tender, about 5 minutes. Place vegetables on serving plate and top with scallop mixture.

SPICED PEPPER STEAK

Servings: 1 Lunch Entrée (4 blocks)

Block Size:	Ingredients:
4 Protein	4 ounces lean beef, thinly sliced
1 Carbohydrate	3 cups mushrooms, sliced
1 Carbohydrate	½ cup Zoned Herb Dressing (see page 716)
1 Carbohydrate	2¼ cups red and green pepper strips
1 Carbohydrate	1 cup onion, sliced
4 Fat	1⅓ teaspoons olive oil

Spices:

⅛ teaspoon Worcestershire sauce
2 tablespoons cider vinegar
⅛ teaspoon garlic powder

Method:
Heat oil in medium nonstick sauté pan. Sprinkle garlic powder onto beef. Sauté beef until cooked. Deglaze pan with Worcestershire sauce and vinegar. Add vegetables and stir-fry 5 to 7 minutes. Combine beef and vegetables in medium bowl and add Zoned Herb Dressing. Toss to coat. Spoon onto plate and serve.

BEEF AND VEGETABLE CASSEROLE

Servings: 1 Lunch Entrée (4 blocks)

Block Size:	Ingredients:
4 Protein	4 ounces lean beef, diced
½ Carbohydrate	1½ cups cabbage, shredded (or coleslaw mix)
½ Carbohydrate	1½ cups mushrooms, sliced
½ Carbohydrate	¼ cup carrots, sliced
½ Carbohydrate	2 teaspoons cornstarch
1 Carbohydrate	1½ cups tomato, chopped
1 Carbohydrate	1 cup onion, chopped
4 Fat	1⅓ teaspoons olive oil

Spices:

2 tablespoons balsamic vinegar
½ teaspoon garlic, minced
⅛ teaspoon celery salt
¼ teaspoon dried cilantro
1 tablespoon Worcestershire sauce
3 tablespoons lime-flavored water

Method:

In a large nonstick sauté pan, lightly sauté beef in hot oil until just browned. Deglaze the pan with vinegar, Worcestershire sauce, and water. Combine all ingredients (except tomato, cornstarch, and cilantro) in pan and cook until tender. Stir in tomatoes and cornstarch and cook, stirring, for 3 to 5 minutes, until tomatoes are heated through and liquid thickens. (Mix cornstarch with a little water to dissolve it before adding to pan.) Spoon onto serving casserole. Sprinkle with cilantro and serve.

ITALIAN-STYLE PORK CUTLET

Servings: 1 Lunch Entrée (4 blocks)

Block Size:	Ingredients:
3 Protein	3 ounces pork cutlet
1 Protein	1 ounce skim milk mozzarella, shredded
1 Carbohydrate	½ cup Zoned Italian Sauce (see page 710)
½ Carbohydrate	1½ cups mushrooms, sliced
1 Carbohydrate	1 cup onion, chopped
1 Carbohydrate	1 cup Italian-style green beans
½ Carbohydrate	½ cup broccoli florets
4 Fat	1⅓ teaspoons olive oil, divided

Spices:

1 tablespoon dry red wine
¼ teaspoon dried oregano
½ teaspoon Worcestershire sauce
⅛ teaspoon dried rosemary
1 tablespoon lemon-flavored water
½ teaspoon garlic, minced
Dash ground thyme
Salt and pepper to taste

Method:
Place cutlet between two pieces of plastic wrap. Pound with a meat mallet until ⅛-inch thick. Heat 1 teaspoon oil in nonstick sauté pan over medium-high heat. Place cutlet in pan and sauté until done. Add Zoned Italian Sauce and simmer 3 to 5 minutes. In second nonstick sauté pan heat remaining oil. Sauté mushrooms, onion, beans, broccoli, wine, oregano, Worcestershire sauce, rosemary, thyme, water, garlic, and salt and pepper. Simmer mixture for 3 to 5 minutes. Spoon vegetables onto serving plate, top with cutlet, sprinkle with cheese, and serve.

TEX-MEX BEEF STIR-FRY

Servings: 1 Lunch Entrée (4 blocks)

Block Size:	Ingredients:
3 Protein	3 ounces lean beef, diced
1 Protein	1 ounce taco cheese, shredded
1 Carbohydrate	1¼ cup tomatoes, chopped
1 Carbohydrate	½ cup salsa*
1 Carbohydrate	¼ cup black beans, rinsed
1 Carbohydrate	2¼ cups red bell pepper strips
4 Fat	1⅓ teaspoons olive oil

Spices:

1 teaspoon chili powder or to taste
½ teaspoon garlic, minced
⅛ teaspoon ground cumin
¼ teaspoon ground red pepper (or
   ⅛ teaspoon hot pepper sauce)
1 tablespoon lemon-flavored water

Method:
In nonstick sauté pan heat oil over medium-high heat. Add beef and stir-fry 2 to 3 minutes. Stir in tomatoes, salsa, black beans, peppers, chili powder, garlic, cumin, red pepper, and water. Simmer until vegetables are tender, about 3 to 5 minutes. Spoon into serving bowl and top with cheese.

*Note: Salsa comes with different levels of heat. Choose one that best fits your family's tastes.

BARBECUE TURKEY TIPS WITH SPINACH SALAD

Servings: 1 Lunch Entrée (4 blocks)

Block Size:	Ingredients:
4 Protein	4 ounces turkey breast, 1-inch cubes
1 Carbohydrate	½ cup Zoned Barbecue Sauce (see page 714)
1 Carbohydrate	½ cup salsa*
½ Carbohydrate	½ cup onion, chopped
1 Carbohydrate	¼ cup chickpeas, rinsed and chopped
½ Carbohydrate	3 cups fresh spinach
4 Fat	1⅓ teaspoons olive oil

Method:

In a medium nonstick sauté pan, heat oil. Add turkey and sauté until cooked through. Blend in Zoned Barbecue Sauce, salsa, and onion. Simmer for 3 to 5 minutes. Arrange spinach on serving plate. Sprinkle spinach with chickpeas. Top spinach with turkey mixture and serve.

*Note: We used medium-heat salsa. Use whatever strength you prefer.

NATIVE AMERICAN CHICKEN WITH VEGETABLES

Servings: 1 Lunch Entrée (4 blocks)

Block Size:	Ingredients:
4 Protein	4 ounces chicken tenderloins, diced
1 Carbohydrate	¼ cup frozen corn kernels
½ Carbohydrate	½ cup onion, diced
1 Carbohydrate	¼ cup cooked black beans, rinsed
½ Carbohydrate	1½ cups mushrooms, sliced
1 Carbohydrate	1 cup whole green beans
4 Fat	1⅓ teaspoons olive oil, divided

Spices:

¼ teaspoon lemon herb seasoning
½ teaspoon Worcestershire sauce
⅛ teaspoon celery seed
½ teaspoon garlic, minced
Salt and pepper to taste

Method:

In a medium nonstick sauté pan, heat ⅔ teaspoon oil. Add chicken and lemon herb seasoning. Sauté until cooked through. In second nonstick sauté pan, heat remaining oil and sauté the corn, onion, black beans, mushrooms, green beans, Worcestershire sauce, celery seed, garlic, and salt and pepper. Cook until vegetables are crisp-tender. Blend chicken with vegetables and serve.

TACO BURGER

Servings: 1 Lunch Entrée (4 blocks)

Block Size:	Ingredients:
1 Protein	1 ounce low-fat jack cheese, shredded
3 Protein	4½ ounces lean (90 percent fat free) ground beef
1 Carbohydrate	1 taco shell, in pieces
1 Carbohydrate	½ cup salsa, divided*
½ Carbohydrate	2 cups lettuce, shredded
1 Carbohydrate	¼ cup cooked black beans, rinsed
½ Carbohydrate	½ cup onion, chopped
4 Fat	1⅓ teaspoons olive oil, divided

Spices:

½ teaspoon garlic, minced
½ teaspoon Worcestershire sauce
⅛ teaspoon celery salt
1 tablespoon lemon- or lime-flavored spring water

Method:
In a small bowl, combine ground beef and ¼ cup salsa. Form into a patty. Heat ⅔ teaspoon oil in a medium nonstick sauté pan and sauté patty until cooked through. In a second nonstick sauté pan, heat remaining oil. Place beans, garlic, ¼ cup salsa, onion, Worcestershire sauce, celery salt, and water in second sauté pan. Cook until heated through. Layer lettuce onto plate. Add patty, sprinkle with taco pieces, and top with bean mixture and cheese.

*Note: We used medium-heat salsa. Use whatever strength you prefer.

PORK AND VEGETABLE POCKET SANDWICH

Servings: 1 Lunch Entrée (4 blocks)

Block Size:	Ingredients:
3 Protein	3 ounces pork cutlet, finely sliced
1 Protein	1 ounce low-fat cheddar cheese, shredded
1 Carbohydrate	½ mini pita pocket
¼ Carbohydrate	¼ cup onion, chopped
¼ Carbohydrate	¼ cup asparagus pieces
¼ Carbohydrate	¾ cup bean sprouts
¼ Carbohydrate	½ tomato, sliced
½ Carbohydrate	¼ cup blueberries
½ Carbohydrate	½ cup raspberries
1 Carbohydrate	¾ cup cantaloupe cubes
1 Fat	1 teaspoon almonds, sliced
3 Fat	1 teaspoon olive oil

Spices:

½ teaspoon garlic, minced
1 teaspoon soy sauce
Dash celery salt
Dash lemon herb seasoning

Method:

Heat oil in medium nonstick sauté pan. Stir-fry pork until lightly browned. Add onion, asparagus, sprouts, garlic, soy sauce, celery salt, and lemon herb seasoning. Cook until asparagus is tender. Stir cheese into pork and blend it in as it melts. Place tomato slices in pita pocket. Spoon in pork mixture and place on serving plate. In a dessert bowl combine melon, berries, and almonds.

ORANGE HERBED CHICKEN STEW

Servings: 1 Lunch Entrée (4 blocks)

Block Size:	Ingredients:
4 Protein	4 ounces chicken tenderloin, diced
1 Carbohydrate	⅓ cup orange juice
2 Carbohydrate	⅔ cup mandarin orange slices
1 Carbohydrate	3 cups mushrooms, sliced
4 Fat	1⅓ teaspoons olive oil, divided

Spices:

1 tablespoon cider vinegar
1 tablespoon parsley, chopped
½ teaspoon garlic, chopped
½ teaspoon pure orange extract
Salt and pepper to taste

Method:

In a medium nonstick sauté pan, heat ⅔ teaspoon oil. Add chicken, vinegar, parsley, garlic, and salt and pepper. In a second nonstick sauté pan heat remaining oil and sauté mushrooms until they soften. Add orange juice, orange slices, and orange extract to the first pan and simmer for 3 minutes. Place mushrooms in a serving bowl and top with chicken mixture.

MARYLAND-STYLE SEAFOOD CHOWDER

Servings: 1 Lunch Entrée (4 blocks)

Block Size:	Ingredients:
1½ Protein	2¼ ounces medium shrimp, large dice*
1½ Protein	2¼ ounces scallops, large dice
1 Protein and 1 Carbohydrate	1 cup 1 percent milk
½ Carbohydrate	½ cup onions, diced
½ Carbohydrate	1 cup celery, diced
½ Carbohydrate	¼ cup water chestnuts, diced
1 Carbohydrate	1¼ cups tomato, chopped
½ Carbohydrate	2 teaspoons cornstarch
4 Fat	1⅓ teaspoons olive oil

Spices:

1 teaspoon garlic, minced
1 cup chicken stock
1 tablespoon parsley
1 tablespoon cilantro
½ teaspoon Worcestershire sauce
Dash hot pepper sauce

Method:
In a medium nonstick sauté pan add oil, onions, water chestnuts, celery, parsley, cilantro, Worcestershire sauce, and hot pepper sauce. Cook until onion and celery are tender, then add shrimp, scallops, and garlic. Cook an additional 3 to 5 minutes, until shrimp are pink and scallops are opaque. Transfer to medium saucepan. Stir in tomato and chicken stock. Bring to a boil, reduce heat, cover and simmer for 7 minutes. Add milk and continue to simmer for 3 minutes. Dissolve

cornstarch in a little of the stock from the pot. Pour into saucepan and continue cooking, stirring frequently, until stock thickens.

Note: Shelled and deveined.

GRILLED SHRIMP SALAD

Servings: 1 Lunch Entrée (4 blocks)

Block Size:	Ingredients:
4 Protein	6 ounces raw shrimp*
½ Carbohydrate	1½ cups green cabbage, shredded
½ Carbohydrate	1½ cups red cabbage, shredded
1 Carbohydrate	1¼ cups chopped tomatoes
½ Carbohydrate	1¼ cups red pepper strips
½ Carbohydrate	1 cup green pepper strips
1 Carbohydrate	¼ cup chickpeas, rinsed
4 Fat	1⅓ teaspoons olive oil, divided

Spices:

½ teaspoon paprika
¼ teaspoon ground coriander
1 teaspoon garlic, minced, divided
1 tablespoon cider vinegar
1 tablespoon fresh parsley
1 tablespoon fresh basil, chopped
Dash cayenne pepper
Salt and pepper to taste

Method:
In a medium nonstick sauté pan add ⅓ teaspoon oil, paprika, coriander, cayenne, parsley, basil, and ½ teaspoon garlic. Heat spices on medium-high heat for 1 minute, then stir in shrimp and coat with seasonings. Stir-fry shrimp in spices until shrimp are pink. In a salad bowl combine

cabbage, tomatoes, peppers, and chickpeas. In small bowl whisk 1 teaspoon oil, vinegar, and remaining garlic. Pour over vegetables and gently toss to coat. Arrange on serving plate and top with shrimp.

Note: Shelled and deveined.

HAWAIIAN-STYLE FILLET OF SOLE SALAD

Servings: 1 Lunch Entrée (4 blocks)

Block Size:	Ingredients:
4 Protein	6 ounce fillet of sole
½ Carbohydrate	3 cups lettuce, shredded
½ Carbohydrate	1½ cups bean sprouts
1 Carbohydrate	2¼ cups red and green pepper strips
½ Carbohydrate	¼ cup carrots, shredded
1½ Carbohydrate	¾ cup pineapple, diced
4 Fat	1⅓ teaspoons olive oil, divided

Spices:

4 teaspoons soy sauce
2 teaspoons garlic, minced, divided
1 tablespoon cilantro
⅛ teaspoon lemon herb seasoning
2 tablespoons scallions, finely diced (for garnish)
2 tablespoons hot chili peppers, finely diced (for garnish)

Method:
In a small nonstick sauté pan, heat ⅓ teaspoon oil. Add 1 teaspoon garlic and cook for 1 minute. Sauté sole in same pan, 2 to 3 minutes per side, until it flakes easily. In salad bowl combine lettuce, sprouts,

peppers, carrots, and pineapple. In a small bowl whisk together remaining oil, garlic, and soy sauce. Pour over vegetables and toss to coat. Flake sole and add to salad. Sprinkle with chopped lemon herb seasoning, scallions, chili peppers, and cilantro.

GARDEN SALAD TOPPED WITH SAUTÉED SCALLOPS AND BACON

Servings: 1 Lunch Entrée (4 blocks)

Block Size:	Ingredients:
1 Protein	1 ounce Canadian bacon, diced
3 Protein	4½ ounces bay scallops
½ Carbohydrate	3 cups lettuce, shredded
1 Carbohydrate	⅓ cup mandarin oranges
½ Carbohydrate	½ cup red onion, diced
1 Carbohydrate	¼ cup kidney beans, rinsed
1 Carbohydrate	¼ cup chickpeas, rinsed
4 Fat	1⅓ teaspoons olive oil, divided

Spices:

1 tablespoon cider vinegar, divided
½ teaspoon fresh mint, chopped
½ teaspoon fresh gingerroot, grated, divided
¼ cup chicken stock

Method:
Heat ⅓ teaspoon oil in medium nonstick sauté pan. Sauté bacon, scallops, 1 teaspoon vinegar, and ¼ teaspoon ginger for 4 minutes on medium-high heat. In a small bowl whisk together remaining oil, mint, ¼ teaspoon ginger, 2 teaspoons vinegar, and chicken stock. Combine remaining ingredients in a salad bowl. Add bacon and scallops. Pour in dressing and toss to coat.

CHINESE SEAFOOD SALAD

Servings: 1 Lunch Entrée (4 blocks)

Block Size:

Ingredients:

1 Protein
1½ ounces small cooked shrimp*

1 Protein
1½ ounces cooked bay scallops

1 Protein
1½ ounces canned salmon, flaked

1 Protein and
½ cup plain low-fat yogurt
1 Carbohydrate

½ Carbohydrate
½ cup scallions, thinly sliced

½ Carbohydrate
3 cups lettuce, shredded

½ Carbohydrate
½ cup tomatoes, diced

½ Carbohydrate
½ cucumber, grated

½ Carbohydrate
1 cup red and green pepper strips

¼ Carbohydrate
½ cup radishes, grated

¼ Carbohydrate
¼ cup snow peas, diced

4 Fat
4 teaspoons light mayonnaise

Spices:

⅛ teaspoon cayenne pepper
1 tablespoon cilantro
⅛ teaspoon dill
Lemon herb seasoning
Dash hot pepper sauce

Method:
In a medium bowl blend shrimp, scallops, salmon, scallions, light mayonnaise, dill, and hot pepper sauce. In second bowl mix together the yogurt, radishes, cucumber, cayenne, and cilantro. Combine yogurt dressing with lettuce, tomatoes, peppers, and snow peas. Top with seafood mixture, sprinkle with lemon herb seasoning, and serve.

*Note: Shelled and deveined.

SMOKED MACKEREL WITH RADISH AND ENDIVE

Servings: 1 Lunch Entrée (4 blocks)

Block Size:	Ingredients:
4 Protein	6 ounces smoked mackerel
½ Carbohydrate	1¼ cups radishes, sliced
½ Carbohydrate	1 cup red and green pepper strips
1 Carbohydrate	½ cup Zoned Herb Dressing (see page 716)
½ Carbohydrate	½ cup red onions, diced
1 Carbohydrate	½ Granny Smith apple, diced
½ Carbohydrate	3½ cups Belgian endive, chopped
4 Fat	1⅓ teaspoons olive oil

Spices:

2 teaspoons cider vinegar
Horseradish, grated (bottled or fresh
to taste)
⅛ teaspoon dill
⅛ teaspoon dry mustard
Salt and pepper to taste

Method:

Combine mackerel, radishes, peppers, onion, apple, and endive in a medium salad bowl. In a blender combine oil, vinegar, horseradish, Zoned Herb Dressing, herbs, and salt and pepper. Pulse until well mixed. Pour over salad and toss gently to coat.

CURRIED TURKEY WITH LENTIL SALAD

Servings: 1 Lunch Entrée (4 blocks)

Block Size:	Ingredients:
3 Protein	4½ ounces deli-style turkey breast, finely chopped
1 Protein and 1 Carbohydrate	½ cup plain low-fat yogurt
1 Carbohydrate	¼ cup lentils, cooked
½ Carbohydrate	1 cup celery, chopped
½ Carbohydrate	½ cup red onion, sliced thinly
¼ Carbohydrate	1½ cups lettuce
¼ Carbohydrate	1½ cups romaine lettuce
¼ Carbohydrate	¾ cup bean sprouts
¼ Carbohydrate	1¼ cups escarole
4 Fat	6 teaspoons slivered almonds

Spices:

⅛ teaspoon curry
⅛ teaspoon cumin
⅛ teaspoon turmeric
⅛ teaspoon coriander
⅛ teaspoon cayenne pepper

Method:
In a medium bowl, combine turkey, yogurt, lentils, and spices. In a salad bowl, combine celery, onion, lettuce, romaine, sprouts, and escarole. Pour on yogurt mixture. Toss to coat and sprinkle with almonds.

GRILLED TURKEY SALAD WITH MANDARIN ORANGES

Servings: 1 Lunch Entrée (4 blocks)

Block Size:	Ingredients:
4 Protein	4 ounces turkey breast
½ Carbohydrate	1 cup celery, finely sliced
½ Carbohydrate	½ cup red onion, finely sliced
¼ Carbohydrate	1½ cups lettuce
¼ Carbohydrate	1½ cups romaine lettuce
1 Carbohydrate	½ cup Zoned French Dressing (see page 717)
1 Carbohydrate	⅓ cup mandarin oranges
½ Carbohydrate	½ peach, diced
4 Fat	1⅓ teaspoons olive oil, divided

Spices:

⅛ teaspoon turmeric
1 tablespoon fresh mint, chopped

Method:
Heat ⅓ teaspoon oil in a small sauté pan. Add turkey and stir-fry until cooked through. In a salad bowl, combine turkey, celery, onion, 1 teaspoon oil, Zoned French Dressing, peach, oranges, turmeric, and mint. Toss lightly to coat. On a lunch plate place lettuce, and top with turkey mixture and serve.

MEDITERRANEAN CHICKEN SALAD WITH ARTICHOKE HEARTS

Servings: 1 Lunch Entrée (4 blocks)

Block Size:	Ingredients:
4 Protein	4 ounces chicken tenderloin, coarsely chopped
1 Carbohydrate	3 small artichoke hearts, chopped*
½ Carbohydrate	½ cup asparagus, 1-inch pieces
¼ Carbohydrate	¼ cup onion, chopped
½ Carbohydrate	1 cup red pepper, chopped
¼ Carbohydrate	½ cup celery, sliced
½ Carbohydrate	½ cup tomatoes, chopped
½ Carbohydrate	¼ cup chickpeas
¼ Carbohydrate	¾ cup lettuce, torn
¼ Carbohydrate	¾ cup romaine lettuce, torn
4 Fat	1⅓ teaspoons olive oil, divided

Spices:

1 tablespoon capers, chopped
1 teaspoon garlic, minced
1 tablespoon balsamic vinegar
1 tablespoon fresh basil, chopped
1 tablespoon fresh parsley, chopped
⅛ teaspoon chili powder
Salt and pepper to taste

Method:
In a medium nonstick sauté pan, sauté chicken in ⅓ teaspoon oil. Place remaining oil, capers, garlic, vinegar, and herbs and spices in a small bowl. Whisk to blend. In medium bowl combine artichokes, asparagus, onion, pepper, celery, and chicken. In a salad bowl combine

the lettuce, romaine, chickpeas, and tomato. Pour dressing over salad and toss gently to coat. Top with chicken mixture and serve.

Note: 3 small artichoke hearts equal 1 medium artichoke.

STIR-FRY CHICKEN AND SNOW PEAS

Servings: 1 Lunch Entrée (4 blocks)

Block Size:	Ingredients:
4 Protein	4 ounces chicken tenderloin
½ Carbohydrate	3 cups spinach
1 Carbohydrate	¼ cup white kidney beans
½ Carbohydrate	1½ cups mushrooms, sliced
1 Carbohydrate	1 cup snow peas
½ Carbohydrate	1½ cups bean sprouts
½ Carbohydrate	½ cup scallions, sliced
4 Fat	1⅓ teaspoons olive oil

Spices:

½ cup chicken stock
2 teaspoons soy sauce
1 teaspoon cider vinegar
2 teaspoons Chinese five-spice
  powder
Hot pepper sauce to taste

Method:
Using a nonstick sauté pan, stir-fry chicken in hot chicken stock for 2 minutes. Add mushrooms and cook 3 minutes. Stir in kidney beans, snow peas, sprouts, and scallions. Cook 2 minutes more. In a small bowl mix oil, soy sauce, vinegar, five-spice powder, and hot sauce. Whisk to blend. In a salad bowl combine spinach, chicken, and vegetables (use slotted spoon to remove from sauté pan). Pour dressing over salad and toss to coat.

GRILLED PORK WITH LENTIL SALAD

Servings: 1 Lunch Entrée (4 blocks)

Block Size:	Ingredients:
3½ Protein	3½ ounces lean pork
½ Protein and	
½ Carbohydrate	¼ cup plain low-fat yogurt
1 Carbohydrate	¼ cup lentils, cooked
½ Carbohydrate	½ cup carrot, shredded
¼ Carbohydrate	½ cup celery, sliced
¼ Carbohydrate	¼ cup red onion, sliced thinly
1 Carbohydrate	⅓ cup mandarin orange sections
¼ Carbohydrate	1 cup romaine lettuce
¼ Carbohydrate	1¼ cups escarole
4 Fat	1⅓ teaspoons olive oil, divided

Spices:

1 teaspoon garlic, minced, divided
½ teaspoon dried oregano
⅛ teaspoon curry powder
1 tablespoon cilantro
½ teaspoon Worcestershire sauce
¼ teaspoon cumin
1 tablespoon cider vinegar
Salt and pepper to taste

Method:

In a medium nonstick sauté pan, heat 1 teaspoon oil. Blend in the curry powder, orange sections, vinegar, ½ teaspoon garlic, oregano, and salt and pepper. Add pork and cook until pork is cooked through. In a small bowl mix yogurt, remaining oil, garlic, cilantro, Worcestershire sauce, and cumin. Place the lettuce, escarole, onion, lentils, carrot, and celery in a salad bowl. Add yogurt mixture and toss to coat. Place salad mixture on a serving plate, top with pork mixture, and serve.

TOMATO BASIL SALAD

Servings: 1 Lunch Entrée (4 blocks)

Block Size:	Ingredients:
4 Protein	4 ounces skim milk mozzarella cheese, shredded
1 Carbohydrate	1¼ cups tomatoes, sliced
1 Carbohydrate	¼ cup chickpeas, rinsed and finely chopped
1 Carbohydrate	4 cups romaine lettuce, chopped
½ Carbohydrate	¼ cup Zoned Herb Dressing (see page 716)
½ Carbohydrate	¼ cup salsa*
4 Fat	1⅓ teaspoons olive oil

Spices:

1 tablespoon red wine vinegar
2 tablespoons fresh basil, chopped
1 tablespoon fresh parsley, chopped
1 teaspoon garlic, minced
¼ teaspoon chili powder

Method:

In a medium bowl combine lettuce, salsa, and Zoned Herb Dressing, then form into a bed on a serving plate. In a second bowl, blend chickpeas, parsley, oil, vinegar, basil, garlic, and chili powder. Alternate slices of tomato and shredded mozzarella on lettuce bed. Pour chickpea dressing over tomatoes and serve.

*Note: We used a medium-heat salsa. Use whatever strength you prefer.

GINGER-GARLIC STIR-FRY

Servings: 1 Lunch Entrée (4 blocks)

Block Size:	Ingredients:
4 Protein	12 ounces extra-firm tofu, ½-inch cubes
1 Carbohydrate	2 cups broccoli florets
½ Carbohydrate	½ cup asparagus spears
½ Carbohydrate	½ cup red onion, thinly sliced
½ Carbohydrate	½ cup scallions, sliced
½ Carbohydrate	1 cup celery, sliced
1 Carbohydrate	⅓ cup water chestnuts, sliced
4 Fat	1⅓ teaspoons olive oil, divided

Spices:

2 teaspoons garlic, minced (or to taste)
1 tablespoon cider vinegar
½ teaspoon Chinese five-spice powder
½ teaspoon Worcestershire sauce
⅛ teaspoon celery salt
2 teaspoons fresh gingerroot, minced
1 tablespoon soy sauce
Salt and pepper to taste

Method:

Heat ⅔ teaspoon oil in medium nonstick sauté pan. When hot, add Worcestershire sauce, celery salt, and tofu. Stir-fry until tofu is browned and crusted on all sides. In second nonstick sauté pan heat remaining oil. Add in broccoli, asparagus, onion, celery, scallions, water chestnuts, garlic, vinegar, five-spice powder, gingerroot, soy sauce, and salt and pepper. Stir-fry until vegetables are crisp-tender, about 5 minutes. Place vegetables on serving plate and top with tofu.

SAUTÉED GREEN BEANS WITH TOFU

Servings: 1 Lunch Entrée (4 blocks)

Block Size:	Ingredients:
4 Protein	12 ounces extra-firm tofu, 1-inch cubes
3 Carbohydrate	3 cups green beans, 2-inch pieces
1 Carbohydrate	1 cup onion, chopped
4 Fat	1⅓ teaspoons olive oil, divided

Spices:

½ teaspoon garlic, minced
½ teaspoon Worcestershire sauce
⅛ teaspoon celery salt
2 teaspoons cider vinegar
⅛ teaspoon nutmeg
⅛ teaspoon cinnamon
⅛ teaspoon lemon herb seasoning
⅛ teaspoon ground double superfine mustard
½ teaspoon soy sauce
Salt and pepper to taste

Method:
Heat ⅔ teaspoon oil in medium nonstick sauté pan. Blend in Worcestershire sauce, celery salt, and tofu. Stir-fry tofu until browned and crusted on all sides. In a second nonstick sauté pan, heat remaining oil and add in green beans, onion, garlic, vinegar, nutmeg, cinnamon, lemon herb seasoning, mustard, soy sauce, and salt and pepper. Cook until beans are crisp-tender. Place beans on serving plate and top with tofu.

MUSTARD-GLAZED BRUSSELS SPROUTS WITH TOFU

Servings: 1 Lunch Entrée (4 blocks)

Block Size:	Ingredients:
4 Protein	12 ounces extra-firm tofu, ½-inch dice
2 Carbohydrate	3 cups brussels sprouts, frozen
1 Carbohydrate	1 cup red onion, chopped
1 Carbohydrate	½ cup Zoned Tarragon Mustard Sauce (see page 720)
4 Fat	1⅓ teaspoons olive oil, divided

Spices:

1 teaspoon garlic, minced
½ teaspoon Worcestershire sauce
⅛ teaspoon celery salt
Salt and pepper to taste

Method:

Heat ⅔ teaspoon oil in a medium nonstick sauté pan. Blend in Worcestershire sauce, celery salt, and tofu. Stir-fry until browned and crusted on all sides. In a medium saucepan cook brussels sprouts according to package directions. Remove from pan and drain. In a second nonstick sauté pan, heat remaining oil and garlic. Stir in sprouts, Zoned Tarragon Mustard Sauce, and onion. Stir-fry until onion is tender. Place sprout mixture on serving plate and top with tofu.

CITRUS TOFU SALAD

Servings: 1 Lunch Entrée (4 blocks)

Block Size:	Ingredients:
4 Protein	12 ounces extra-firm tofu, ½-inch dice
1 Carbohydrate	1 cup asparagus spears, 1-inch pieces
½ Carbohydrate	1 cup celery, sliced
½ Carbohydrate	1½ cups romaine lettuce
2 Carbohydrate	⅔ cup mandarin orange segments
4 Fat	1⅓ teaspoons olive oil, divided

Spices:

½ teaspoon garlic, minced
Dash hot pepper sauce
½ teaspoon paprika
⅛ teaspoon lemon herb seasoning
½ teaspoon Worcestershire sauce
⅛ teaspoon celery salt
½ teaspoon dried dill
Salt and pepper to taste

Method:

In a medium nonstick sauté pan, heat ⅔ teaspoon oil. Blend in Worcestershire sauce, celery salt, and tofu. Stir-fry until browned and crusted on all sides. In a second nonstick sauté pan, heat remaining oil and stir-fry the asparagus, celery, garlic, hot pepper sauce, paprika, lemon herb seasoning, dill, and salt and pepper until vegetables are crisp-tender. Place lettuce on serving plate. Distribute orange segments over lettuce. Top first with vegetable mixture, then with tofu.

CANADIAN-STYLE SPINACH SALAD

Servings: 1 Lunch Entrée (4 blocks)

Block Size:	Ingredients:
4 Protein	4 ounces Canadian bacon, diced
½ Carbohydrate	3 cups spinach*
1 Carbohydrate	1 cup canned mushrooms, sliced
½ Carbohydrate	½ cup scallions, sliced (white and green parts)
1 Carbohydrate	½ cup Zoned Herb Dressing (see page 716)
1 Carbohydrate	½ Granny Smith apple, cored and chopped
4 Fat	1⅓ teaspoons olive oil, divided

Spices:

2 teaspoons balsamic vinegar
½ teaspoon Dijon mustard
Salt and pepper to taste

Method:
In a nonstick sauté pan, heat ⅓ teaspoon oil. Lightly brown the Canadian bacon in the oil. Blend 1 teaspoon oil, balsamic vinegar, mustard, and salt and pepper into the Zoned Herb Dressing. Combine spinach, mushrooms, scallions, apple, and bacon in serving bowl. Add dressing, toss to coat, and serve.

*Note: Fresh spinach needs to be cleaned very well, because of its tendency to have sand in it, so be sure to soak spinach in water to remove any sand or dirt before using.

GRILLED SOLE WITH LEEKS

Servings: 1 Lunch Entrée (4 blocks)

Block Size:	Ingredients:
4 Protein	6 ounces fillet of sole
3 Carbohydrate	3 cups leeks, sliced
1 Carbohydrate	4 ounces Johannesburg Riesling
4 Fat	1⅓ teaspoons olive oil, divided

Spices:

1 teaspoon garlic, minced
1 shallot, minced*
½ teaspoon lemon herb seasoning
1 teaspoon dill
Salt and pepper to taste

Method:
Brush a medium baking dish with oil. Layer bottom of dish with leeks. Place sole on top. In a medium bowl combine wine, garlic, shallot, dill, and salt and pepper. Gently pour wine mixture into baking dish. Sprinkle with lemon herb seasoning. Tightly cover baking dish and place in a preheated 375 degree Fahrenheit oven. Bake for 25 to 30 minutes and serve.

*Note: Shallots are available in most supermarkets and have a purple-white appearance. Shallots provide dishes with both an onion and garlic flavor.

FRUIT SALAD WITH PEPPER RELISH

Servings: 1 Lunch Entrée (4 blocks)

Block Size:	Ingredients:
4 Protein	1 cup low-fat cottage cheese
1 Carbohydrate	½ Granny Smith apple, cored and chopped
1 Carbohydrate	⅓ cup mandarin orange sections
½ Carbohydrate	2 cups romaine lettuce
½ Carbohydrate	1½ teaspoons raisins
1 Carbohydrate	¾ cup Zoned Pepper Relish (see page 719)
4 Fat	4 macadamia nuts, chopped

Spices:

Salt and pepper to taste

Method:

Form a bed of romaine on a serving plate. Top with Zoned Pepper Relish. In a medium bowl, combine cheese, apple, orange sections, raisins, and salt and pepper. Mix well. Mound cheese on top of lettuce and sprinkle with nuts.

GINGER TURKEY WITH ORIENTAL VEGETABLES

Servings: 1 Lunch Entrée (4 blocks)

Block Size:	Ingredients:
3 Protein	4½ ounces lean ground turkey
1 Protein	2 egg whites
1 Carbohydrate	⅓ cup water chestnuts, finely chopped
½ Carbohydrate	½ cup scallions, finely chopped, divided
1 Carbohydrate	1 cup canned mushrooms, minced, divided
½ Carbohydrate	1½ cups cabbage, shredded
½ Carbohydrate	1½ cups bean sprouts
½ Carbohydrate	1 cup celery, sliced
4 Fat	1⅓ teaspoons olive oil, divided

Spices:

¼ teaspoon curry powder
½ teaspoon chili powder
½ teaspoon garlic, minced
2 tablespoons lemon- and lime-flavored water
2 teaspoons cilantro, chopped
4 teaspoons soy sauce
Salt and pepper to taste

Method:

In a small bowl combine turkey, egg white, 1 teaspoon soy sauce, ¼ cup mushrooms, ¼ cup scallions, water chestnuts, and salt and pepper. Mix well and form into a patty. Heat ⅓ teaspoon oil in a small nonstick sauté pan. Sauté patty until cooked through. In a medium-sized nonstick sauté pan heat remaining oil. Add ¼ cup scallions, ¾ cup mushrooms, cabbage, bean sprouts, celery, curry powder, chili powder, garlic, cilantro, 3 teaspoons soy sauce, lemon- and lime-water, and salt and pepper. Cook until crisp-tender. Spoon vegetables onto serving plate and top with patty.

ITALIAN-STYLE CHICKEN

Servings: 1 Lunch Entrée (4 blocks)

Block Size:	Ingredients:
4 Protein	4 ounces chicken tenderloin, sliced diagonally
1 Carbohydrate	1 cup onion, chopped
1 Carbohydrate	¼ cup chickpeas, rinsed
1 Carbohydrate	1¼ cups plum tomatoes, chopped
1 Carbohydrate	6 cups spinach, chopped
4 Fat	1⅓ teaspoons olive oil, divided

Spices:

½ cup chicken stock
½ teaspoon Worcestershire sauce
1 teaspoon garlic, chopped
1½ teaspoons dried oregano
Salt and pepper to taste

Method:
In a medium nonstick sauté pan, heat ⅔ teaspoon oil. Add chicken, ½ cup onion and Worcestershire sauce. In a second nonstick sauté pan heat remaining oil. Stir in ½ cup onion, chickpeas, plum tomatoes, spinach, stock, garlic, oregano, and salt and pepper. Sauté until spinach begins to wilt. Place vegetable mixture on serving plate and top with chicken.

STIR-FRY CHICKEN WITH GINGER VEGETABLES

Servings: 1 Lunch Entrée (4 blocks)

Block Size:	Ingredients:
4 Protein	4 ounces chicken tenderloin, ½-inch cubes
½ Carbohydrate	1½ cups mushrooms, sliced
1 Carbohydrate	1½ cups cabbage, shredded
½ Carbohydrate	½ cup snow peas
1 Carbohydrate	⅓ cup water chestnuts
½ Carbohydrate	½ cup scallion, ¼-inch pieces
½ Carbohydrate	½ cup cauliflower florets
4 Fat	1⅓ teaspoons olive oil, divided

Spices:

1 tablespoon soy sauce
¼ cup chicken broth
2 teaspoons fresh gingerroot, minced, divided
1 teaspoon garlic, minced, divided

Method:

Heat ⅔ teaspoon oil in a medium nonstick sauté pan. Add chicken, ½ teaspoon ginger, and ½ teaspoon garlic. Stir-fry until chicken is cooked and garlic is lightly browned. In a second nonstick sauté pan heat remaining oil and stir in mushrooms. Cook for 2 minutes. Add cabbage, snow peas, water chestnuts, scallions, cauliflower, soy sauce, broth, and remaining ginger and garlic. Stir-fry until cabbage and cauliflower are tender. Place vegetables on serving dish and top with chicken.

BAKED CHICKEN AND ITALIAN VEGETABLE PACKAGES

Servings: 1 Lunch Entrée (4 blocks)

Block Size:	Ingredients:
4 Protein	4 ounces chicken tenderloin, finely diced
1 Carbohydrate	1 cup zucchini, ⅛-inch slices
1 Carbohydrate	1 cup onion, thinly sliced
1 Carbohydrate	⅓ cup red potato, thinly sliced
1 Carbohydrate	1¼ cup tomato, seeded and chopped
4 Fat	1⅓ teaspoons olive oil

Spices:

1 tablespoon balsamic vinegar
2 teaspoons garlic, minced
1 teaspoon dried thyme
1 teaspoon dried oregano
4 tablespoons parsley, chopped
Salt and pepper to taste

Method:

Preheat oven to 425 degrees Fahrenheit. Combine chicken and vegetables in a medium bowl. In a small bowl whisk together olive oil, vinegar, garlic, thyme, oregano, parsley, and salt and pepper. Pour over chicken-vegetable mixture. Toss to coat. Cut a piece of aluminum foil large enough to wrap mixture. Place foil on baking tray and fill with mixture. Fold foil up around the mixture and seal it. Leave a small steam vent on the top of the package. Bake for 25 to 30 minutes. When done, cut open foil (be careful of escaping steam) and spoon mixture onto serving dish.

THAI TURKEY SOUP

Servings: 1 Lunch Entrée (4 blocks)

Block Size:	**Ingredients:**
4 Protein	6 ounces ground turkey
½ Carbohydrate	1½ cups bean sprouts
½ Carbohydrate	½ cup scallions, sliced
½ Carbohydrate	2 cups spinach leaves
1 Carbohydrate	¼ cup cooked fine egg noodles
1½ Carbohydrate	¾ cup fruit cocktail
4 Fat	1⅓ teaspoons olive oil

Spices:

3 teaspoons garlic, minced
½ teaspoon fresh gingerroot, grated
2 tablespoons soy sauce
2½ cups chicken stock
1 tablespoon hot chili pepper, finely diced

Method:
Combine turkey, sprouts, scallions, oil, garlic, gingerroot, soy sauce, stock, and chili pepper in a medium saucepan. Bring to a boil, reduce heat, and simmer for 15 minutes. Add spinach and noodles. Simmer for 1 minute. Spoon into serving bowl and serve with fruit cocktail as a side dish, in a second serving bowl.

VEGETABLE STEW

Servings: 1 Lunch Entrée (4 blocks)

Block Size:	Ingredients:
4 Protein	4 soy hot dogs, sliced
½ Carbohydrate	1 cup celery, sliced
1 Carbohydrate	1 cup scallions, sliced
1 Carbohydrate	½ cup carrots, finely diced
1 Carbohydrate	1¼ cups tomato, chopped
½ Carbohydrate	1½ cups mushrooms, sliced
4 Fat	1⅓ teaspoons olive oil

Spices:

2 teaspoons garlic, minced
3 cups beef stock
2 tablespoons cider vinegar
⅛ teaspoon Worcestershire sauce
⅛ teaspoon dried oregano
Salt and pepper to taste

Method:

Combine all ingredients in a large saucepan. Bring to a boil, then simmer for 35 to 40 minutes, stirring occasionally until all vegetables are tender. Place mixture in serving dish, and serve immediately.

DINNER

CHICKEN CREOLE

Servings: 1 Dinner Entrée (4 blocks)

Block Size:	Ingredients:
4 Protein	4 ounces chicken tenderloins, ½-inch cubes
1 Carbohydrate	1 cup onions, chopped
1 Carbohydrate	½ cup Zoned Italian Sauce (see page 710)
½ Carbohydrate	1½ cups mushrooms, sliced
½ Carbohydrate	1¼ cups celery, sliced
1 Carbohydrate	2¼ cups red and green pepper strips
4 Fat	1⅓ teaspoons olive oil

Spices:

1 teaspoon chili powder
½ teaspoon dry red wine
1 teaspoon garlic, minced
Hot pepper sauce to taste
(optional)

Method:

Heat oil in medium nonstick sauté pan. Add chicken, onion, mushrooms, celery, pepper strips, chili powder, wine, and garlic. Stir-fry until chicken is cooked and vegetables are tender. Stir in Zoned Italian Sauce and cook an additional 3 minutes. Spoon onto plate and serve.

MUSHROOM SAUCE STEAK WITH MIXED VEGETABLES

Servings: 1 Dinner Entrée (4 blocks)

Block Size:	Ingredients:
4 Protein	4 ounces lean beef, thinly sliced
1 Carbohydrate	1 cup Zoned Mushroom Sauce (see page 708)
1 Carbohydrate	1 cup asparagus pieces
½ Carbohydrate	½ cup onion, chopped
½ Carbohydrate	1 cup cauliflower florets
1 Carbohydrate	1 cup whole green beans
4 Fat	1⅓ teaspoons olive oil

Spices:

1 teaspoon garlic, minced
½ teaspoon Worcestershire sauce

Method:
Sauté beef and garlic in hot oil until cooked. Add Zoned Mushroom Sauce and Worcestershire sauce. Simmer for 3 minutes, until heated through. Steam vegetables until crisp-tender (4 to 5 minutes). Place vegetables on one side of serving plate and spoon saucy beef onto the other.

SHEPHERD'S PIE

Servings: 1 Dinner Entrée (4 blocks)

Block Size:	Ingredients:
3 Protein	4½ ounces lean ground beef
1 Protein	¼ cup egg substitute
½ Carbohydrate	¼ cup tomato puree
½ Carbohydrate	1½ cups mushrooms, sliced
1 Carbohydrate	¼ cup frozen corn kernels
1 Carbohydrate	1 cup turnip, diced
½ Carbohydrate	½ cup green beans
½ Carbohydrate	½ cup onion, chopped
4 Fat	1⅓ teaspoons olive oil, divided

Spices:

2 tablespoons beef stock, divided
1 teaspoon Worcestershire sauce
⅛ teaspoon celery seed
⅛ teaspoon dried marjoram
1 tablespoon balsamic vinegar
⅛ teaspoon lemon herb seasoning
1 cup water
Salt and pepper to taste

Method:
In a medium nonstick sauté pan heat ⅓ teaspoon of oil. Add ground beef, egg substitute, ½ teaspoon Worcestershire sauce, and celery seed. Stir-fry until cooked. Blend in tomato puree and marjoram. Cook an additional 3 minutes. In a second nonstick sauté pan heat 1 teaspoon oil, mushrooms, corn, green beans, onion, vinegar, ½ teaspoon Worcestershire sauce, 1 tablespoon beef stock, lemon herb seasoning, and salt and pepper. While the beef mixture and mushroom mixture are cooking, place diced turnip and 1 cup of water in a saucepan and

cook until turnip softens. Drain water from saucepan and mash turnip. Layer a small casserole dish with beef mixture. Sprinkle with 1 tablespoon beef stock. Add mushroom mixture on top of beef mixture and place a layer of turnip on mushroom mixture. Brown casserole in broiler and serve.

Note: This recipe is simple to prepare and reheats well in a microwave or toaster oven.

OLD-FASHIONED ITALIAN PIE

Servings: 1 Dinner Entrée (4 blocks)

Block Size:	Ingredients:
1 Protein	¼ cup egg substitute
1 Protein	2 ounces skim milk ricotta cheese (approximately ¼ cup)
2 Protein	3 ounces lean ground beef
1 Carbohydrate	½ cup Zoned Italian Sauce (see page 710)
½ Carbohydrate	¼ cup tomato puree
½ Carbohydrate	½ cup onion, chopped
1 Carbohydrate	1½ cups broccoli florets
1 Carbohydrate	1 cup frozen asparagus pieces
4 Fat	1⅓ teaspoons olive oil, divided

Spices:

½ teaspoon garlic, minced
⅛ teaspoon dried marjoram
⅛ teaspoon dried oregano
Dash ground nutmeg
¼ teaspoon lemon herb seasoning
½ teaspoon Worcestershire sauce
Salt and pepper to taste

Method:

In a medium nonstick sauté pan heat ⅔ teaspoon of oil, beef, cheese, egg substitute, Worcestershire sauce, garlic, marjoram, oregano, nutmeg, salt and pepper until beef is cooked. In a second nonstick sauté pan heat ⅔ teaspoon oil and sauté the onion, broccoli, asparagus, and lemon herb seasoning. Cook until vegetables are crisp-tender. Add Zoned Italian Sauce and tomato puree. Simmer 3 to 5 minutes. In a small casserole dish alternate layers of meat and vegetables. Place in microwave and heat through.

GERMAN BEEF SALAD

Servings: 1 Dinner Entrée (4 blocks)

Block Size:	Ingredients:
4 Protein	4 ounces cooked lean beef, thinly sliced
1 Carbohydrate	1 cup onion, thinly sliced
½ Carbohydrate	3 cups fresh spinach
½ Carbohydrate	1 cup celery, sliced
1 Carbohydrate	1 cup sauerkraut, drained
1 Carbohydrate	½ cup Zoned Herb Dressing (see page 716)
4 Fat	1⅓ teaspoons olive oil

Spices:

½ teaspoon Worcestershire sauce

Method:

In small nonstick sauté pan heat oil. Add beef and brown. Stir in Zoned Herb Dressing and Worcestershire sauce. Remove from heat. On serving plate, layer spinach, sauerkraut, celery, and onion. Top with meat mixture and serve.

SPICED BEANS WITH MUSHROOMS

Servings: 1 Dinner Entrée (4 blocks)

Block Size:	Ingredients:
4 Protein	12 ounces extra-firm tofu, ½-inch cubes
½ Carbohydrate	½ cup green beans
1 Carbohydrate	3 cups mushrooms, sliced
½ Carbohydrate	½ cup onions, chopped
1 Carbohydrate	½ cup Zoned Herb Dressing (see page 716)
1 Carbohydrate	¼ cup cooked black beans, rinsed
4 Fat	1⅓ teaspoons olive oil, divided

Spices:

⅛ teaspoon celery salt
½ teaspoon Worcestershire sauce
1 tablespoon balsamic vinegar
¼ teaspoon lemon and herb seasoning

Method:
Heat ⅔ teaspoon oil in a medium nonstick sauté pan. Sauté tofu, celery salt, and Worcestershire sauce until well browned and crusted on all sides. In a second nonstick sauté pan, heat remaining oil. Add green beans, mushrooms, onions, black beans, balsamic vinegar, and lemon and herb seasoning. Sauté until vegetables are crisp-tender, about 3 to 5 minutes. Mix tofu with vegetables. Add Zoned Herb Dressing, heat through, and serve.

SWEET AND SOUR SHRIMP SALAD

Servings: 1 Dinner Entrée (4 blocks)

Block Size:	Ingredients:
4 Protein	6 ounces cooked shrimp
1 Carbohydrate	½ cup canned pineapple, cubed
1 Carbohydrate	1 cup snow peas, 1-inch pieces
½ Carbohydrate	½ cup onion, chopped
½ Carbohydrate	¾ cup canned bean sprouts
1 Carbohydrate	½ cup Zoned Barbecue Sauce (see page 714)
4 Fat	1⅓ teaspoons olive oil

Spices:

½ teaspoon garlic, minced
2 tablespoons lemon-flavored water

Method:
Heat oil in a medium nonstick sauté pan. Add snow peas, onion, and sprouts. Sauté until crisp-tender. Stir in pineapple, water, Zoned Barbecue Sauce, and garlic. Cook an additional 3 to 5 minutes. Add shrimp and heat through. Spoon into a medium bowl and serve.

SHRIMP GUMBO

Servings: 1 Dinner Entrée (4 blocks)

Block Size:	Ingredients:
4 Protein	6 ounces small shrimp*
½ Carbohydrate	1 cup celery, sliced
1 Carbohydrate	1 cup onion, chopped
1 Carbohydrate	1¼ cups tomatoes, chopped
½ Carbohydrate	½ cup frozen okra, sliced
1 Carbohydrate	¼ cup frozen corn kernels
4 Fat	1⅓ teaspoons olive oil

Spices:

½ teaspoon hot pepper sauce (or to taste)
½ teaspoon garlic, minced
¼ teaspoon chili powder
⅛ teaspoon celery seed
⅓ cup lemon- and lime-flavored water
½ teaspoon lemon herb seasoning
¼ teaspoon paprika

Method:
Heat oil in a medium nonstick sauté pan. Add celery, onion, tomatoes, okra, corn, hot pepper sauce, garlic, chili powder, and celery seed. Cook until vegetables are tender. Mix in the shrimp, paprika, lemon herb seasoning, and water. Simmer 3 to 5 minutes until the shrimp are cooked. Spoon into a medium bowl and serve.

Note: Shelled and deveined.

WARMED DILL TUNA SALAD

Servings: 1 Dinner Entrée (4 blocks)

Block Size:	Ingredients:
4 Protein	4 ounces albacore tuna, canned in water
½ Carbohydrate	5½ cups alfalfa sprouts
1 Carbohydrate	½ cup salsa*
½ Carbohydrate	½ cup tomato, chopped
½ Carbohydrate	3 cups lettuce, shredded
½ Carbohydrate	½ cup onion, chopped, divided
1 Carbohydrate	½ cup Zoned Herb Dressing (see page 716)
4 Fat	1⅓ teaspoons olive oil

Spices:

1 teaspoon dill

Method:

Heat oil in a medium nonstick sauté pan. In a medium bowl combine tuna, sprouts, salsa, and dill. Add to sauté pan. Sauté until heated through and lightly browned. On a serving plate, form the lettuce into a bed and top with tomato and onion. Spoon on tuna mixture and sprinkle with Zoned Herb Dressing.

*Note: We used a medium-heat salsa. Use whatever strength you prefer.

STIR-FRY SALMON WITH SNOW PEAS

Servings: 1 Dinner Entrée (4 blocks)

Block Size:	Ingredients:
3 Protein	4½ ounces canned salmon
1 Protein	1 whole egg
½ Carbohydrate	½ cup onion, chopped
1 Carbohydrate	1 cup fresh snow peas
1 Carbohydrate	⅓ cup water chestnuts, sliced
1 Carbohydrate	½ cup salsa*
½ Carbohydrate	1½ cups mushrooms, sliced
4 Fat	1⅓ teaspoons olive oil, divided

Spices:

1 teaspoon dill
1 teaspoon Worcestershire sauce
1 tablespoon balsamic vinegar
⅛ teaspoon celery seed
⅛ teaspoon dry ground double
   superfine mustard

Method:

Heat ⅔ teaspoon oil in a medium nonstick sauté pan. Combine salmon, egg, salsa, and dill. Sauté until heated through. Heat remaining oil in a second pan. Add onion, snow peas, water chestnuts, mushrooms, Worcestershire sauce, vinegar, celery seed, and mustard. Sauté until vegetables are tender. Combine salmon mixture with vegetables and serve.

*Note: We used a medium-heat salsa. Use whatever strength you prefer.

GOURMET GARDENBURGERS

Servings: 1 Dinner Entrée (4 blocks)

Block Size:	Ingredients:
4 Protein	6 ounces lean ground beef
1 Carbohydrate	1 cup Zoned Mushroom Sauce (see page 708)
1 Carbohydrate	3 cups bean sprouts, divided
½ Carbohydrate	2 cups cucumber, peeled, seeded, and chopped
1 Carbohydrate	¼ cup kidney beans, rinsed
½ Carbohydrate	½ cup onion, chopped
4 Fat	1⅓ teaspoons olive oil, divided

Spices:

1 teaspoon Worcestershire sauce
½ teaspoon garlic, minced
⅛ teaspoon dried oregano
⅛ teaspoon celery seed
Dash chili powder
⅛ teaspoon lemon herb seasoning
Salt and pepper to taste

Method:

Heat ⅔ teaspoon olive oil in a medium nonstick sauté pan. In a medium bowl combine the beef, 1½ cups sprouts, Worcestershire sauce, garlic, celery seed, oregano, and chili powder. Form into four small patties. Sauté patties in hot oil until cooked. Add in Zoned Mushroom Sauce and heat through. In a second nonstick sauté pan, heat remaining oil. Add 1½ cups sprouts, cucumber, kidney beans, onion, and lemon herb seasoning. Sauté until the vegetables start to soften. Drain excess liquid from vegetables. Spoon into a small serving bowl. Place burgers onto a serving dish with more Zoned Mushroom Sauce.

STIR-FRY PORK WITH TARRAGON-MUSTARD SAUCE

Servings: 1 Dinner Entrée (4 blocks)

Block Size:	Ingredients:
4 Protein	4 ounces pork strips, thinly sliced
1 Carbohydrate	½ cup Zoned Tarragon Mustard Sauce (see page 720)
1 Carbohydrate	1 cup onion, chopped
1 Carbohydrate	¼ cup kidney beans, rinsed
1 Carbohydrate	2¼ cups frozen red and green bell pepper strips
4 Fat	1⅓ teaspoons olive oil, divided

Spices:

2 teaspoons Worcestershire sauce
1 tablespoon lemon-flavored water

Method:

Heat ⅔ teaspoon oil in a medium sauté pan. Add pork and water to pan and stir-fry until meat is cooked. Spoon in Zoned Tarragon Mustard Sauce and heat through. In second nonstick sauté pan, heat remaining oil. Place onion, beans, peppers, and Worcestershire sauce in second pan and stir-fry until tender. Place vegetables on a serving plate. Top with meat mixture and serve.

PORK CUTLET TUSCAN-STYLE

Servings: 1 Dinner Entrée (4 blocks)

Block Size:	Ingredients:
4 Protein	4 ounces pork cutlets
1 Carbohydrate	1 cup onion, chopped
½ Carbohydrate	¼ cup tomato puree
1 Carbohydrate	½ cup Zoned Herb Dressing, divided (see page 716)
1 Carbohydrate	¼ cup canned chickpeas, chopped
½ Carbohydrate	1½ cups mushrooms, sliced
4 Fat	1⅓ teaspoons olive oil, divided

Spices:

½ teaspoon ground double superfine mustard
⅛ teaspoon black pepper
1 teaspoon Worcestershire sauce
2 tablespoons lemon- or lime-flavored water

Method:

Blend mustard, pepper, Worcestershire sauce, and ¼ cup Zoned Herb Dressing in a small bowl. Heat ⅔ teaspoon oil in a nonstick sauté pan. Add mustard mixture and water to pan. Place cutlets and onion in pan. Make sure to coat both sides of cutlets with mustard mixture. In a second nonstick pan heat remaining oil. Add chickpeas and mushrooms. Cook for 3 to 5 minutes. Stir in tomato puree and ¼ cup Zoned Herb Dressing. Simmer for an additional 2 minutes. Combine vegetables and pork. Blend well and spoon onto a serving plate.

SOUTH AMERICAN CHILI SOUP

Servings: 1 Dinner Entrée (4 blocks)

Block Size:	Ingredients:
4 Protein	4 ounces chicken tenderloin, chopped
1 Carbohydrate	2¼ cups frozen red and green pepper strips
1 Carbohydrate	½ cup salsa*
1 Carbohydrate	1¼ cups tomatoes, chopped
½ Carbohydrate	½ cup onion, chopped
½ Carbohydrate	2 teaspoons cornstarch
4 Fat	1⅓ teaspoons olive oil

Spices:

1 teaspoon Worcestershire sauce
1 tablespoon balsamic vinegar
⅛ teaspoon hot pepper sauce
1 cup chicken stock
½ teaspoon garlic, minced
¼ teaspoon chili powder

Method:
In a nonstick sauté pan heat oil. Sauté chicken, onion, peppers, salsa, Worcestershire sauce, vinegar, and hot pepper sauce until lightly browned. In large saucepan combine chicken mixture, tomatoes, chicken stock, garlic, chili powder, and cornstarch. (Mix cornstarch with chicken stock before adding to saucepan.) Bring mixture to a simmer, stirring constantly, for 3 to 5 minutes. Spoon into bowl and serve.

*Note: We used medium-heat salsa. Use whatever strength you prefer.

DEVILED STEAK WITH MIXED VEGETABLES

Servings: 1 Dinner Entrée (4 blocks)

Block Size:

4 Protein

1 Carbohydrate
1 Carbohydrate
1 Carbohydrate
½ Carbohydrate
½ Carbohydrate

4 Fat

Ingredients:

4 ounces lean beef

3 cups mushrooms, sliced
¼ cup frozen corn kernels
1 cup asparagus cuts
½ cup onion, chopped
¼ cup tomato puree

1⅓ teaspoons olive oil

Spices:

½ teaspoon Worcestershire sauce
1 tablespoon balsamic vinegar
Dash ground cloves
1 teaspoon ground double superfine
    mustard
2 tablespoons lemon- and lime-
    flavored water
⅛ teaspoon celery salt

Method:

In a medium nonstick sauté pan, combine oil, Worcestershire sauce, vinegar, cloves, mustard, and water. Stir to mix well. Add meat to pan and sprinkle the meat with the celery salt. Cook 3 to 5 minutes. Add mushrooms, corn, asparagus, and onion. Sauté until vegetables are tender. Add tomato puree and simmer 3 to 5 minutes. Spoon onto plate and serve.

SWISS-STYLE CHICKEN

Servings: 1 Dinner Entrée (4 blocks)

Block Size:	Ingredients:
2 Protein	2 ounces chicken tenderloin, diced
1 Protein	1 ounce low-fat Swiss cheese, shredded
1 Protein and 1 Carbohydrate	½ cup plain low-fat yogurt
½ Carbohydrate	½ cup onion, chopped
½ Carbohydrate	3 cups spinach
1 Carbohydrate	1¼ cups tomato, diced
1 Carbohydrate	⅓ cup mandarin orange slices
4 Fat	1⅓ teaspoons olive oil, divided

Spices:

Dash celery salt
2 tablespoons lemon- and lime-
   flavored water
½ teaspoon Worcestershire sauce
1 teaspoon parsley flakes
1 teaspoon garlic, minced
1 tablespoon cider vinegar
Dash ground nutmeg

Method:

In a medium nonstick sauté pan combine ⅓ teaspoon oil, yogurt, and celery salt. Add chicken, onion, Worcestershire sauce, parsley, and water. Simmer for 3 to 5 minutes. In second pan heat remaining oil. Add spinach, tomato, garlic, vinegar, and nutmeg. Sauté until spinach has wilted and tomato softened slightly. Sprinkle cheese over chicken and let melt. Spoon spinach onto serving plate and top with chicken. Garnish with orange segments and serve.

PORK TENDERLOIN WITH APPLE COMPOTE

Servings: 1 Dinner Entrée (4 blocks)

Block Size:	Ingredients:
4 Protein	4 ounces pork tenderloin
2 Carbohydrate	1 Granny Smith apple, cored and chopped
1 Carbohydrate	⅓ cup unsweetened applesauce
1 Carbohydrate	3 cups mushrooms, sliced
4 Fat	1⅓ teaspoons olive oil, divided

Spices:

2 tablespoons cider vinegar
⅛ teaspoon celery salt
⅛ teaspoon cinnamon
2 tablespoons lemon- and lime-flavored water
¼ teaspoon lemon herb seasoning

Method:

Heat ⅔ teaspoon of oil in a medium nonstick sauté pan. Sauté pork loin until cooked through and lightly browned. Add apple, applesauce, vinegar, celery salt, cinnamon, water, and lemon herb seasoning. Simmer for 3 to 5 minutes. In second nonstick sauté pan, heat remaining oil. Add mushrooms and cook for 3 to 5 minutes. Spoon mushrooms onto a serving plate. Top with pork mixture and serve.

HUNGARIAN CHICKEN

Servings: 1 Dinner Entrée (4 blocks)

Block Size:	Ingredients:
4 Protein	4 ounces chicken tenderloin, cut in large chunks
1 Carbohydrate	1¼ cups tomatoes, chopped
1 Carbohydrate	2¼ cups green and red pepper strips
1 Carbohydrate	1 cup onion, chopped
1 Carbohydrate	¼ cup chickpeas, rinsed
4 Fat	1⅓ teaspoons olive oil, divided

Spices:

Dash hot red pepper sauce
  (optional)
1 tablespoon paprika
1 teaspoon Worcestershire sauce
½ teaspoon garlic, minced
⅛ teaspoon celery seed
Salt and pepper to taste

Method:

Heat ⅔ teaspoon oil in a medium nonstick sauté pan. Add chicken, sprinkle with salt and pepper. Cook chicken until lightly browned. In a second nonstick sauté pan, heat remaining oil and cook tomatoes, pepper strips, onion, chickpeas, hot pepper sauce, paprika, Worcestershire sauce, garlic, and celery seed. Sauté vegetables and seasonings for 3 to 5 minutes, until they begin to soften. Spoon vegetables onto a serving dish and top with chicken.

CHICKEN MEXICALI SALAD

Servings: 1 Dinner Entrée (4 blocks)

Block Size:	Ingredients:
3 Protein	3 ounces chicken tenderloin, large dice
1 Protein and 1 Carbohydrate	½ cup plain low-fat yogurt
1 Carbohydrate	½ cup salsa*
½ Carbohydrate	1½ cups cabbage, shredded (¾ cup red cabbage and ¾ cup green cabbage)
½ Carbohydrate	¼ cup Zoned Herb Dressing (see page 716)
1 Carbohydrate	3 cups mushrooms, sliced
4 Fat	1⅓ teaspoons olive oil, divided

Spices:

1 tablespoon cider vinegar
⅛ teaspoon hot pepper sauce
Celery salt and black pepper
   to taste

Method:

In a medium nonstick sauté pan add ⅔ teaspoon oil, chicken, mushrooms, and salsa and cook 3 to 5 minutes stirring occasionally. Add vinegar, hot pepper sauce, and Zoned Herb Dressing to chicken mixture, stirring constantly, heating throughout. Remove from heat and stir in the yogurt and raw cabbage. Spoon onto serving plate and sprinkle lightly with celery salt and black pepper.

*Note: We used medium-heat salsa. Use whatever strength you prefer.

SUMMER VEGETABLES WITH GARLIC STIR-FRY

Servings: 1 Dinner Entrée (4 blocks)

Block Size:	Ingredients:
4 Protein	12 ounces extra-firm tofu, diced
1 Carbohydrate	1¼ cups tomato, chopped
½ Carbohydrate	1 cup celery, sliced
1 Carbohydrate	1½ cups zucchini, large dice
½ Carbohydrate	½ cup scallion, 1-inch pieces
1 Carbohydrate	½ cup Zoned Italian Sauce (see page 710)
4 Fat	1⅓ teaspoons olive oil, divided

Spices:

½ teaspoon parsley flakes
½ teaspoon Worcestershire sauce
⅛ teaspoon celery salt
⅛ teaspoon lemon herb seasoning
⅛ teaspoon dried oregano
1 tablespoon dry red wine
Dash ground thyme
1 tablespoon lemon-flavored water
1 tablespoon garlic, minced
Salt and pepper to taste

Method:
In a medium nonstick sauté pan heat ⅔ teaspoon oil. Add Worcestershire sauce and celery salt. Stir in tofu and stir-fry until tofu is browned and crusted on all sides. In a second nonstick sauté pan heat remaining oil and sauté tomato, celery, zucchini, scallion, Zoned Italian Sauce, parsley, lemon herb seasoning, oregano, wine, thyme, water, garlic, and salt and pepper. Cook vegetables until they are tender. Place browned tofu in bottom of serving bowl and spoon vegetables on top.

PEPPER STIR-FRY

Servings: 1 Dinner Entrée (4 blocks)

Block Size:	Ingredients:
4 Protein	12 ounces extra-firm tofu, diced
½ Carbohydrate	2 teaspoons cornstarch
1 Carbohydrate	1¼ cups tomatoes, chopped
1 Carbohydrate	2¼ cups red and yellow bell peppers, chopped
½ Carbohydrate	½ cup onion, chopped
1 Carbohydrate	¼ cup chickpeas, rinsed
4 Fat	1⅓ teaspoons olive oil, divided

Spices:

⅛ teaspoon celery salt
½ teaspoon Worcestershire sauce
1 teaspoon garlic, minced
1 tablespoon cider vinegar
Dash hot pepper sauce
⅛ teaspoon paprika
⅓ cup lemon- and lime-flavored water
Dash lemon herb seasoning

Method:
In a medium nonstick sauté pan, heat ⅔ teaspoon of oil. Add tofu, celery salt, and Worcestershire sauce and stir-fry until browned and crusted on all sides. In a second pan heat remaining oil. Add peppers, onion, chickpeas, garlic, vinegar, hot pepper sauce, and paprika. Cook until the vegetables are tender. Add tomatoes, water, and cornstarch. (Mix cornstarch with water to dissolve it before adding to sauté pan.) Combine tofu and vegetable mixture. Spoon onto serving plate and sprinkle with lemon herb seasoning.

COUNTRY-STYLE TURKEY WITH GREEN BEANS

Servings: 1 Dinner Entrée (4 blocks)

Block Size:	Ingredients:
4 Protein	6 ounces lean ground turkey
½ Carbohydrate	1 cup celery, finely diced, divided
1 Carbohydrate	1 cup green beans, 2-inch pieces
1 Carbohydrate	1¼ cups cherry tomatoes, halved
½ Carbohydrate	½ cup leeks, finely diced
1 Carbohydrate	1 cup Zoned Country-Style Chicken Gravy (see page 709)
4 Fat	1⅓ teaspoons olive oil, divided

Spices:

½ teaspoon Worcestershire sauce
½ teaspoon garlic, minced, divided
⅛ teaspoon parsley, minced
Dash black pepper
⅛ teaspoon chili powder

Method:

In a medium mixing bowl, combine turkey, ½ cup celery, leeks, Worcestershire sauce, and parsley. Form into ½-inch meatballs. Coat a baking dish with ⅔ teaspoon oil. Place meatballs in baking dish. Bake in a preheated 370-degree Fahrenheit oven for 15 minutes. In a medium nonstick sauté pan heat remaining oil. Add remaining celery, green beans, cherry tomatoes, garlic, black pepper, and chili powder. Cook until vegetables are tender. Stir in Zoned Country-Style Chicken Gravy. Heat through and serve.

CHICKEN ZUCCHINI ITALIANO

Servings: 1 Dinner Entrée (4 blocks)

Block Size:

1 Protein	1 ounce skim milk mozzarella, shredded
3 Protein	3 ounces chicken tenderloin, finely diced
2 Carbohydrate	3 cups zucchini, sliced
1 Carbohydrate	½ cup Zoned Italian Sauce (see page 710)
½ Carbohydrate	1½ cups mushrooms, diced
½ Carbohydrate	½ cup onion, chopped
4 Fat	1⅓ teaspoons olive oil

Spices:

1 tablespoon fresh basil, chopped
2 teaspoons garlic, minced
⅛ teaspoon dried oregano

Method:
In a medium nonstick sauté pan add oil, chicken, zucchini, mushrooms, onion, basil, garlic, and oregano. Sauté until vegetables are tender, then add Zoned Italian Sauce. Spoon into serving bowl and top with cheese.

POLYNESIAN-STYLE SHRIMP AND FRUIT STEW

Servings: 1 Dinner Entrée (4 blocks)

Block Size:	Ingredients:
4 Protein	6 ounces cooked shrimp
1 Carbohydrate	½ cup pineapple, cubed
½ Carbohydrate	2 teaspoons cornstarch
½ Carbohydrate	3 cups kale
1 Carbohydrate	½ cup honeydew melon, cubed
1 Carbohydrate	⅓ cup mandarin orange segments
4 Fat	1⅓ teaspoons olive oil, divided

Spices:

½ cup lemon- and lime-flavored
water
½ teaspoon lemon extract
½ teaspoon orange extract
¼ teaspoon Worcestershire sauce
1 teaspoon cider vinegar
Dash lemon herb seasoning

Method:

Heat ⅔ teaspoon oil in a medium nonstick sauté pan. Add kale and cook until just wilted. Remove to serving bowl. In a second pan heat remaining oil and stir in the shrimp, pineapple, melon, orange segments, water, lemon extract, orange extract, Worcestershire sauce, vinegar, and lemon herb seasoning. Sauté until orange breaks up. Mix cornstarch with a little water to dissolve it and add to sauté pan, stirring constantly, until liquid thickens slightly. On large lunch plate spoon shrimp and fruit mixture over kale and serve.

PORTUGUESE-STYLE PORK WITH CLAMS

Servings: 1 Dinner Entrée (4 blocks)

Block Size:	Ingredients:
3 Protein	3 ounces pork loin, sliced ⅛-inch thick
1 Protein	1½ ounces clams
½ Carbohydrate	½ cup onions, sliced
1 Carbohydrate	¾ Zoned Pepper Relish (see page 719)
1 Carbohydrate	¼ cup chickpeas, diced
1 Carbohydrate	2 cups celery, sliced
½ Carbohydrate	½ cup white wine
4 Fat	1⅓ teaspoons olive oil

Spices:

2 teaspoons garlic
1 tablespoon parsley flakes
Dash hot pepper sauce
⅛ teaspoon paprika
2 teaspoons cider vinegar

Method:
In a glass bowl, combine the vinegar, oil, and garlic. Add pork and turn in liquid to coat. Cover and refrigerate for 30 minutes. When pork is marinated add pork and liquid to a medium nonstick sauté pan. Stir in remaining ingredients and sauté until pork is cooked through. Spoon onto dish and serve.

PORK MEDALLIONS WITH PEAR AND BLUEBERRY COMPOTE

Servings: 1 Dinner Entrée (4 blocks)

Block Size:	Ingredients:
4 Protein	4 ounces pork loin, sliced ⅛-inch thick
1½ Carbohydrate	1½ pears, diced
½ Carbohydrate	2 cups romaine lettuce, shredded
1 Carbohydrate	2 teaspoons brown sugar, divided
½ Carbohydrate	¼ cup blueberries
½ Carbohydrate	½ cup scallion, shredded
4 Fat	1⅓ teaspoons olive oil, divided

Spices:

½ teaspoon soy sauce
1 tablespoon lemon- and lime-flavored water
2 teaspoons mint, minced
2 teaspoons Dijon mustard
1 tablespoon cider vinegar
2 tablespoons red wine vinegar
⅛ teaspoon celery salt
⅛ teaspoon black pepper

Method:

In a glass bowl, combine ⅔ teaspoon oil, mustard, cider vinegar, and 1 teaspoon brown sugar. Add pork and turn to coat. Cover and refrigerate for 30 minutes. When pork is done marinating add the mixture to a medium nonstick sauté pan. Sauté until the pork is cooked through. Stir in the pears, blueberries, 1 teaspoon brown sugar, mint, and water. In a medium bowl mix together the ⅔ teaspoon oil, soy sauce, red wine vinegar, scallions, romaine, celery salt, and black pepper. Spoon vegetable mixture onto serving plate and top with pork and fruit mixture.

HOT AND SOUR STIR-FRY PORK AND CABBAGE

Servings: 1 Dinner Entrée (4 blocks)

Block Size:	**Ingredients:**
4 Protein	4 ounces lean pork loin, large dice
¼ Carbohydrate	1 teaspoon cornstarch
¼ Carbohydrate	½ cup cauliflower pieces
½ Carbohydrate	½ cup onion, sliced
½ Carbohydrate	½ cup scallions, chopped
½ Carbohydrate	1½ cups cabbage, shredded
2 Carbohydrate	1 pear, cored and sliced
4 Fat	1⅓ teaspoons olive oil

Spices:

½ cup chicken stock
1 tablespoon soy sauce
⅛ teaspoon black pepper
2 tablespoons jalapeño peppers, diced
1 tablespoon cider vinegar
2 teaspoons minced garlic
2 teaspoons fresh gingerroot, minced

Method:
In a medium glass bowl combine the oil, pork, stock, cornstarch, soy sauce, vinegar, scallions, and spices. Cover and refrigerate for 30 minutes. When the pork is done marinating, place mixture in a medium nonstick sauté pan. Sauté pork until browned on both sides, then add vegetables and continue cooking until vegetables are tender. Place pork and vegetables on a large dinner plate, garnished with pear slices. Serve immediately.

SPICED GROUND LAMB WITH
SPRING VEGETABLES

Servings: 1 Dinner Entrée (4 blocks)

Block Size:	Ingredients:
4 Protein	6 ounces lean ground lamb
½ Carbohydrate	½ cup scallions, finely chopped
½ Carbohydrate	½ cup red onion, chunks
½ Carbohydrate	1½ cups mushrooms
1 Carbohydrate	1¼ cups tomatoes, diced
½ Carbohydrate	½ cup green beans, diced
1 Carbohydrate	⅕ cup cooked brown rice
4 Fat	1⅓ teaspoons olive oil

Spices:

1 teaspoon cider vinegar
1 tablespoon cilantro
2 teaspoons gingerroot, minced
¼ teaspoon cumin
¼ teaspoon coriander
⅛ teaspoon black pepper
½ teaspoon celery salt
⅛ teaspoon cinnamon

Method:

In a small glass bowl combine lamb, rice, vinegar, and spices. Cover and refrigerate for 30 minutes. Heat the oil in a medium nonstick sauté pan. Add meat mixture and vegetables. Cook, breaking meat up as it cooks, until lamb is cooked through and the vegetables are tender. Spoon onto plate and serve.

LAMB WITH SPICED BEANS

Servings: 1 Dinner Entrée (4 blocks)

Block Size:	Ingredients:
3 Protein	3 ounces lean lamb, finely diced
1 Protein and 1 Carbohydrate	½ cup plain low-fat yogurt
½ Carbohydrate	½ cup onions, thinly sliced
1 Carbohydrate	3 cups cabbage, shredded
1 Carbohydrate	¼ cup cooked white kidney beans
½ Carbohydrate	3¾ cups escarole, chopped
4 Fat	1⅓ teaspoons olive oil

Spices:

2 teaspoons garlic, minced
½ teaspoon paprika
¼ teaspoon ground cumin
⅛ teaspoon cayenne pepper
⅛ teaspoon celery salt

Method:
In a glass bowl combine lamb, yogurt, paprika, cumin, garlic, cayenne, and celery salt. Mix well to coat. Cover and refrigerate for 4 hours. Heat oil in medium nonstick sauté pan. Add meat mixture and vegetables. Cook until lamb is cooked through and vegetables are tender.

BRAISED LAMB WITH KALE AND BEANS

Servings: 1 Dinner Entrée (4 blocks)

Block Size:	Ingredients:
4 Protein	4 ounces lean lamb, small dice
1 Carbohydrate	1 cup onions, sliced
1 Carbohydrate	1¼ cups kale, torn
1 Carbohydrate	½ Granny Smith apple, roughly chopped
1 Carbohydrate	¼ cup white kidney beans
4 Fat	1⅓ teaspoons olive oil

Spices:

½ cup lemon- and lime-flavored water
½ teaspoon ground cinnamon
⅛ teaspoon cayenne pepper
Salt and pepper to taste

Method:

In a small pan sauté lamb and onion in hot oil until lightly browned. Add water, cinnamon, cayenne, and salt and pepper. Cover, reduce heat, and simmer for 10 minutes. Add kale, apple, and beans. Bring to a boil, reduce heat, cover, and simmer for 2 minutes to heat through. Place lamb on serving dish, and using a slotted spoon, arrange vegetables on dish.

BRAISED BEEF WITH MIXED VEGETABLES

Servings: 1 Dinner Entrée (4 blocks)

Block Size:	Ingredients:
4 Protein	4 ounces lean beef, small dice
1 Carbohydrate	1 cup onion, roughly chopped
1 Carbohydrate	1 cup green beans, 2-inch pieces
½ Carbohydrate	1 cup celery, roughly chopped
½ Carbohydrate	1½ cups mushrooms, sliced
1 Carbohydrate	6 ounces beer (flat beer is acceptable)
4 Fat	1⅓ teaspoons olive oil

Spices:

¼ cup beef stock
⅛ teaspoon celery salt
⅛ teaspoon dried thyme
⅛ teaspoon Worcestershire sauce
⅛ teaspoon dried rosemary
1 teaspoon garlic, minced
⅛ teaspoon dried oregano
½ tablespoon fresh parsley, chopped

Method:
Combine ingredients in a medium saucepan. Bring to a boil, reduce heat and simmer, covered, 25 to 30 minutes. Place mixture in a large soup bowl and serve.

GRILLED STEAK WITH SPICED MUSHROOM SALAD

Servings: 1 Dinner Entrée (4 blocks)

Block Size:	Ingredients:
4 Protein	4 ounces lean beef
1 Carbohydrate	⅓ cup cooked potato, thinly sliced
½ Carbohydrate	½ cup red onion, thinly sliced
½ Carbohydrate	1½ cups mushrooms, thinly sliced
½ Carbohydrate	1 cup red pepper, thinly sliced
1 Carbohydrate	1 cup asparagus spears, chopped
½ Carbohydrate	½ cup scallions, chopped
4 Fat	1⅓ teaspoons olive oil, divided

Spices:

4 tablespoons balsamic vinegar, divided
2 tablespoons Dijon mustard, divided
½ teaspoon garlic, minced
1 teaspoon Worcestershire sauce
Salt and pepper to taste

Method:

In a medium bowl combine beef, ⅔ teaspoon oil, 2 tablespoons vinegar, mustard, and ½ teaspoon Worcestershire sauce. Turn meat to cover with mixture. Cover bowl and refrigerate for 4 hours. Heat remaining oil in a medium nonstick sauté pan. Sauté beef until cooked through. In a small bowl whisk together remaining vinegar, remaining Worcestershire sauce, garlic, salt and pepper. In another medium bowl combine the potato, onion, mushrooms, pepper, asparagus, and scallions. Pour on dressing and toss to coat. Spoon salad onto serving dish and top with meat.

HERB-MARINATED BEEF WITH SUMMER VEGETABLES

Servings: 1 Dinner Entrée (4 blocks)

Block Size:	Ingredients:
4 Protein	4 ounces lean beef, diced
1 Carbohydrate	2¼ cups red and green pepper strips
½ Carbohydrate	½ cup zucchini, chunks
½ Carbohydrate	½ cup yellow squash, chunks
½ Carbohydrate	1½ cups mushrooms, quartered
1 Carbohydrate	1¼ cups tomato, chopped
½ Carbohydrate	2 ounces dry red wine
4 Fat	1⅓ teaspoons olive oil, divided

Spices:

1 tablespoon balsamic vinegar
1 teaspoon Worcestershire sauce
1 teaspoon garlic, minced
1 tablespoon fresh basil, chopped
1 tablespoon fresh mint, chopped
1 tablespoon fresh parsley, chopped
Salt and pepper to taste

Method:
Combine ⅔ teaspoon oil with wine, vinegar, Worcestershire sauce, garlic, basil, mint, parsley, and salt and pepper. Add meat, turn to coat, cover, and refrigerate 4 hours. Heat remaining oil in medium nonstick sauté pan. Sauté beef, pepper, zucchini, squash, mushrooms, and tomatoes until beef is cooked through and vegetables are tender.

BEEF WITH PEACHES AND ROOT VEGETABLES

Servings: 1 Dinner Entrée (4 blocks)

Block Size:	Ingredients:
4 Protein	4 ounces lean beef, thinly sliced
1 Carbohydrate	1 cup onion, finely chopped
1 Carbohydrate	½ cup carrot, thinly sliced
1½ Carbohydrate	1½ peaches, large dice
½ Carbohydrate	1 cup celery, chopped
4 Fat	1⅓ teaspoons olive oil

Spices:

1 tablespoon red wine vinegar
1 tablespoon Dijon mustard
1 teaspoon garlic, minced
⅛ teaspoon celery salt
⅛ teaspoon dried thyme
⅛ teaspoon cayenne pepper

Method:

Heat oil in a medium nonstick sauté pan. Add beef, onion, carrot, peaches, celery, and seasonings. Stir-fry until beef is cooked through and vegetables are tender.

TOFU-EGGPLANT GUMBO

Servings: 1 Dinner Entrée (4 blocks)

Block Size:	Ingredients:
4 Protein	12 ounces extra-firm tofu, 1-inch cubes
½ Carbohydrate	½ cup onion, chopped
½ Carbohydrate	½ cup scallion, chopped
½ Carbohydrate	1¼ cups green pepper, chopped
½ Carbohydrate	¾ cup okra, sliced
½ Carbohydrate	1 cup celery, sliced
1 Carbohydrate	1¼ cups tomato, crushed
½ Carbohydrate	¾ cup eggplant, diced
4 Fat	1⅓ teaspoons olive oil, divided

Spices:

2 cups beef stock
2 teaspoons garlic, chopped
½ teaspoon dried thyme
⅛ teaspoon cayenne pepper
2 teaspoons Worcestershire sauce, divided
⅛ teaspoon celery salt
¼ cup fresh parsley, chopped

Method:
In a medium nonstick sauté pan heat ⅔ teaspoon oil. Stir in ½ teaspoon Worcestershire sauce and celery salt. Add tofu and stir-fry until browned and crusted on all sides. In a second nonstick sauté pan heat remaining oil. Place onion, scallion, green peppers, celery, tomato, and eggplant in pan. Sprinkle with remaining Worcestershire sauce and remaining spices. Cook vegetables until just tender. Add okra and beef stock. Continue cooking until liquid thickens. Spoon into serving bowl and top with tofu.

SPICY TOFU-VEGETABLE STIR-FRY

Servings: 1 Dinner Entrée (4 blocks)

Block Size:	Ingredients:
4 Protein	12 ounces extra-firm tofu
½ Carbohydrate	1½ cups mushrooms, sliced
¼ Carbohydrate	¼ cup onion, thinly sliced
1 Carbohydrate	1½ cups zucchini, sliced
½ Carbohydrate	1½ cups bean sprouts
½ Carbohydrate	2 teaspoons cornstarch
¼ Carbohydrate	½ cup red bell pepper, diced
¼ Carbohydrate	¼ cup scallions, 1-inch pieces
½ Carbohydrate	1 cup celery, chopped
¼ Carbohydrate	½ cup radishes, sliced
4 Fat	1⅓ teaspoons olive oil, divided

Spices:

⅛ teaspoon celery salt
½ teaspoon Worcestershire sauce
1 tablespoon soy sauce
1 teaspoon garlic, crushed
1 teaspoon gingerroot, grated
1 tablespoon cider vinegar
¼ teaspoon chili powder
1 cup lemon- and lime-flavored
water

Method:

In a medium nonstick sauté pan heat ⅔ teaspoon oil. Stir in Worcestershire sauce and celery salt. Add tofu and stir-fry until browned and crusted on all sides. In another nonstick sauté pan cook vegetables in remaining oil until tender, then add ½ cup water and cover to steam sauté. In saucepan add ½ cup water, soy sauce, spices, and cornstarch. (Mix cornstarch with water to dissolve it before adding to saucepan.) Heat sauce to a light boil while constantly stirring, then add diced tofu to sauce and heat. Add tofu and sauce to vegetables, stir, and simmer for 2 to 3 minutes. On a large dinner plate place tofu-vegetable mixture and serve.

GINGER-GRILLED TUNA

Servings: 1 Dinner Entrée (4 blocks)

Block Size:	Ingredients:
4 Protein	4 ounces tuna steak
3 Carbohydrate	3 cups asparagus
1 Carbohydrate	½ cup Zoned Herb Dressing (see page 716)
4 Fat	1⅓ teaspoons olive oil, divided

Spices:

4 teaspoons cider vinegar
2 teaspoons soy sauce
1½ tablespoons scallions, sliced
1 tablespoon gingerroot, minced
1 teaspoon garlic, minced
Coarse ground black pepper to taste

Method:
In the bottom of a small baking dish place ⅔ teaspoon oil, then place tuna steak. In a small bowl combine remaining oil, vinegar, soy sauce, scallions, ginger, garlic, and pepper. Pour spice mixture over tuna. Cover and bake in a preheated 350-degree Fahrenheit oven for 30 to 35 minutes. Steam the asparagus until crisp-tender. Place asparagus on one side of a serving plate. Pour Zoned Herb Dressing over it. Remove tuna from baking dish and place on serving plate.

SWORDFISH WITH PEACH-CUCUMBER SALSA

Servings: 1 Dinner Entrée (4 blocks)

Block Size:	Ingredients:
4 Protein	4 ounces swordfish steak
1 Carbohydrate	1 peach, chopped
1 Carbohydrate	½ cup salsa*
½ Carbohydrate	2 cups cucumber, chopped
½ Carbohydrate	2 cups romaine lettuce
½ Carbohydrate	½ cup shallots, diced
½ Carbohydrate	¼ cup dry white wine
4 Fat	1⅓ teaspoons olive oil

Spices:

½ teaspoon dill
1 teaspoon lemon- and lime-
flavored water
½ teaspoon lemon herb
seasoning
Salt and pepper to taste

Method:

Place swordfish in a baking dish. Drizzle with water, oil, and wine. Sprinkle with dill, salt and pepper, and lemon herb seasoning. Cover and bake in a preheated 350-degree Fahrenheit oven for 30 to 35 minutes. In a small bowl combine chopped peaches, salsa, cucumber, and shallots. Place lettuce on one side of a large dinner plate. Spoon salsa mixture on top of lettuce, then place swordfish on the other side of plate and serve.

*Note: We used medium-heat salsa. Use whatever strength you prefer.

CIOPPINO

Servings: 1 Dinner Entrée (4 blocks)

Block Size:	Ingredients:
1 Protein	1½ ounces cherrystone clams
1 Protein	1½ ounces sole
1 Protein	1½ ounces small shrimp*
1 Protein	1½ ounces baby bay scallops
½ Carbohydrate	½ cup onion, chopped
½ Carbohydrate	1 cup green pepper, chopped
1 Carbohydrate	1 cup canned tomato, chopped
1 Carbohydrate	3 cups mushrooms, chopped
1 Carbohydrate	4 ounces dry red wine
4 Fat	1⅓ teaspoons olive oil

Spices:

1 teaspoon garlic, minced
½ cup lemon- and lime-flavored water
1 tablespoon parsley, chopped (for garnish)
¼ teaspoon dried oregano
¼ teaspoon dried basil
⅛ teaspoon cayenne pepper
Salt and pepper to taste

Method:
In a medium saucepan combine oil, vegetables, spices, water, and wine. Bring to a boil, reduce heat and bring to a simmer. Add seafood, cover, and simmer for 5 to 7 minutes. Spoon into a bowl and serve.

*Note: Shelled and deveined.

INDIAN SHRIMP WITH APPLES AND YOGURT

Servings: 1 Dinner Entrée (4 blocks)

Block Size:	Ingredients:
3 Protein	4½ ounces cooked small shrimp*
1 Protein and	
1 Carbohydrate	½ cup plain low-fat yogurt
½ Carbohydrate	½ cup onion, minced
2 Carbohydrate	1 Granny Smith apple, diced
½ Carbohydrate	2 cups romaine lettuce
4 Fat	1⅓ teaspoons olive oil

Spices:

⅛ teaspoon fresh gingerroot, minced
½ teaspoon garlic, minced
1 tablespoon cilantro
2 teaspoons cider vinegar
Dash hot pepper sauce
¼ teaspoon turmeric
⅛ teaspoon ground coriander
⅛ teaspoon ground cumin

Method:
Heat the oil in a medium nonstick sauté pan. Add shrimp and spices. Cook 1 to 2 minutes. In a second nonstick sauté pan heat yogurt, apple, and onion. When heated through, add shrimp mixture. Stir to mix. Form a bed of romaine on a serving plate and top with shrimp mixture.

Note: Shrimp should be deveined and shelled.

BAKED SALMON WITH FRUIT SALSA

Servings: 1 Dinner Entrée (4 blocks)

Block Size:	Ingredients:
4 Protein	6 ounces salmon steak
1 Carbohydrate	¾ cup blackberries
1 Carbohydrate	½ cup salsa*
1 Carbohydrate	1 kiwi fruit, peeled and diced
1 Carbohydrate	½ Granny Smith apple, diced
4 Fat	1⅓ teaspoons olive oil

Spices:

2 teaspoons soy sauce
1 teaspoon gingerroot, chopped
½ teaspoon dill
Dash hot pepper sauce

Method:
Brush baking dish with oil; place salmon steak in baking dish. Sprinkle with soy sauce, gingerroot, dill, and hot pepper sauce. Cover and bake in a preheated 350-degree Fahrenheit oven for 30 to 35 minutes. In a medium bowl combine salsa and fruit. Place fish on one side of a serving plate and salsa beside it.

*Note: We used a medium heat salsa. Use whatever strength you prefer.

SAUTÉED SCALLOPS WITH WINE-FLAVORED VEGETABLES

Servings: 1 Dinner Entrée (4 blocks)

Block Size:	Ingredients:
4 Protein	6 ounces baby bay scallops
½ Carbohydrate	¼ cup white wine
½ Carbohydrate	½ cup asparagus, chopped
2 Carbohydrate	6 small artichoke hearts, chopped*
½ Carbohydrate	1 cup red pepper, sliced
½ Carbohydrate	¼ cup Zoned French Dressing (see page 717)
4 Fat	1⅓ teaspoons olive oil, divided

Spices:

½ teaspoon garlic, minced
1 tablespoon fresh parsley, chopped
½ teaspoon Worcestershire sauce
Salt and pepper to taste

Method:
In a medium nonstick sauté pan heat ⅔ teaspoon oil. Add scallops, garlic, parsley, and Worcestershire sauce. Sauté until scallops are cooked through. In a second nonstick sauté pan add remaining oil, asparagus, artichokes, red pepper, and Zoned French Dressing. Cook until vegetables are crisp-tender. Add scallops and wine. Sauté an additional 3 to 5 minutes and spoon onto a serving dish. Salt and pepper to taste.

*Note: 3 small artichoke hearts equal 1 medium artichoke.

SAUTÉED TURKEY WITH APPLE-CHILI PEPPER RELISH

Servings: 1 Dinner Entrée (4 blocks)

Block Size:	Ingredients:
4 Protein	4 ounces turkey breast, diced (boneless, skinless)
1 Carbohydrate	1 cup red onion, chopped
1 Carbohydrate	¾ cup Zoned Pepper Relish (see page 719)
2 Carbohydrate	1 Granny Smith apple, chopped
4 Fat	1⅓ teaspoons olive oil

Spices:

1 tablespoon cider vinegar
½ teaspoon garlic, minced
⅛ teaspoon sweet paprika
¼ teaspoon chili powder
Salt and pepper to taste

Method:

In a medium nonstick sauté pan heat the oil. Add turkey, onion, vinegar, garlic, paprika, and salt and pepper. Sauté until cooked through. In a medium bowl combine Zoned Pepper Relish, apple, and chili powder. Spoon relish onto serving plate and top with turkey.

TURKEY SCALOPPINI WITH MUSHROOMS

Servings: 1 Dinner Entrée (4 blocks)

Block Size:	Ingredients:
4 Protein	4 ounces turkey breast, sliced in strips
½ Carbohydrate	½ cup onion, finely chopped
1 Carbohydrate	3 cups mushrooms, thinly sliced
2 Carbohydrate	⅔ cup unsweetened applesauce
½ Carbohydrate	2 teaspoons cornstarch
4 Fat	1⅓ teaspoons olive oil, divided

Spices:

2 teaspoons cider vinegar
1 teaspoon orange extract
⅛ teaspoon dill
¼ teaspoon cinnamon
1 cup lemon- and lime-flavored water
⅛ teaspoon lemon herb seasoning

Method:

Heat ⅔ teaspoon oil in medium nonstick sauté pan. Sauté turkey with onion, cider vinegar, and lemon herb seasoning. Sauté until turkey is cooked through, about 1 to 2 minutes. In second sauté pan heat remaining oil and sauté mushrooms for 3 to 5 minutes. Add remaining ingredients and sauté until liquid is thickened. (Mix cornstarch with a little water to dissolve it before adding to saucepan.) Spoon mushroom mixture onto serving plate and top with turkey.

TURKEY WITH LENTILS AND SPINACH

Servings: 1 Dinner Entrée (4 blocks)

Block Size:	Ingredients:
4 Protein	6 ounces lean ground turkey
¼ Carbohydrate	½ cup celery, chopped
¼ Carbohydrate	¼ cup onion, chopped
1 Carbohydrate	½ cup Zoned Italian Sauce (see page 710)
½ Carbohydrate	3 cups spinach, chopped
2 Carbohydrate	½ cup cooked lentils
4 Fat	1⅓ teaspoons olive oil

Spices:

1 teaspoon garlic, chopped
1 tablespoon fresh parsley, chopped
Dash fresh grated nutmeg
Salt and pepper to taste

Method:
Heat oil in a medium nonstick sauté pan. Add turkey, celery, onion, garlic, parsley, nutmeg, salt and pepper. Cook until turkey is cooked through and vegetables are slightly softened. Stir in Zoned Italian Sauce, lentils, and spinach. Heat through and spoon into a medium serving bowl.

CORDON BLEU CHICKEN STUFFED WITH HAM

Servings: 1 Dinner Entrée (4 blocks)

Block Size:	Ingredients:
3 Protein	3 ounces chicken breast (boneless, skinless)
½ Protein	¾ ounce deli-style ham, diced
½ Protein	½ ounce low-fat Swiss cheese
1 Carbohydrate	1 cup leeks, sliced (white part only)
1 Carbohydrate	¾ cup Zoned Espagnol (Brown) Sauce (see page 715)
½ Carbohydrate	1 cup celery, sliced
½ Carbohydrate	1½ cups mushrooms, quartered
1 Carbohydrate	1 cup green beans, 2-inch pieces
4 Fat	1⅓ teaspoons olive oil, divided

Spices:

⅛ teaspoon dried thyme
¼ teaspoon parsley, chopped
Salt and pepper to taste

Method:
Flatten chicken breast until ¼-inch thick. Place ham and cheese in the center of the flattened chicken breast and sprinkle with thyme, parsley, salt and pepper. Roll up chicken breast around filling and secure with toothpicks. Brush ⅓ teaspoon oil onto a baking dish. Place rolled chicken in dish and cover tightly. Bake in a preheated 350-degree Fahrenheit oven for 15 to 20 minutes. Heat remaining oil in a medium nonstick sauté pan, then add leeks, celery, mushrooms, and green beans and cook for 3 to 5 minutes. When the vegetables are tender blend in Zoned Espagnol Sauce and heat through. Spoon vegetables onto serving plate and top with rolled chicken breast.

SOUTHWESTERN CHICKEN WITH PEPPER AND BEAN SALSA

Servings: 1 Dinner Entrée (4 blocks)

Block Size:	Ingredients:
4 Protein	4 ounces chicken tenderloin, diced
1 Carbohydrate	½ cup salsa*
½ Carbohydrate	½ cup onion, chopped
1 Carbohydrate	¼ cup kidney beans, rinsed
½ Carbohydrate	3 cups spinach
1 Carbohydrate	¼ cup black beans, rinsed
4 Fat	1⅓ teaspoons olive oil

Spices:

1 tablespoon garlic, minced
⅛ teaspoon celery salt
2 teaspoons chili powder
Black pepper to taste

Method:

Heat oil in a medium nonstick sauté pan and add chicken and garlic. Sauté until chicken is cooked through and slightly browned. Add salsa, onion, kidney beans, black beans, chili powder, celery salt, and pepper and heat through. Form spinach into a bed on serving plate. Top with chicken mixture and serve.

*Note: We used a medium-heat salsa. Use whatever strength you prefer.

SPICY TOFU WITH SCALLIONS AND RADISHES

Servings: 1 Dinner Entrée (4 blocks)

Block Size:	Ingredients:
4 Protein	12 ounces extra-firm tofu, 1-inch cubes
1 Carbohydrate	1½ cups jalapeño and red bell pepper, finely diced (mixed to desired heat)
½ Carbohydrate	2 cups fresh spinach, torn
¼ Carbohydrate	½ cup radishes, thinly sliced
1 Carbohydrate	1 cup tomatoes, seeded and diced
½ Carbohydrate	½ cup scallions, chopped
¾ Carbohydrate	¾ cup canned mushroom slices
4 Fat	1⅓ teaspoons olive oil

Spices:

1 tablespoon lemon juice
1 tablespoon water
4 teaspoons soy sauce
½ tablespoon white wine
¾ teaspoon gingerroot, minced
¼ teaspoon garlic, minced
Salt and pepper to taste

Method:
Heat oil and ¼ teaspoon gingerroot in medium sauté pan. Stir-fry tofu until browned on all sides. Whisk lemon juice, water, soy sauce, wine, garlic, salt, pepper, and remaining gingerroot together in a small bowl. Combine vegetables in a medium bowl and pour in soy sauce mixture. Toss to coat. Add in tofu and spoon onto serving dish.

MUSHROOM TENDERLOIN WITH
ARTICHOKE HEARTS

Servings: 1 Dinner Entrée (4 blocks)

Block Size:	Ingredients:
4 Protein	4 ounces beef tenderloin
1 Carbohydrate	1 cup Zoned Mushroom Sauce (see page 7088)
1 Carbohydrate	1 cup onions, chopped
2 Carbohydrate	6 small artichoke hearts, diced*
4 Fat	1⅓ teaspoons olive oil

Method:

In a nonstick sauté pan add oil, onion, artichoke hearts, and beef. Cook until beef is done and vegetables are tender. Add Zoned Mushroom Sauce and heat through. Place mixture on a large dinner plate and serve immediately.

*Note: 3 small artichoke hearts equal 1 medium artichoke.

ITALIAN-STYLE STEAK AND PEPPERS

Servings: 1 Dinner Entrée (4 blocks)

Block Size:	Ingredients:
3 Protein	3 ounces lean beef
1 Protein	1 ounce skim milk mozzarella, shredded
1 Carbohydrate	½ cup Zoned Italian Sauce (see page 710)
2 Carbohydrate	2¼ cups red and green pepper strips
1 Carbohydrate	1 cup onion, diced
4 Fat	1⅓ teaspoons olive oil

Method:

In a nonstick sauté pan, place oil, beef, and vegetables. Cook until beef is done and vegetables are tender. Add Zoned Italian Sauce and heat through. Top with cheese and serve.

CONDIMENTS AND SAUCES

ZONED MUSHROOM SAUCE

Servings: Four 1-cup servings, 1 Carbohydrate Block each*

Block Size:

1½ Carbohydrate
2½ Carbohydrate

Ingredients:

4½ cups mushrooms, sliced
10 teaspoons cornstarch

Spices:

3 cups strong beef stock
⅛ teaspoon Worcestershire sauce
1 tablespoon red wine
⅛ teaspoon chili powder
½ teaspoon garlic, chopped
1 tablespoon dried parsley flakes
Salt and pepper to taste

Method:

Combine all ingredients in a small saucepan to form a sauce. (Mix cornstarch with a little cold water to dissolve it before adding to saucepan.) Heat sauce to a simmer, constantly stirring until mixture thickens. Transfer sauce mixture to a storage container, let cool, and refrigerate.** Each time you make a Zone-favorable meal use this sauce as a replacement for 1 Carbohydrate Zone Block.

*Note: Each cup of Zoned Mushroom Sauce contains 1 Carbohydrate Zone Block. There are no Protein or Fat Blocks in this sauce recipe. This recipe is used as a component in other Zone Recipes.

**Note: This sauce may be refrigerated for up to 5 days, or if you prefer the sauce may be frozen and defrosted for later use. Although the sauce is freeze-thaw stable, after sauce has been frozen and defrosted it may need to be stirred to reincorporate the small amount of moisture that forms on the sauce during the freezing and thawing process.

ZONED COUNTRY-STYLE CHICKEN GRAVY

*Servings: Four 1-cup servings, 1 Carbohydrate Block each**

Block Size:	**Ingredients:**
2 Carbohydrate	2 cups onions, sliced
2 Carbohydrate	8 teaspoons cornstarch

Spices:

2½ cups strong chicken stock
1 tablespoon white wine
½ teaspoon garlic, chopped
½ teaspoon celery salt
1 teaspoon dried parsley flakes
Salt and pepper to taste

Method:

Combine all ingredients in a small saucepan to form a sauce. (Mix cornstarch with a little cold water to dissolve it before adding to saucepan.) Heat sauce to a simmer, constantly stirring until mixture thickens. Transfer sauce mixture to a storage container, let cool and refrigerate.** Each time you make a Zone-favorable meal use this sauce as a replacement for 1 Carbohydrate Zone Block.

Note: Each cup of Zoned Country-Style Chicken Gravy contains 1 Carbohydrate Zone Block. There are no Protein or Fat Blocks in this sauce recipe. This recipe is used as a component in other Zone Recipes.

**Note: This sauce may be refrigerated for up to 5 days, or if you prefer the sauce may be frozen and defrosted for later use. Although the sauce is freeze-thaw stable, after sauce has been frozen and defrosted it may need to be stirred to reincorporate the small amount of moisture that forms on the sauce during the freezing and thawing process.*

ZONED ITALIAN SAUCE

Servings: Four ½-cup servings, 1 Carbohydrate Block each*

Block Size:

3 Carbohydrate
1 Carbohydrate

Ingredients:

1½ cups tomato puree
4 teaspoons cornstarch

Spices:

1 cup strong chicken stock
1 tablespoon red wine
1 teaspoon dried parsley flakes
1 teaspoon dried oregano
1 teaspoon dried basil
⅛ teaspoon ground dried thyme
⅛ teaspoon ground nutmeg
1½ teaspoons garlic, chopped

Method:
Combine all ingredients in a small saucepan to form a sauce. (Mix cornstarch with a little cold water to dissolve it before adding to saucepan.) Heat sauce to a simmer, constantly stirring with a whip until mixture thickens. Transfer sauce mixture to a storage container, let cool, and refrigerate.** Each time you make a Zone-favorable meal use this sauce as a replacement for 1 Carbohydrate Zone Block.

*Note: Each ½ cup of Zoned Italian Sauce contains 1 Carbohydrate Zone Block. There is no Protein or Fat Blocks in this sauce recipe. This recipe is used as a component in other Zone Recipes.

**Note: This sauce may be refrigerated for up to 5 days, or if you prefer the sauce may be frozen and defrosted for later use. Although the sauce is freeze-thaw stable, after sauce has been frozen and defrosted it may need to be stirred to reincorporate the small amount of moisture that forms on the sauce during the freezing and thawing process.

ZONED WHITE SAUCE

Servings: Four ½-cup servings, 1 Protein Block and
1 Carbohydrate Block each*

Block Size:	Ingredients:
1 Protein	1 envelope Knox unflavored gelatin
1 Protein	1 ounce white low-fat cheddar cheese, shredded
2 Protein and 2 Carbohydrate	2 cups 1 percent milk
1½ Carbohydrate	6 teaspoons cornstarch
½ Carbohydrate	½ cup onion, finely minced or pureed in a blender

Spices:

½ cup low-fat chicken stock
⅛ teaspoon celery salt
⅛ teaspoon Worcestershire sauce
White pepper to taste

Method:
Combine all ingredients in a small non-aluminum saucepan to form a sauce. (Mix cornstarch with a little cold water to dissolve it before adding to saucepan.) Heat sauce to a simmer, constantly stirring with a whip until mixture thickens. Transfer sauce mixture to a storage container, let cool, and refrigerate.** Each time you make a Zone-favorable meal use this sauce as a replacement for 1 Carbohydrate Zone Block.

*Note: Each ½ cup of Zoned White Sauce contains 1 Protein Zone Block and 1 Carbohydrate Zone Block. There are no Fat Blocks in this sauce recipe. This recipe is used as a component in other Zone Recipes.

**Note: This sauce may be refrigerated for up to 5 days, or if you prefer the sauce may be frozen and defrosted for later use. Although the sauce is

freeze-thaw stable, after sauce has been frozen and defrosted it may need to be stirred to reincorporate the small amount of moisture that forms on the sauce during the freezing and thawing process.

ZONED FINE HERB CHEESE SAUCE

Servings: Four ½-cup servings, 1 Protein Block and 1 Carbohydrate Block each*

Block Size:	Ingredients:
2 Protein	2 ounces yellow low-fat cheddar cheese
2 Protein and 2 Carbohydrate	2 cups 1 percent milk
1½ Carbohydrate	6 teaspoons cornstarch
½ Carbohydrate	½ cup onion, finely minced or pureed in a blender

Spices:

½ tablespoon dry sherry
⅛ teaspoon dried parsley
⅛ teaspoon dried chives
⅛ teaspoon dried basil
1 teaspoon paprika
⅛ teaspoon chili powder
⅛ teaspoon Worcestershire sauce
⅛ teaspoon celery salt
1 teaspoon garlic, minced
½ teaspoon lemon herb seasoning

Method:
Combine all ingredients in a small non-aluminum saucepan to form a sauce. (Mix cornstarch with a little cold water to dissolve it before adding

to saucepan.) Heat sauce to a simmer, constantly stirring with a whip until mixture thickens. Transfer sauce mixture to a storage container, let cool, and refrigerate.** Each time you make a Zone-favorable meal use this sauce as a replacement for 1 Carbohydrate Zone Block.

*Note: Each ½ cup of Zoned Fine Herb Cheese Sauce contains 1 Protein Zone Block and 1 Carbohydrate Zone Block. There are no Fat Blocks in this sauce recipe. This recipe is used as a component in other Zone Recipes.

**Note: This sauce may be refrigerated for up to 5 days, or if you prefer the sauce may be frozen and defrosted for later use. Although the sauce is freeze-thaw stable, after sauce has been frozen and defrosted it may need to be stirred to reincorporate the small amount of moisture that forms on the sauce during the freezing and thawing process.

ZONED BARBECUE SAUCE

Servings: Four ½-cup servings, 1 Carbohydrate Block each*

Block Size:	**Ingredients:**
1 Carbohydrate	4 teaspoons cornstarch
2 Carbohydrate	1 cup tomato puree
1 Carbohydrate	⅓ cup unsweetened applesauce

Spices:

1 tablespoon liquid smoke flavoring
4 teaspoons garlic, minced
1 teaspoon Worcestershire sauce
¾ cup strong chicken stock
3 tablespoons cider vinegar
¼ teaspoon chili powder

Method:
Combine all ingredients in a small saucepan to form a sauce. (Mix cornstarch with a little cold water to dissolve it before adding to saucepan.) Heat sauce to a simmer, constantly stirring with a whip until mixture thickens. Transfer sauce mixture to a storage container, let cool, and refrigerate.** Each time you make a Zone-favorable meal use this sauce as a replacement for 1 Carbohydrate Zone Block.

*Note: Each ½ cup of Zoned Barbecue Sauce contains 1 Carbohydrate Zone Block. There are no Protein or Fat Blocks in this sauce recipe. This recipe is used as a component in other Zone Recipes.

**Note: This sauce may be refrigerated for up to 5 days, or if you prefer the sauce may be frozen and defrosted for later use. Although the sauce is freeze-thaw stable, after sauce has been frozen and defrosted it may need to be stirred to reincorporate the small amount of moisture that forms on the sauce during the freezing and thawing process.

ZONED ESPAGNOL (BROWN) SAUCE

Servings: Four ¾-cup servings, 1 Carbohydrate Block each*

Block Size:

1 Carbohydrate
¼ Carbohydrate
2¾ Carbohydrate

Ingredients:

½ cup tomato puree
¼ cup onion, finely diced
11 teaspoons cornstarch

Spices:

3 cups strong beef stock
⅛ teaspoon Worcestershire sauce
1 tablespoon red wine
2 teaspoons garlic, chopped
⅛ teaspoon dried oregano
1 teaspoon dried parsley flakes
Salt and pepper to taste

Method:

Combine all ingredients in a small saucepan to form a sauce. (Mix cornstarch with a little cold water to dissolve it before adding to saucepan.) Heat sauce to a simmer, constantly stirring with a whip until mixture thickens. Transfer sauce mixture to a storage container, let cool, and refrigerate.** Each time you make a Zone-favorable meal use this sauce as a replacement for 1 Carbohydrate Zone Block.

*Note: Each ¾ cup of Zoned Espagnol (Brown) Sauce contains 1 Carbohydrate Zone Block. There are no Protein or Fat Blocks in this sauce recipe. This recipe is used as a component in other Zone Recipes.

**Note: This sauce may be refrigerated for up to 5 days, or if you prefer the sauce may be frozen and defrosted for later use. Although the sauce is freeze-thaw stable, after sauce has been frozen and defrosted it may need to be stirred to reincorporate the small amount of moisture that forms on the sauce during the freezing and thawing process.

ZONED HERB DRESSING

Servings: Four ½-cup servings, 1 Carbohydrate Block each*

Block Size:

1 Carbohydrate
1 Carbohydrate

2 Carbohydrate

Ingredients:

1 cup onion, finely minced
¼ cup chickpeas, canned, minced finely
8 teaspoons cornstarch

Spices:

1¾ cups water
¼ cup cider vinegar
2 tablespoons balsamic vinegar
⅛ teaspoon Worcestershire sauce
1 teaspoon dried tarragon
1 teaspoon dried oregano
1 teaspoon parsley flakes
2 teaspoons garlic, minced
1 teaspoon dried basil
⅛ teaspoon chili powder
½ teaspoon celery salt
1 teaspoon dried dill

Method:
Combine all ingredients in a small saucepan to form a thickened dressing. (Mix cornstarch with a little cold water to dissolve it before adding to saucepan.) Heat dressing to a simmer, constantly stirring until mixture thickens. Transfer dressing mixture to a storage container, let cool, and refrigerate.** Each time you make a Zone-favorable meal use this dressing as a replacement for 1 Carbohydrate Zone Block.

*Note: Each ½ cup of Zoned Herb Dressing contains 1 Carbohydrate Zone Block. There are no Protein or Fat Blocks in this sauce recipe. This recipe is used as a component in other Zone Recipes.

**Note:* This dressing may be refrigerated for up to 5 days, or if you pre-fer the dressing may be frozen and defrosted for later use. Although the dressing is freeze-thaw stable, after dressing has been frozen and defrosted it may need to be stirred to reincorporate the small amount of moisture that forms on the dressing during the freezing and thawing process.*

ZONED FRENCH DRESSING

*Servings: Four ½-cup servings, 1 Carbohydrate Block each**

Block Size:	Ingredients:
½ Carbohydrate	½ cup onion, finely minced
½ Carbohydrate	¼ cup tomato puree
2 Carbohydrate	8 teaspoons cornstarch
1 Carbohydrate	¼ cup kidney beans, canned, rinsed, and minced

Spices:

1¾ cups water
¼ cup cider vinegar
2 tablespoons balsamic vinegar
⅛ teaspoon Worcestershire sauce
1 teaspoon dried tarragon
1 teaspoon dried oregano
1 teaspoon dried parsley flakes
3 teaspoons garlic, minced
1 teaspoon dried basil
½ teaspoon chili powder
2 teaspoons paprika
1 teaspoon dried dill

Method:
Combine all ingredients in a small saucepan to form a thickened dressing. (Mix cornstarch with a little cold water to dissolve it before

adding to saucepan.) Heat dressing to a simmer, constantly stirring until mixture thickens. Let dressing cool for about 10 to 15 minutes, then place dressing in a food processor and blend for 2 to 3 minutes until a smooth consistency forms. Transfer dressing mixture to a storage container, let cool, and refrigerate.** Each time you make a Zone-favorable meal use this dressing as a replacement for 1 Carbohydrate Zone Block.

*Note: Each ½ cup of Zoned French Dressing contains 1 Carbohydrate Zone Block. There are no Protein or Fat Blocks in this sauce recipe. This recipe is used as a component in other Zone Recipes.

**Note: This dressing may be refrigerated for up to 5 days, or if you prefer, the dressing may be frozen and defrosted for later use. Although the dressing is freeze-thaw stable, after dressing has been frozen and defrosted it may need to be stirred to reincorporate the small amount of moisture that forms on the dressing during the freezing and thawing process.

ZONED PEPPER RELISH

Servings: Four ¾-cup servings, 1 Carbohydrate Block each*

Block Size:	Ingredients:
1½ Carbohydrate	3½ cups frozen red and green bell pepper strips
½ Carbohydrate	½ cup frozen onions, chopped
1 Carbohydrate	½ cup tomato puree
½ Carbohydrate	½ cup tomato, chopped
½ Carbohydrate	2 teaspoons cornstarch

Spices:

¼ cup water
1 tablespoon cider vinegar
2 teaspoons pickling spice
½ teaspoon lemon herb seasoning
⅛ teaspoon celery salt

Method:

Combine all ingredients in a small saucepan to form the pepper relish. (Mix cornstarch with a little cold water to dissolve it before adding to saucepan.) Heat relish to a simmer, constantly stirring until mixture thickens. Simmer for 3 to 5 minutes until entire mixture is hot. Transfer relish mixture to a storage container, let cool, and refrigerate.** Each time you make a Zone-favorable meal use this dressing as a replacement for 1 Carbohydrate Zone Block.

*Note: Each ¾ cup of Zoned Pepper Relish contains 1 Carbohydrate Zone Block. There are no Protein or Fat Blocks in this sauce recipe. This recipe is used as a component in other Zone Recipes or used as a condiment to other Zone Recipes.

**Note: This relish may be refrigerated for up to 5 days, or if you prefer the relish may be frozen and defrosted for later use. Although the relish is freeze-thaw stable, after relish has been frozen and defrosted it may need to be stirred to reincorporate the small amount of moisture that forms on the relish during the freezing and thawing process.

ZONED TARRAGON MUSTARD SAUCE

Servings: Four ½-cup servings, 1 Carbohydrate Block each*

Block Size:	Ingredients:
2 Carbohydrate	½ cup chickpeas, canned, minced finely
2 Carbohydrate	8 teaspoons cornstarch

Spices:

2 cups chicken stock
2 tablespoons cider vinegar
½ teaspoon Worcestershire sauce
2 teaspoons dried tarragon
2 teaspoons ground mustard
¼ teaspoon turmeric
2 teaspoons garlic, minced

Method:

Combine all ingredients in a small saucepan to form a sauce. (Mix cornstarch with a little cold water to dissolve it before adding to saucepan.) Heat sauce to a simmer, constantly stirring with a whip until mixture thickens. Transfer sauce mixture to a storage container, let cool, and refrigerate.** Each time you make a Zone-favorable meal use this sauce as a replacement for 1 Carbohydrate Zone Block.

*Note: Each ½ cup of Zoned Tarragon Mustard Sauce contains 1 Carbohydrate Zone Block. There are no Protein or Fat Blocks in this sauce recipe. This recipe is used as a component in other Zone Recipes.

**Note: This sauce may be refrigerated for up to 5 days, or if you prefer the sauce may be frozen and defrosted for later use. Although the sauce is freeze-thaw stable, after sauce has been frozen and defrosted it may need to be stirred to reincorporate the small amount of moisture that forms on the sauce during the freezing and thawing process.

ZONED CHINESE PICKLED VEGETABLES

Servings: Four ½-cup servings, 1 Carbohydrate Block each*

Block Size:	Ingredients:
1 Carbohydrate	1½ cups frozen broccoli florets
1 Carbohydrate	⅓ cup canned water chestnuts, sliced
1 Carbohydrate	2 teaspoons sugar
½ Carbohydrate	1½ cups cabbage, shredded (or coleslaw mix)
½ Carbohydrate	1 cup frozen cauliflower florets

Spices:

1 teaspoon garlic, minced
1 tablespoon Worcestershire sauce
1 tablespoon soy sauce
¼ teaspoon celery salt
1 teaspoon pickling spice
2 cups water
⅛ teaspoon hot red pepper flakes (optional)

Method: Combine all ingredients in a saucepan and bring to a boil. Reduce heat and simmer for 10 minutes. Transfer mixture to a storage container, let cool, and refrigerate. Each time you make a Zone-favorable meal use these pickled vegetables as a replacement for 1 Carbohydrate Zone Block.

*Note: Each ½ cup of Zoned Chinese Pickled Vegetables contains 1 Carbohydrate Zone Block. There are no Protein or Fat Blocks in this sauce recipe. This recipe is used as a component in other Zone Recipes.

DESSERTS AND SNACKS

FROZEN YOGURT ALASKA JUBILEE

Servings: 8 Serving Dishes (1 block each)

Block Size:	Ingredients:
3 Protein	3 envelopes Knox unflavored gelatin
1 Protein	2 egg whites, uncooked
4 Protein and	
4 Carbohydrate	2 cups plain low-fat yogurt
3 Carbohydrate	1½ cups canned pitted tart cherries, in water
1 Carbohydrate	2 teaspoons sugar
8 Fat	8 teaspoons almonds, slivered and toasted

Spices:

2 teaspoons cherry extract
½ teaspoon vanilla extract
⅛ teaspoon powdered ginger

Method:

In saucepan, combine yogurt, gelatin, fruit, extracts, and ginger. Heat until mixture becomes thoroughly warm, no more than 180 degrees. Set aside yogurt mixture and let cool. In a mixing bowl, whip egg whites and sugar until firm. When the mixture in the saucepan has cooled, combine mixture with whipped egg whites and chopped almonds. Place mixture in a pan and place in freezer or add mixture to an ice cream maker and blend. When mixture is frozen, scoop into eight small serving dishes.

HOMEMADE CINNAMON APPLESAUCE WITH YOGURT

Servings: 8 Serving Dishes (1 block each)

Block Size:	Ingredients:
4 Protein	4 envelopes Knox unflavored gelatin
4 Protein and 4 Carbohydrate	2 cups plain low-fat yogurt
4 Carbohydrate	2 Granny Smith apples, cored and diced in ½-inch cubes
8 Fat	8 teaspoons almonds, slivered and toasted

Spices:

1 teaspoon ground cinnamon
½ teaspoon pure lemon extract

Method:

In a medium bowl, combine yogurt, gelatin, fruit, almonds, cinnamon, and extract. Blend well, chill, and serve in 8 serving bowls.

POACHED PEAR WITH CHEESE

Servings: 8 Serving Dishes (1 block each)

Block Size:	Ingredients:
8 Protein	2 cups low-fat cottage cheese
6 Carbohydrate	3 pears, halved, cored, and sliced in thin strips
1 Carbohydrate	4 ounces Johannesburg Riesling
½ Carbohydrate	2 teaspoons cornstarch
½ Carbohydrate	¼ cup blueberries
8 Fat	8 teaspoons almonds, slivered

Spices:

½ teaspoon orange extract
½ teaspoon lemon extract
Dash of ground cloves

Method:
In a small nonstick sauté pan, combine wine, extracts, and cornstarch. (Mix cornstarch in wine before adding to sauté pan.) Add pears to the sauté pan and bring to a simmer. Simmer for 3 to 5 minutes, stirring frequently, until the pears soften and the juices reduce and thicken. As the mixture cooks add cloves. Divide cottage cheese into the bottom of 8 serving bowls. Place warm pears on top of cottage cheese. Sprinkle with almonds and blueberries and serve.

PEACHES WITH A AND A TOPPING

Servings: 8 Serving Dishes (1 block each)

Block Size:	Ingredients:
8 Protein	2 cups low-fat cottage cheese
4½ Carbohydrate	4½ peaches, halved and pitted
2 Carbohydrate	⅔ cup unsweetened applesauce
½ Carbohydrate	2 teaspoons cornstarch
1 Carbohydrate	4 ounces Johannesburg Riesling
8 Fat	8 teaspoons almonds, finely chopped

Spices:

2 tablespoons water
½ teaspoon orange extract
½ teaspoon lemon extract
Dash ground cloves
⅛ teaspoon ground ginger
Dash ground cinnamon

Method:

In a small nonstick sauté pan, combine wine, water, extracts, cloves, ginger, and cornstarch. (Mix cornstarch in wine before adding to sauté pan.) Add peaches to the sauté pan and bring to a simmer. Simmer for 3 to 5 minutes, stirring frequently, until the peaches soften and the juices reduce and thicken. In a small bowl whip together applesauce, almonds, and cinnamon. Divide cottage cheese into the bottom of 8 serving bowls. Place warm peaches on top of cottage cheese. Spoon on almonds and applesauce topping and serve.

GLAZED SPICED APPLE

Servings: 4 Serving Dishes (1 block each)

Block Size:	Ingredients:
4 Protein	4 ounces low-fat cheddar cheese, shredded
2 Carbohydrate	1 red Delicious apple, cored and cut into 1-inch cubes
1 Carbohydrate	1 peach, halved, pitted, and finely diced
½ Carbohydrate	1 teaspoon brown sugar
½ Carbohydrate	2 teaspoons cornstarch
4 Fat	4 teaspoons almonds, sliced and toasted

Spices:

½ cup water
3 tablespoons cider vinegar
¼ teaspoon lemon extract
⅛ teaspoon ground cinnamon
Dash celery salt

Method:
Combine all ingredients (except cheese) in a small saucepan. Stirring constantly, over medium heat, cook until the apple is thoroughly coated and a sauce forms. Continue simmering 3 to 5 minutes until flavors are blended. Spoon into bowls, top with shredded cheese, and serve hot.

SHRIMP AND VEGETABLE PLATTER

Servings: 4 Serving Dishes (1 block each)

Block Size:	Ingredients:
4 Protein	6 ounces baby shrimp
1 Carbohydrate	2 cups broccoli florets
1 Carbohydrate	1 cup celery, julienne
1 Carbohydrate	1 cup cherry tomatoes
1 Carbohydrate	½ cup Zoned Herb Dressing (see page 716)
4 Fat	12 black olives

Method:
Place Zoned Herb Dressing into 4 small serving dishes, and place on center of 4 serving plates. Arrange an equal amount of vegetables, olives, and shrimp around the edge of each plate.

BLUSHING PEAR

Servings: 8 Serving Dishes (1 block each)

Block Size:	Ingredients:
8 Protein	8 ounces low-fat cottage cheese
6 Carbohydrate	3 pears, cored, halved, and sliced into thin strips
1 Carbohydrate	4 ounces white Zinfandel
½ Carbohydrate	2 teaspoons cornstarch
½ Carbohydrate	½ cup raspberries
8 Fat	8 teaspoons almonds, finely chopped

Spices:

½ teaspoon orange extract
½ teaspoon lemon extract
Dash of ground cloves

Method:
In a small nonstick sauté pan, combine wine, extracts, and cornstarch. (Mix cornstarch in wine before adding to sauté pan.) Add pears to the sauté pan and bring to a simmer. Simmer for 3 to 5 minutes, stirring frequently, until the pears soften and the juices reduce and thicken. As the mixture cooks, add cloves. Divide cottage cheese into the bottom of 8 serving bowls. Place warm pears on top of cottage cheese. Sprinkle with raspberries and almonds and serve.

BLUEBERRY CUSTARD JUBILEE

Servings: 4 Serving Dishes (1 block each)

Block Size:	Ingredients:
2 Protein	2 whole eggs
2 Protein and	
2 Carbohydrate	2 cups 1 percent milk
1 Carbohydrate	½ cup blueberries
1 Carbohydrate	2 teaspoons sugar

Spices:

⅛ teaspoon vanilla extract or lemon zest

Method:

Beat eggs until they are light and fluffy; then put eggs, milk, vanilla extract, and sugar in a nonstick saucepan. Heat mixture to a simmer, but not boiling. Pour mixture into 4 serving dishes and refrigerator to cool. After mixture has cooled for 20 minutes divide blueberries into 4 serving dishes and return to refrigerator. Serve when custard has set.

TANGY FRUIT FLUFF

Servings: 4 Serving Dishes (1 block each)

Block Size:	Ingredients:
3 Protein	6 egg whites
1 Protein	1 envelope Knox unflavored gelatin
2 Carbohydrate	1 cup blueberries
1 Carbohydrate	1 cup raspberries
1 Carbohydrate	¾ cup blackberries

Method:

In a mixing bowl whip egg whites and gelatin until a fluffy mixture with stiff peaks forms. Slowly fold berries into whipped egg whites. Equally divide mixture into 4 serving dishes and sprinkle with almonds. Place serving dishes in freezer until set.

MELON SMOOTHIE

Servings: 4 Glasses (1 block each)

Block Size:	Ingredients:
1 Protein	1/3 ounce protein powder
2 Protein and 2 Carbohydrate	2 cups 1 percent milk
1 Protein and 1 Carbohydrate	1/2 cup plain low-fat yogurt
1 Carbohydrate	3/4 cup cantaloupe chunks
4 Fat	4 teaspoons almonds, slivered

Method:
Place all ingredients except protein powder in blender. Blend until smooth, then add protein powder. Pour into four glasses and serve immediately.

RASPBERRY-LIME SMOOTHIE

Servings: 4 Glasses (1 block each)

Block Size:	Ingredients:
2 Protein	⅔ ounce protein powder
1 Protein and 1 Carbohydrate	1 cup 1 percent milk
1 Protein and 1 Carbohydrate	½ cup plain low-fat yogurt
1 Carbohydrate	1 cup raspberries
1 Carbohydrate	Juice of 1 lime
4 Fat	4 teaspoons almonds, slivered

Method:
Place all ingredients except protein powder in blender. Blend until smooth, then add protein powder. Pour into four glasses and serve immediately.

STRAWBERRY-ORANGE SMOOTHIE

Servings: 4 Glasses (1 block each)

Block Size:	Ingredients:
2 Protein	⅔ ounce protein powder
1 Protein and 1 Carbohydrate	1 cup 1 percent milk
1 Protein and 1 Carbohydrate	½ cup plain low-fat yogurt
1 Carbohydrate	1 cup strawberries
1 Carbohydrate	⅓ cup mandarin orange segments
4 Fat	4 teaspoons almonds, slivered

Method:

Place all ingredients except protein powder in blender. Blend until smooth, then add protein powder. Pour into four glasses and serve immediately.

ZONE-PERFECT GOURMET MEALS

Let's face it. Gourmet meals are called gourmet meals because they are difficult to prepare and take more time to present. But there will be those occasions when you will want to take the time to prepare a gourmet meal, and of course you want to make it Zone-Perfect.

Fortunately, some of the best chefs in America have already done the work for you. This meal comes from La Bocage, which is one of the top French restaurants in the Greater Boston area. For a recent meeting of the Boston Culinary Society, Susanna Harwell-Tolini and Ed Tolini prepared the following Zone meal, consisting of chicken consommé with chicken quenelles, poached Atlantic salmon with asparagus coulis, baked tomatoes stuffed with spinach using a tomato sauce, and strawberry mousse. Here's how to make this gourmet Zone meal for a party of six:

CHICKEN STOCK

Ingredients:

1 large stewing fowl
1½–2 gallons cold water
1 cup carrots (diced)
1 cup onions (diced)
1 cup celery (diced)
1 cup leeks (diced)
¼ cup loosely packed fresh parsley
2 bay leaves
1 teaspoon thyme

Method:
In a large pot, place the stewing fowl and cover with cold water; then add the vegetables and herbs. Bring the water to a boil, and skim off the fat and impurities. Add the spices and simmer 4 to 5 hours. Strain the broth and cool, then refrigerate.

CHICKEN CONSOMMÉ

Ingredients:

1½ quarts chilled chicken stock
½ cup carrots (coarsely chopped)
½ cup onions (coarsely chopped)
½ cup fresh tomato (chopped)
½ cup egg whites (lightly beaten)
½ pound chicken meat (ground skinless chicken breast with
    no fat)
2 bay leaves
2 sprigs fresh thyme
1 teaspoon black peppercorns (crushed)
1 teaspoon salt

Method:
Puree the vegetables in a food processor fitted with a steel blade. Combine the vegetables with the ground chicken meat and mix with the lightly beaten egg whites. Add the herbs and seasonings. Marinate and chill for 1 hour. Place the ingredients in a stockpot with the chilled chicken stock. Stir well to incorporate. Stir until the stock has come to a slow boil. Simmer 2 to 3 hours. The raft should be well formed on the top of the consommé.* Do not boil rapidly, as this will cause the raft to break and fall. After simmering, strain through a fine strainer with cheesecloth. Serve with chicken quenelles (see following page) in a warmed soup bowl.

*Note: A raft is the culinary term used to describe the solid mass formed by the vegetables, egg whites, and spices to remove impurities from stock.

CHICKEN QUENELLES

Ingredients:

8 ounces skinless chicken breast
1 tablespoon egg whites
2 teaspoons light cream
2 ounces chicken stock
½ nutmeg (freshly ground)
1 pint chicken broth
Salt and white pepper to taste

Method:

Puree chicken breast in a food processor. Add the light cream, egg whites, and 2 ounces chicken broth while the processor is on. Be sure to emulsify all of the liquid ingredients into the chicken. Season with salt, pepper, and nutmeg. Heat the pint of chicken broth in a small pan to boiling point. Test one or two quenelles for flavor and texture by dropping a small ball of the chicken mixture in the stock. Taste and correct the seasonings if needed. Cook the remaining quenelles by taking soupspoons and dropping round or oval shapes into the stock (about 2 full teaspoons each). Serve 1½ ounces per person.

POACHED ATLANTIC SALMON WITH ASPARAGUS COULIS

Servings: 6

Ingredients:

6 4½-ounce each Atlantic salmon fillets (skins removed)
1 bunch asparagus (peeled and stems removed)

Court Bouillon:

1 quart water
1 cup dry white wine
1 small white onion, peeled
½ cup leek greens, diced
2 ribs celery
3 large bay leaves
1 teaspoon black peppercorns
½ cup parsley stems

Asparagus Coulis (may need additional asparagus for the coulis):

3 large shallots, peeled and cut in quarters
1 large white leek (diced)
¾ cup chicken stock
1 pound asparagus trimmings (stems and reserved peelings)
1 cup chicken stock
¼ bunch sorrel
¼ bunch watercress

Method:
Peel and cut the woody stems from the asparagus. Reserve the peelings and stems. Blanch the asparagus in boiling water. Immediately cool

and reserve for final presentation. Combine the ingredients for the court bouillon in a medium skillet or saucepan and simmer for 45 minutes.

For the Coulis:
Simmer the shallots and leek white in the ¾ cup of chicken stock for 20 minutes. Add the asparagus trimmings and the additional cup of chicken stock. Slowly braise the trimmings for 45 minutes, or until all the greens are tender (retaining the brilliant green color). Stir in the sorrel and watercress and immediately remove from the stove. Strain off half the chicken stock and reserve. Puree the asparagus greens in a blender and strain through a fine sieve. The reserved cooking liquid may be used to correct the body of the coulis.

To finish the plate:
Poach the salmon in the simmering court bouillon 10 minutes per inch of thickness. Heat up the blanched asparagus in the reserved cooking liquid from the coulis recipe. Heat up the coulis (do not boil), check for the seasoning, and add salt and white pepper to taste.
Place the salmon on a plate on the coulis and finish with 2 or 3 asparagus spears placed over the salmon.

TOMATO SAUCE

Yield: approximately 2 quarts

Ingredients:

3 cloves of garlic (peeled)
1 large Spanish onion (chopped)
½ cup carrots (chopped)
½ cup celery (chopped)
½ cup leeks (chopped)
1 tablespoon olive oil
2 pounds plum tomatoes (chopped)
1 cup chicken stock
Basil and thyme to taste (optional)

Method:

Sauté the onion, garlic, carrots, celery, and leeks over high heat in the olive oil for approximately 10 minutes, or until tender. Add the plum tomatoes and chicken stock. Simmer for 1 hour. Strain the sauce through a fine sieve. Chill the sauce and reserve for cooking the baked spinach stuffed tomato (see following page). The remainder of the sauce may be used in other vegetable preparations, such as ratatouille.

BAKED TOMATOES STUFFED WITH SPINACH

Ingredients:

3 large tomatoes
1 tablespoon olive oil
6 cups loosely packed fresh spinach (diced)
6 cups loosely packed broccoli (diced)
1 medium onion (finely chopped)
½ cup tomato sauce (see page 739)
½ cup low-fat cottage cheese (puree in a food processor)
2 teaspoons salt
½ teaspoon white pepper
Bread crumbs

Method:
Prepare the tomatoes by removing the stems, cutting them in half, and scooping out the pulp. In a large sauté pan, sauté the onion in the olive oil over medium heat for about 5 minutes. Add the washed spinach and broccoli. Cover and steam sauté the vegetables for 8 minutes. Add the tomato sauce, cottage cheese, salt, and pepper. Cook for 5 more minutes. Generously stuff the tomato halves with spinach filling and top with the bread crumbs. Bake at 400 degrees Fahrenheit for 10 to 15 minutes, until the bread crumbs are well browned.

STRAWBERRY MOUSSE

Ingredients:

3 cups fresh strawberries (the sweetest available)
2 tablespoons brown sugar
½ cup Neufchâtel cheese
1 cup low-fat cottage cheese
4 tablespoons "Just Whites" (mixed with water according to directions on the package)*
1 package plain Knox gelatin, dissolved in water

Garnish (per serving):
6 teaspoons plain low-fat yogurt
6 fresh strawberries (cut in a fan presentation)

Method:
Clean and core the strawberries, blend with the brown sugar, and let marinate for two hours. In a food processor fitted with a steel blade, puree the strawberries. Add the Neufchâtel cheese and process until the cheese is uniformly pureed with the strawberries. Then add the cottage cheese and puree again. Add the "Just Whites" and puree for uniformity. Finally add the dissolved gelatin, then pulse until thoroughly combined. Pour into 6 chilled wineglasses. Cover each with plastic wrap and refrigerate until the mousse is set. Top with the plain yogurt and strawberries when ready to serve.

Obviously, gourmet Zone-Perfect meals are not made in minutes, but they do show you how a truly gourmet meal can be created that keeps you firmly in the center of the Zone.

Note: "Just Whites" are powdered egg whites.

QUICK ZONE SNACKS

One of the biggest problems for people is finding easy-to-prepare one-block Zone snacks. Here are number of delicious choices:

LOW-FAT COTTAGE CHEESE AND FRUIT

¼ cup low-fat cottage cheese
1 block canned light fruit
1 macadamia nut or 3 almonds

TOMATO SALAD AND LOW-FAT CHEESE

3 tomatoes, diced
1 clove garlic, minced
⅓ teaspoon chopped fresh basil leaves
1 ounce low-fat cheese
⅓ teaspoon olive oil

Add balsamic vinegar to taste, then combine and mix well.

WALDORF SALAD

1 cup celery, sliced
¼ apple, diced
1 teaspoon light mayonnaise
1 pecan, crushed
1 ounce low-fat cheese

Combine and mix well.

LOW-FAT YOGURT AND NUTS

½ cup plain low-fat yogurt
1 teaspoon slivered almonds or 1 crushed macadamia nut

Sprinkle the nuts over the yogurt.

LOW-FAT COTTAGE CHEESE AND TOMATO

¼ cup low-fat cottage cheese
3 tomatoes, sliced
1 tablespoon avocado

CHEF SALAD SNACK

1½ ounces deli-style turkey or ham
1 tossed garden salad:
    2 cups shredded lettuce
    ¼ sliced tomato
    ¼ green bell pepper
    ¼ raw cucumber
    1 teaspoon olive oil and balsamic vinegar dressing:
        ⅓ teaspoon olive oil
        ⅔ teaspoon balsamic vinegar

TACO SALAD

1½ ounces ground turkey cooked with small amounts nonfat cooking spray and a small amount taco seasoning powder
1 tablespoon salsa
1 tossed green salad:
    2 cups shredded lettuce
    ¼ sliced tomato
    ¼ green bell pepper
    ¼ raw cucumber
    1 tablespoon avocado

Assemble the salad and top with cooked ground turkey and avocado.

HAM AND FRUIT

4 slices 97 percent fat-free deli ham
½ apple (or any other 1-block fruit serving)
1 macadamia nut (or any other 1-block fat)

APPLESAUCE AND LOW-FAT CHEESE

⅓ cup applesauce
1 ounce low-fat cheese
1 tablespoon avocado

BERRIES, LOW-FAT CHEESE, AND NUTS

½ cup blueberries
1 ounce low-fat cheese
1 pecan half

CHEESE AND GRAPES

1 ounce part-skim mozzarella string cheese
½ cup grapes
6 peanuts

FAT-FORTIFIED SKIM MILK

6 ounces skim milk
2 macadamia nuts or 6 almonds or 12 peanuts

COTTAGE CHEESE AND FRUIT

¼ cup low-fat cottage cheese
½ cup pineapple, diced
1 teaspoon slivered almonds

WINE AND CHEESE

4 ounces wine (or 6 ounces beer or 1 ounce distilled spirits)
1 ounce cheese

HOT DOG

1 soy hot dog
1 6-inch corn tortilla
1 teaspoon light mayonnaise or 1 tablespoon guacamole

1 PERCENT MILK

6 ounces 1 percent milk
6 peanuts

MINI PITA PIZZA

½ mini pita pocket topped with:
    1 tablespoon tomato sauce
    ⅓ teaspoon olive oil
    1 ounce part-skim mozzarella cheese

QUICK PIZZA

1 Wasa cracker topped with:
    ⅓ teaspoon olive oil
    1 ounce low-fat cheese

Top the Wasa cracker with the olive oil and low-fat cheese and microwave on high for 30 seconds.

SPINACH SALAD

1 hard boiled egg white, sliced
1 spinach salad:
   3 cups raw spinach
   ¼ raw onion
   ¼ cup raw mushrooms
   ¼ raw tomato
   ⅓ teaspoon olive oil
   Balsamic vinegar to taste

CRABMEAT SALAD SANDWICH

1½ ounces crabmeat
1 teaspoon light mayonnaise
½ mini pita pocket cut into triangles

VEGGIES AND DIP

3 ounces firm tofu blended with ⅓ teaspoon olive oil and some
   dry onion soup mix
3 green bell peppers, sliced for dipping

CHIPS AND SALSA

½ ounce baked tortilla chips
1 tablespoon salsa
1 ounce low-fat jack cheese
1 tablespoon avocado

To make even more 1-block Zone snacks, try combinations of the following:

Proteins (choose one):
¼ cup low-fat cottage cheese
1 ounce low-fat cheese
1 ounce mozzarella cheese made with skim milk
2½ ounces ricotta cheese

Fats (choose one):
3 olives
3 hazelnuts
3 almonds
1 macadamia nut
6 peanuts
¼-inch slice of avocado

Carbohydrates (choose one):
½ apple
½ grapefruit
½ cup grapes
3 apricots
½ cup cubed honeydew melon
¾ cup cubed cantaloupe
¼ cantaloupe
¾ cup cherries
1 kiwi
½ orange
½ nectarine
1 tangerine
½ pear
1 plum
½ cup fruit cocktail
⅓ cup peaches
½ cup crushed pineapple

1 cup strawberries
1 cup raspberries
¾ cup blackberries
¾ cup blueberries

With meals ranging from quick Zone meals to gourmet Zone-Perfect meals to simple-to-prepare Zone snacks, you now have all the tools to enter the Zone with remarkable ease. The following chapters will give you even more tools to make your stay in the Zone a permanent one.

7

ZONING YOUR KITCHEN

Staying in the Zone becomes even easier if you take the time to Zone your kitchen so that you can quickly and easily make Zone-Perfect meals any time of the day.

Try to visualize your new Zone kitchen as your food pharmacy. Every time you open the refrigerator door you'll be pulling out a drug as powerful as any you will ever encounter. So the first thing you want to do is to temporarily remove all the potentially dangerous drugs from your kitchen that will drive you out of the Zone. Take all the pasta, rice, pancake and cookie mixes, breads, and bagels and put them in a bag. Then put the bag in the trash or in a dark corner of your basement where you aren't likely to venture in the next few weeks. Do the same for all the breadmakers and juicers you own. (It's not that juicers are bad, but they remove fiber from the fruit and make it easier to overconsume fruit in the form of juice.) Put them in the attic. That's step one, and it takes only a few minutes.

Zone-Perfect meals are primarily based on low-fat protein, fruits, and vegetables, which means grocery shopping will be a key to your success. So here's a helpful Zone hint: Buy protein, fruits, and vegetables two to three times a week. It's amazing that with all the grocery stores and automobiles available to Americans, for many of us buying food is in the same category as making a trek to Outer Mongolia. Go to the store two to three times a week to buy perishables like protein, fruits, and vegetables. Buy only what you need for the next couple of days of Zone-Perfect meals, which means you are less likely to throw out any once-fresh food bought one or two weeks earlier.

PROTEIN

Always choose low-fat sources such as chicken, turkey, very lean cuts of beef, fish, low-fat cottage cheese, or soybean-based food products. This is desirable because you are always going to add some monounsaturated fat back to your meal. Always try to have some protein already prepared in your refrigerator for easy snacking. This might include sliced turkey, cottage cheese, string cheese, tuna salad, or even a tofu dip.

CARBOHYDRATES

The carbohydrate foundation of the Zone Diet is built upon fruits and vegetables. If you think that fresh fruit and vegetables are too expensive compared to pasta, then consider using frozen fruit and vegetables. They won't taste as good, but, surprisingly, they are actually more nutritious than the fresh variety. By the time "fresh" food reaches your home, it's been on the road for a long time. It has to be picked, packed, and trucked to the distribution center. Then it is trucked again to the supermarket, where it sits until you buy it. Then you transport it to your home, where it sits again until you eat it. The longer it sits, the more nutrition (especially vitamins) is lost.

Frozen fruits and vegetables, on the other hand, lead a different life. Usually only the best food picked is quick-frozen, and this is done within hours after harvesting. The end result is that frozen fruit and vegetables will usually have a higher vitamin content by the time they get to your home than fresh fruit or vegetables.

Of course you can always purchase canned fruits and vegetables, but these are a different story nutritionally. They will be the most inexpensive, but there will be a significant drop-off in their vitamin and mineral content (and in their taste, for that matter). Yet no matter how much nutrition canned fruits and vegetables have lost, they will still have more nutrients than the freshest bagel or fanciest pasta.

FATS

Of all the basic components of the Zone Diet, fats have the longest shelf life, and cooking oils can almost be considered Zone staples because you don't have to shop continually for them to maintain their freshness.

There are three good reasons to use oils in cooking. First, the fat found in oils acts like soluble fiber to slow down the rate of entry of any carbohydrate into the bloodstream. Second, fat also sends a hormonal signal to the brain to say stop eating. Finally, fat makes food taste better and enhances the flavors of the food. Since fat has no effect on insulin, make it your ally, not your enemy, in your Zone kitchen.

Another key to Zone cooking is using oils instead of butter when you cook. Not just any type of oil, however, will do. The best oil is olive oil, because it's rich in monounsaturated fats. This type of fat has absolutely no effect on insulin, and thus will be an integral partner in your battle against obesity. Surprisingly, the best type of olive oil to cook with is not the premium extra virgin olive oil, but the considerably less expensive refined olive oil.

The terms *extra virgin* and *virgin* denote the amount of contaminants of free fatty acids (which have a bitter taste) in the olive oil. *Extra virgin* means the oil has less than 0.5 percent by weight of free fatty acids, whereas *virgin* indicates less than 1.0 percent by weight. Olive oil containing more than 2 percent of free fatty acids has to be refined, which will reduce the amount of the free fatty acid to 0 percent. That's right, a big zero. Unfortunately, refining also removes many of the components that give premium olive oil its unique flavor characteristics. Therefore, refined olive oil won't have the zesty zing with all the flavor of the more expensive brands, but as far as cooking in the Zone goes, it is the ideal one to use. Keep in mind that oils do not have an indefinite shelf life. Never keep an oil more than six months, and store it in a cool location that is not exposed to light.

FROZEN FOODS

Frozen foods should be an ideal component in a Zone kitchen because of their long shelf-life. The only problem is the taste. Freezing pulls water from the cells so that food loses its plumpness at the cellular level. As a result, food loses its texture. In addition, the formation of ice crystals in the food can damage cells and cause the loss of flavor and nutrients. This happens because water expands when it freezes and the ice crystals can act as microscopic blades. Vegetables tend to freeze better than meats, seafood, and fruit. Some vegetables, such as peas, spinach, and lima beans, usually retain a reasonable texture after thawing. On the other hand, broccoli and cauliflower don't hold up well during freezing and lose the most texture.

Here are some Zone tips on buying frozen foods. If there is any frost on the package, it means that it has been partially thawed and some of the water has escaped and has refrozen on the outside of the package. Avoid those packages. Also, take your frozen food from deep inside the freezer, since the temperature is likely to be cooler with less chance of thawing.

ZONE STAPLES

Plan to restock your kitchen with Zone staples. These are items that make Zone cooking and snacking incredibly easy. Since Zone staples have a long shelf life, measured in months, you won't have to buy these as often.

The first Zone staple to buy is oatmeal, the only grain I really recommend on the Zone Diet. It's rich in soluble fiber (known as beta-glucan) that slows down the absorption of carbohydrate, and it contains an essential fatty acid (gamma linolenic acid, or GLA) that is found in mother's breast milk. (Not surprisingly, it's also what your grandmother told you to eat for breakfast.) Oats are rich in soluble fiber, as are many fruits (like apples) and vegetables (like black beans and kidney beans). But oat manufacturers have better marketing people, so that's why the Food and Drug Administration has given them permission to label their products with the following message: "Soluble fiber from oatmeal, as part of a low saturated fat, low cholesterol diet, may reduce the risk of heart disease." Too bad the apple lobby and black bean lobby are not as powerful or as savvy as the oat lobby.

Not all oatmeals are the same, and you pay a real hormonal price for convenience. Additional processing to raw oatmeal to make it faster to cook results in less insulin control. All oatmeals start with the whole grain known as the groat. The groat is then steamed to soften the oats. Without a doubt, these are the best oats for cooking: thick, coarse oats that take about thirty minutes to cook. These oats are also known as Scottish oats or Irish oatmeal and are the kind that I most highly recommend.

What if you don't have thirty minutes to cook oatmeal in the morning? The next best choice is old-fashioned oats, which have been steamed and rolled between large steel rollers to flatten them. These oats take about five minutes to cook, and they still retain their chewy texture.

Further processing gives you quick oats, which are simply old-fashioned oats that have been cut to allow them to cook faster (in about one minute). Unfortunately, the faster cooking time also means that the carbohydrates in the oatmeal will enter your bloodstream faster. A further significant step down in insulin control are instant oats, which are cut even finer than quick oats, and need only boiling water and a little stirring to prepare.

However, even the worst type of oatmeal (instant oats) is still superior to any other type of typical cold breakfast cereal in slowing down the rate of entry of carbohydrates into the bloodstream because of the soluble fiber content. (The typical cold breakfast cereal has only insoluble fiber, which has no effect on carbohydrate entry into the bloodstream.) The slower the entry rate of carbohydrates into the blood, the less insulin you produce and the less likely it is that you'll move out of the Zone with that meal.

One protein source can be considered a Zone staple because of its very long shelf life. That source is isolated protein powder, which can be used to fortify a meal with adequate protein. Although there are many types of isolate protein powders, hormonally speaking the best is soybean isolate, as it has the least effect on insulin and the greatest effect on glucagon. Unfortunately, soybean isolates don't taste as good as other isolated protein sources such as whey, milk, or egg proteins. As with oatmeal, there will be a compromise between taste and hormonal benefits.

Another important Zone staple is nuts. Before people learned how to extract oil from olives or seeds some 5,000 years ago, they ate nuts for fat. Nuts are a great storage tank for oils. Realize that once you extract an oil from a seed or nut, it begins to go rancid very quickly. In fact, the shelf-life of a typical isolated oil under the best conditions (no exposure to air, no exposure to light, and maintained at room temperature) is only six months. Therefore the oils in nuts are much more resistant to rancidity. Your best choices are nuts rich in monounsaturated fats, like macadamia nuts and almonds. This is why slivered almonds are a great condiment to any meal. Other good choices in nuts rich in monounsaturated fats are cashews and pistachios.

Peanuts are also a readily available monounsaturated fat source, although not quite as rich in monounsaturated fat as the nuts discussed above. Although many people would like to think of peanut butter as a source of protein, in reality it's primarily a fat (although a pretty good fat). A better Zone choice would be almond butter. Using nuts or nut butters are great ways to add monounsaturated fat to Zone-Perfect meals.

The last Zone staples you definitely want in your Zone kitchen are spices. Remember, it was during the quest for cheaper access to spices that America was discovered. Spices were so highly sought because they make food taste better. The more spices you use, the greater the taste sensations. And spices have no effect on insulin. Life is good.

8

ZONE TOOLS

Now that you have Zoned your kitchen, you still need some basic Zone tools for cooking Zone-Perfect meals. Let's start with the most important—knives. A good sharp knife is your greatest Zone tool— the sharper the edge, the faster you can prepare Zone-Perfect meals.

KNIVES

By far and away the best raw material for making knives is carbon steel. Unfortunately, this material is attacked by acids (found in lemons and citrus fruits) that can stain the knife. These knives have to be wiped clean right after use to prevent staining. If you are truly a gourmet cook, carbon steel knives are your choice.

The next step down in blade sharpness are high-carbon knives. The cutting edge will not be as sharp as the edge of carbon steel knives, but these knives will not stain when exposed to acid. However, these knives are the most expensive. Companies like Henckels and Forshmer manufacture these knives.

Lower in quality and sharpness of edge is a stainless steel knife. Unlike carbon steel knives, these knives will become dull very quickly. And the duller the edge of the knife, the more effort involved in food preparation. Finally, some knives are super stainless steel. These are advertised as never needing sharpening. This is because they *can't* be sharpened. Stay away from these knives. Since a good knife should last a lifetime, make an appropriate investment for your Zone kitchen.

Once you decide which type of material you plan to choose for your knives, determine what type of knives you need. The four basic knives needed in any Zone kitchen include: a paring knife (three to four inches in length), a utility knife (six inches in length), a chef's knife (eight inches in length), and a slicing or carving knife (usually ten inches in length). The chef's knife is thicker than a slicing knife because the extra weight produces chopping power. On the other hand, the slicing knife is narrower and gives thinner slices, which is a major advantage in Zone cooking.

Now that you have the knives, buy a knife sharpener. Unless you keep the edges beveled to improve the ease of cutting (regardless of the material), you're more likely to revert to using prepared meals as it becomes more difficult and time-consuming to prepare the basic ingredients required for Zone-Perfect meals.

Keeping your knives sharp actually makes your kitchen a much safer place. Surprisingly, dull knives are more dangerous than sharp knives. First, you're likely to be more careful using a sharp knife than a dull one. Second, a sharp knife is less likely to slip since you have to apply less pressure to cut food than with a dull knife. A sharper knife also means more efficiency and quicker preparation time in the kitchen. You also minimize tearing and ripping of your protein source or vegetables, and the thinner slices mean less cooking time.

POTS AND PANS

Your next most important Zone kitchen tools are your pots and pans. Preparing the raw ingredients for Zone-Perfect meals is one thing, cooking them is another. You need the appropriate pots and pans to increase heat transfer and cook the food with the least amount of vitamin and mineral loss.

The secret of Zone cooking is not spending much time in the

kitchen, and this includes cleanup. Therefore, nonstick pans will be your greatest ally. Teflon is the first type of pan that comes to mind, but as most of you know, the Teflon coating can be easily scratched. A better choice for longevity would be Silverstone, since it lasts longer and therefore becomes less expensive in the long run. Anodized aluminum pans are another potential choice. The surface of these pans has been oxidized to prevent food from adhering, which provides them with a "nonsticky" surface.

But the reason you use metal pans is to get good, uniform heat transfer from your range to the food. When it comes to heat transfer, copper and aluminum are among the best metals. The trouble with copper is that it needs constant cleaning to prevent oxide formation, which reduces heat transfer. Stainless steel is less efficient, and glass and earthenware are the least desirable for efficient heat transfer. Stainless steel pans with a copper bottom may appear to be a good compromise, but the copper coating is actually very thin and it still needs constant cleaning and attention.

The thicker the pan, the better and more uniform the heat transfer to the food. This is why cast-iron skillets are often used by gourmet chefs. Probably the most reasonable choice in cookware is what is called a multi-ply pan. These pans have a layer of aluminum sandwiched between two layers of stainless steel. This gives you good heat transfer with a minimum of cleaning, a very important Zone kitchen feature.

In your Zone kitchen, the primary pan will be a frying or sauté pan. A sauté pan has a high vertical wall (about two and a half inches), which reduces the amount of splattering. This is different from a skillet, which has sloping walls to help slide food out of the pan. Other essential pans are various sizes of saucepans so that you can cook for one as well as for a family.

One other key item to consider for your Zone kitchen is a hanging fruit basket. Fruit will last longer if you allow air to circulate totally around the fruit. Fruits are still alive and consume oxygen even after harvesting. If oxygen is restricted, then the fruit at the cellular level switches to anaerobic (in the absence of oxygen) metabolism, causing a buildup of alcohol. This in turn causes brown spots below the skin of the fruit and brown cores within the fruit. Besides making fruit last longer, fruit baskets look great hanging from the ceiling.

ZONE COOKING TIPS

Now that you have Zoned your kitchen and have all your Zone tools together, here are some helpful hints for making Zone cooking an integral part of your life.

RANGES AND OVENS

As far as cooking itself goes, I believe that gas ranges and electric ovens are best for preparing Zone meals. Gas ranges will give you more control when cooking (especially in turning down the heat) than electric ranges. This is especially true if you plan to do any stir-frying. On the other hand, electric ovens provide a more constant temperature than gas ovens. A third type of oven is the convection oven, which circulates the heated air, giving even more uniform temperature control and cutting down on cooking time by about one-third. Although they are more expensive, so is your time in the kitchen.

But what about microwave ovens? Microwave cooking was invented in 1947 and represents the first major breakthrough in cooking technology in several centuries. Microwaves cook the food through excitation of the water molecules in the food. This is the most efficient heating process known and can cut your cooking time by up to 75 percent, because you are cooking the food from within as opposed to heating the outer surface and transferring the heat more slowly to the center of the food. Unfortunately, you pay a culinary price for such speed because microwave cooking can give food a dry, mushy texture. If food doesn't look good or taste good, what's the use of eating it?

Although there are drawbacks to microwave cooking as mentioned above, it has a real place in your Zone kitchen. Cook several Zone-Perfect meals on the weekend, and then freeze them. Heat them in the microwave during the week. High technology is your best friend in a Zone kitchen, especially since virtually everyone can operate a microwave oven.

COOKING PROTEIN

At the molecular level, meat is a combination of muscle fibers held together by collagen (collagen is basically like the wires that hold together a bale of cotton). As you heat protein, the collagen begins to liquefy into gelatin as the temperature of the meat increases. The secret of preparing meat perfectly is to detach the muscle fibers from one another (giving a tender taste and texture), but to retain enough of the collagen superstructure to prevent the protein from falling apart and becoming mushlike. Therefore cooking becomes the art of compromise.

This is why many people find fish so difficult to cook. It contains very little collagen compared to meat, and fish collagen turns to gelatin at a much lower temperature than the collagen in meat. Under ideal conditions, perfectly cooked fish flakes very easily (the muscle fibers are easily dissociated). However, slightly overcooking fish gives it that mushlike effect that makes even the experienced cook shudder.

The toughness of a cut of meat is determined by how much collagen it contains. Highly active muscles (like those of any good athlete) are rich in collagen. Also, the older the animal, the greater amount of collagen a piece of meat contains. Therefore the less active the animal, and the younger the animal before slaughter, the more tender the meat.

COOKING CARBOHYDRATES

The amount of protein you plan to prepare determines the amount of carbohydrate to be consumed at the same time. On the Zone Diet, this means eating primarily fruits and vegetables as your source of carbohydrates.

Fruits are easy to prepare. Just wash them, peel if necessary, and eat. A piece of fresh fruit or a fruit cocktail is a great dessert to complete a meal. Even adding a small dollop of whipped cream will have very little effect on insulin.

Vegetables, because of their low carbohydrate density, are always an excellent source of carbohydrates, but their preparation is somewhat different. Frankly, raw vegetables get tiresome after a little while. The best way to prepare vegetables is to lightly steam them. This preserves most of the vitamins and minerals while also making the vegetables more digestible since the steaming process has begun to break down the cell walls. Steaming also leaves very little mess to clean up (a very important feature in Zone cooking).

Although steaming is the best way to prepare vegetables, many people still will not eat them. I have found that the best way to ensure people (even your kids) will eat vegetables is to sauté them in olive oil. It will take some time, but it works.

Finally, keep the grains, starches, and breads to a minimum on the Zone Diet. These foods have such a dense carbohydrate content that they will cause a rapid increase in your insulin levels when eaten in excess. Although they are much cheaper than fruits and vegetables, you will actually see your food bills decrease once you start to use these high-density carbohydrates as condiments rather than as the base of your meals. Why? Because you won't be as hungry and your carbohydrate cravings will be dramatically reduced, if not eliminated, which means spending less money on snack foods.

COOKING WITH FAT

Because you are using low-fat protein sources, you can now add back the fat of your choice as a sauce or dressing, using your favorite monounsaturated fat source (like olive oil), or as condiments including olives, guacamole, macadamia nuts, or almonds. If you stir-fry tofu, for example, leave the oil in the meal when you serve it. The fat will carry the flavor of the spices and seasonings with the tofu.

ZONE COOKING

Regardless of your type of stove or oven, there are two ways to cook any food: using dry heat or using moist heat. These cooking methods have not really changed to any great extent over the centuries. Dry heat cooks the food through the air. While air is not a very good conductor of heat (this is why you can put your hand into an oven at 400 degrees Fahrenheit and not get immediately burned), you can heat it to a pretty high temperature. Obviously the earliest form of dry heating was roasting over an open fire. A more recent innovation (starting about 5,000 years ago) was baking using an oven to retain the heat. In both cases you are heating the air around the food to cook it.

Broiling is an even faster way to create heat transfer, as the surface of the heating elements can become extremely hot (3,000 degrees Fahrenheit for gas burners and 2,000 degrees Fahrenheit for electric burners), and the protein is usually only six inches away from the heating element. Not surprisingly, it is easy to overcook food when broiling, and therefore this method is used only with relatively thin and tender protein (i.e., that containing less connective tissue).

A variation of dry heating is pan-frying or sautéing. To prevent the protein from sticking to the pan, you add some oil. Since oil transfers heat very well, the addition of cooking oil can decrease the cooking time. But like broiling, less cooking time with higher heat means you run the risk of undercooking the interior of the protein while overcooking the exterior. This is why food preparation using a sharp knife to keep the food very thin and very tender is ideal for sautéing.

Stir-frying is simply sautéing with a different type of pan (with higher sloping walls and a deeper well), and is primarily used for cooking vegetables instead of protein. As in sautéing, you add a small amount of oil to prevent the food from sticking and to aid in heat transfer. In fact, the only difference between sautéing and stir-frying is the type of pan used. One reason that very little cooking oil is used in stir-frying was that until recently cooking oil was extremely expensive, whereas vegetables were very cheap. It therefore made good economic sense not to use much cooking oil. As a result, constant stirring was necessary to maintain contact of the vegetables with the thin film of oil.

Moist heating uses water instead of air to transfer the heat to the food. Although water cannot be heated as hot as air, it conducts heat much more effectively (imagine if you were to stick one hand in boiling water and the other hand in a heated oven at 400 degrees Fahrenheit) and therefore is usually used with tougher cuts of meat or very fiber-rich vegetables. Since you can't heat water beyond 212 degrees Fahrenheit, it also becomes hard (but not impossible) to overcook food (unless you boil away all the water), although you may have to cook it for a long time to break down the collagen. The less experienced a cook you are, or the cheaper the cuts of protein you use, the more I recommend that you use moist heat to cook your foods.

Boiling is the most common form of moist heat as you are surrounding the entire food with water. Unfortunately, this is also the best way to leach out all the vitamins and minerals from the food into the surrounding water. Other forms of moist cooking include simmering and stewing. Simmering simply means keeping the temperature of the liquid less than 212 degrees Fahrenheit, usually around 195 degrees Fahrenheit, whereas in stewing the meat is cut into smaller pieces and usually overcooked so the connective tissue is completely broken down, making it "fork tender."

You can also decrease the cooking time using moist heat by increasing the pressure of the water. Steaming or pressure cooking are two ways to achieve this goal, as they allow you to get to a higher temperature, and therefore cook food faster.

Braising is a compromise between stewing and sautéing because a small amount of water is added to a closed pan. This allows longer cooking without the danger of overcooking. Braising is usually used with large cuts of meat that have a lot of connective tissue, such as a rump roast.

Then there is deep-frying. This is basically boiling with oil instead of water. Now you can reach a much higher temperature (nearly 400 degrees Fahrenheit) and have great heat transfer to the food because of the intimate contact of the heated oil with the food. This is why French fries get cooked so quickly using deep-frying compared to the time it takes to bake a potato. But of course your food is now drenched in fat. While the Zone Diet recommends more fat in the diet, even I draw the line at deep-frying.

MAKING FOOD TASTE BETTER

The secret of French cooking has always been the sauces. Why do sauces make food taste better? It's the fat. Fat not only gives food a better mouth feel, but also carries flavors better, since most flavors are fat-soluble.

The best French sauces are essentially emulsified fat. Examples of natural emulsified fats are butter and milk. Butter is called a water-in-fat emulsion (since most of the weight is fat, with a small amount of emulsified water), whereas milk is a water-in-oil emulsion (most of the weight is water, with a small amount of emulsified fat).

The most common manmade emulsified sauce is mayonnaise. As the name suggests, mayonnaise originated in France and is often considered the poor relative of sauces, since it is used for adding fat to everything from a turkey sandwich to potato salad. More complex fat emulsions include hollandaise sauce used for vegetables like artichokes, asparagus, and broccoli, and béarnaise sauce used for meat. In fact, béarnaise sauce is actually hollandaise sauce to which tarragon leaves and tarragon vinegar have been added. Frankly, any Zone meal is going to taste better when you use these more complex fat emulsions in your meal.

Why were sauces first developed? Because food (especially protein) tasted pretty bad within a couple of days without refrigeration, and a century ago there was no refrigeration. Let a piece of beef sit out at room temperature for a couple of days and you see why sauces were so important. The best way to cover up the foul odor of rancid meat is to use a sauce of great flavor. Béarnaise sauce does a great job for steak. The fat in the sauce also adds mouth feel to your taste buds (remember that before grain was fed to livestock, most meat was very lean). Furthermore, fat holds flavor better, as most flavors are actually fat-soluble chemicals. In a fat-rich environment provided by the sauce, flavors blend together much better and retain their unique sensory impact.

Small wonder that once the French learned how to cover up rancid meat with sauces it took little time to realize that vegetables would also taste better by adding sauces to them.

When you think of sauces, like béarnaise and hollandaise, you usually envision a tub of melted butter used in the preparation of the sauce. Zone sauces are a little different. Rather than using massive amounts of butter, replace the butter with refined olive oil. Now you have the right type of monounsaturated fat that is heart healthy and has all of the flavor benefits of a classic French sauce. Combine these Zone sauces with Zone meals, and you are really cooking.

Salad dressings, like vinaigrette, are also emulsions. The emulsified oil (ideally olive oil) in the dressing will not be repulsed by the water on the surface of the lettuce in the salad, and mixes nicely.

Can sauces be used with fruits? Of course. Probably the easiest sauce for fruit is whipped cream. Whipped cream is also an emulsion. If you are going to whip the cream yourself, use the freshest possible cream, as any lactic acid (the off-flavor in milk) will tend to destroy the emulsion.

How do you make an emulsified Zone sauce in minutes? The easiest way is to buy a prepared dry hollandaise or béarnaise sauce mix at any grocery store. Take the dry mix, add one or two tablespoons of olive oil to it, and stir until the oil is fully blended in (this takes about fifteen seconds). Then add the right amount of low-fat milk to it, and stir in a saucepan near boiling for about one to two minutes until the sauce thickens. Then pour the appropriate amount over the vegetables or the protein. Just as the French did more than two centuries ago, and are still doing today.

Although the Zoned sauces in Chapter 6 are easy to make, if you are feeling a little more adventuresome, you can try your hand at some variations of sauce recipes with the addition of other ingredients. For example, add julienne vegetables to the Zoned Espagnol Sauce to create Jardiniere Sauce. However, to make complex emulsified sauces, like hollandaise or béarnaise from scratch, you need to know a little food chemistry, and you often need a lot of luck. Once you try to make your own emulsified sauces, you realize that those packages of dry mixes are actually a pretty good idea.

If sauces are the secret of French cooking, spices and herbs can't be too far behind. Since the flavors of spices and herbs are heat-sensitive, the best time to add seasoning to a meal is just at the end of sautéing the meat or vegetables because prolonged exposure to heat will dissipate the flavors of the seasonings.

While sauces and seasonings add flavor and zest to any meal, there is one anti-spice. It's called monosodium glutamate, or MSG. The Japanese learned long ago that adding seaweed to a meal tended to increase the flavor. The active ingredient in seaweed? It's MSG. If you are really a poor cook or use inferior quality materials, MSG is your spice of choice. Whatever flavor is actually in the food will be enhanced. Unfortunately for many people, there will be a price for using this spice, because many react violently to its presence in food, probably due to MSG's potential neurotoxic effects on the central nervous system. For this reason alone, you should never use MSG, and you should steer clear of any food that may contain it.

Finally there is the ubiquitous seasoning—sugar. Sweetness is one of the four types of receptors on our taste buds. The other three are receptors for bitterness, hot, and cold. Since many plants make poisonous alkaloids as a defense, having a bitter taste receptor makes good evolutionary sense to keep you from eating such toxic plants. If a food had a sweet taste, you could be pretty sure that it was safe to eat.

Today, however, those same sweet receptors increase your likelihood of eating more food. So if you are a food manufacturer, the more sugar you put into the food, the more likely the consumer will be to eat it.

The key to staying in the Zone is to use natural sweeteners that have the least impact on insulin. This means fructose, which is about 33 percent sweeter for the same amount of carbohydrate found in table sugar. In addition, fructose enters the bloodstream very slowly as glucose because it must be converted to glucose by an enzyme (phosphofructose kinase) found in the liver. Because of the slow entry rate, it has a very limited effect on insulin secretion. This makes it the ideal Zone sweetener for any Zone kitchen. Always try to use the type of natural sweetener that has the greatest sweetness for the least amount of carbohydrate. Just for reference, although fructose is slightly sweeter than table sugar, it is twice as sweet as pure glucose (the most potent stimulator of insulin), three times as sweet as maltose, and six times as sweet as lactose (the sugar found in milk). Where do you find fructose? In every supermarket in America.

Artificial sweeteners are a different story. Saccharine is an intensely sweet-tasting compound that has been used since the 1920s to sweeten food. Although it is 700 times sweeter than sugar, it leaves a slight aftertaste that doesn't make it a very good sweetener. Unfortunately, since the 1980s saccharine has all but been replaced by a newer food additive, aspartame. This sweetener is actually two amino acids linked together to form a very small protein that interacts with the sweet taste receptors in your mouth, to generate the sensation of sweetness. Although aspartame has become ubiquitous in our society, I still have strong reservations about its massive use because of continual adverse reports to the FDA about some individuals who seem to be sensitive to it. If you can, try to avoid aspartame whenever possible.

However, there is a new sweetener that is actually an old one. It's called stevia, and it's an herbal preparation that is 300 times sweeter than sugar. Long used in Asia, it is now available in many health food stores in this country as a nutritional supplement. If you want to use an artificial sweetener, consider stevia your best bet.

11

KIDS IN THE ZONE

If you think being in the Zone is important for you, it's even more important for your kids. While adult obesity has increased by 32 percent in the last decade, the extent of childhood obesity has doubled. It's a literal epidemic, and yet no one seems to care.

I am the first to admit that kids are incredibly picky eaters. But more to your advantage, they are even worse cooks. And to top it off, they are incredibly lazy in the kitchen. You can use these realities to get your kids into the Zone. If you do, you will suddenly begin to look like the Ward and June Cleaver of your block because your kids will maintain better blood sugar levels, which means they actually begin to listen to you and their mood swings will be highly moderated. They might even start to clean up their rooms. (Maybe not!)

The easiest way to get kids in the Zone is to make Zone desserts. This isn't as hard as you think. In fact, your grandmother did it all the time using a dessert that wiggled. That dessert was natural gelatin with some fruit embedded in it. Protein from the gelatin, carbohydrate from the fruit. And the fat? Add a dab of whipped cream to it.

If you are a little more adventuresome with your desserts, try adding some protein powder to pudding. When you check the pudding package for its nutritional labeling, you come to realize that most puddings are virtually pure carbohydrate. Blend in enough protein powder to balance out the carbohydrates as you make the pudding, and presto it becomes Zone-Perfect. Again, don't be afraid to add a little whipped cream to it.

One of the biggest problems for parents is getting kids to eat protein. Well, there is one protein source that virtually every kid will eat, and it's called string cheese. String cheese is popular with kids because it looks like junk food. It also matches their cooking ability, which usually stops with opening a wrapper. String cheese may be a little high in saturated fat, but it's a very convenient and user-friendly way of getting some protein into your child. A good compromise is string cheese made from skim milk or low-fat milk. The ideal snack for many kids would be a piece of string cheese plus some carbohydrate like a cup of grapes (they don't need much preparation either).

Another trick parents can use is to make blended drinks that have the correct protein-to-carbohydrate ratio. Actually, we have one that has been around for nearly 8,000 years. It's called milk. Although it enters the bloodstream faster than solid food (and therefore will not have an optimal effect on insulin secretion), it's a great source of calcium and it's easy to make (just pour). Unfortunately, a good number of kids are lactose intolerant. This means they can't digest the carbohydrate in milk. In these cases, try soy milk, which is devoid of any lactose but still contains the correct protein-to-carbohydrate ratio.

To make milk more of a treat, think about malted milk. The malt is extra carbohydrate, so this means you have to add some extra protein powder to it to keep the drink in the Zone. But if your child is more likely to drink it, then it's worth the extra effort.

A variation on this theme is making a fruit smoothie to which you add some extra protein powder. Since a fruit smoothie requires a blender, this seemingly small task is well beyond the cooking skills of most kids. But you can make a protein-fortified fruit smoothie for your children and keep it in the refrigerator so all they have to do is pour. Now this is definitely within the range of their cooking skills.

Yogurt seems like a logical snack choice for most kids. But very few kids like natural yogurt. Food manufacturers realize this and therefore load up commercial yogurts with massive amounts of carbohydrates (either extra fruit or simply extra sugar) to make the yogurt taste better. Unfortunately, the end result for children when they eat these carbohydrate-heavy "healthy" yogurts is that they fall right out of the Zone. Frozen yogurt is even worse, because it is almost pure carbohydrate. It is simply politically correct cotton candy, especially if it's fat-free, and should be avoided unless you're having a protein chaser with it.

The food choices above are the easy part. The next step is to begin to teach your kids to eat the foods they were designed to eat—fruits and vegetables. Fruits should be great for kids since they require no cooking. But fruits can be intimidating for kids because they have to be peeled. So start your kids out with the easy fruits: grapes, apples, and pears. These don't require a lot of work on their part. But even here, if you precut the fruits for your kids, you will dramatically increase the likelihood that they will actually eat them. The same is true of oranges that have to be peeled, which for many kids is the equivalent of climbing Mount Everest. Here's the solution, but you have to do a little preparation because you will actually have to cut these fruits yourself (do you think your kids will?). Every couple of days, cut up a lot of strawberries, oranges, and melons and put them in a bowl in the refrigerator. As soon as your kids come home after school, put the bowl out and let them eat from it. What they don't eat, put back into the refrigerator. Use your kids' laziness to your advantage. Faced with the challenge of opening a package of potato chips or simply eating prepared fruit waiting for them when they come home should be a no-brainer for your child. Just make sure to have some string cheese waiting too.

The same is true with breakfast. Before they leave for school, take out the same bowl of precut fruit for them to eat. For a little variety, you can add some precut apples, pears, or other fruits that tend to oxidize quickly. Squirt a little lemon juice on the cut fruit to prevent oxidation. Nothing turns off a kid more than brown fruit. You will have to make a new fruit bowl every other day, but it sure beats buying a six-pack of potato chips or other snack goodies every week.

Regardless of the fruit you provide for your children, make sure they have easy access to a protein chaser to balance the carbohydrates in the fruit. Try your old standby of string cheese. Keep it in the wrapper, because if your kid doesn't eat it, you can always put it back into the refrigerator.

To make life easier for you, simply ask your children to make a list of what kinds of protein they will eat. It might be a very short list, but at least it's a beginning. That list might include Canadian bacon or egg-white omelettes in the morning, sliced turkey or string cheese at lunch, and chicken, fish, or very lean cuts of beef at dinner. And if your child is a vegetarian, then try soybean imitation meat products like soybean sausages for breakfast, soybean hot dogs for lunch, and soybean hamburger patties for dinner.

Of course, the greatest challenge for a parent is getting kids to eat vegetables. It was also the greatest challenge for your grandmother. One solution is to put vegetables in a soup or stew. Just make sure that you have adequate protein at the same time. Another way is to sauté vegetables in olive oil and add some spices like oregano to them. The more olive oil you use to sauté the vegetables, the more likely your kids are going to eat them. And herein lies the secret with vegetables: added fat. Sautéing vegetables in olive oil is one way. The other method is to do what the French learned to do centuries ago: add sauces. As discussed in the last chapter, the best sauces are nothing but emulsified fat that adds great taste to any vegetable or food. Even canned vegetables that have been sitting in your pantry for the past three years will taste pretty good once you put some sauces over them. And the better the quality of the sauce, the more likely that your kids will eat their vegetables without a big production at lunch or dinner.

ZONE SUPPLEMENTS

Macronutrients (protein, carbohydrate, and fat), not micronutrient (vitamin and mineral) supplements, are your passport to the Zone. Are supplements important for the Zone? A few are, but never let the tail wag the dog. Used properly, they can enhance the hormonal benefits of being in the Zone, but they will never get you to the Zone by themselves.

It is commonly reported that today's food supply is adulterated with pesticides, herbicides, hormones, and antibiotics. I agree. And if you are really concerned about your health, you should take every opportunity to use only organically grown fruits and vegetables, and range-fed chicken and beef. However, Americans want it both ways: safe food and cheap food. The cheapest food on the face of the earth is only made possible by using the very same substances that cause everyone justifiable concern. So while organic fruits and vegetables are available, recognize that you are going to have to pay a much higher price for them and you may have to spend much more time searching out these items. The same is true of range-fed and hormone-free chicken and beef.

I strongly recommend using unadulterated food whenever possible. Since the Zone is all about hormonal control, it doesn't take a genius to figure out that if food sources contain hormones, herbicides, or pesticides, they can have adverse hormonal effects that can push you out of the Zone. If you opt for cheaper food, then plan to pay even closer attention to the protein-to-carbohydrate ratio at every meal, which should help counteract the effects of the other substances that have been creeping into our food supply over the past fifty years.

And what about vitamins and minerals? Isn't our food poorer in these essential micronutrients than it was fifty years ago? The answer is probably yes. Why? Because fifty years ago, most of the fruits and vegetables came from your backyard or just outside town at the nearby farm. Now they come from all over the world and can be stored for months after being harvested. Vitamins are incredibly sensitive to heat, light, and storage time. Minerals are more stable, but they are very sensitive to processing and cooking technologies. The first casualties in the war for cheap food will always be the vitamin and mineral content of that food. So should you spend a good chunk of your food budget down at the local health food store? No, but you can use nutritional supplements wisely to get the most Zone bang for the buck.

ESSENTIAL SUPPLEMENTS

As I mentioned in *The Zone,* only two supplements are essential for the Zone Diet: purified fish oils and vitamin E. Both are supported by compelling research about their health benefits, and their cost is relatively inexpensive.

Let's talk about fish oil first, since your grandmother probably used this in the form of cod liver oil. Cod liver oil is rich in vitamin A and vitamin D, and two generations ago fear of a disease called rickets, caused by a deficiency of vitamin D, was still fresh in many minds. Cod liver oil was the best source for these vitamins, even though it was (and probably still is) one of the most disgusting foods known to man. Disgusting or not, its daily consumption was a given in your grandmother's day.

It turns out the real reason that cod liver oil was so beneficial was not because of the vitamins it contained, but because of a rare fatty acid called eicospentaenoic acid, or EPA. EPA turns out to be a key factor in controlling insulin levels. So even though your grandmother was forcing your parents to take cod liver oil for the wrong biochemical reason, she was doing an excellent job of controlling insulin in the process.

Just as the balance of protein to carbohydrate is critical for maintaining the Zone, so is the balance of certain types of fats called essential fats. These essential fats come in two distinct groups, Omega–6 and Omega–3. EPA is a long-chain Omega–3 fat that keeps this balance in sync. Fish are very efficient concentrators of EPA (which is made by plankton) since they are at the end of the food chain that begins with these single-celled organisms.

Although humans evolved from the sea, the need for these Omega–3 fatty acids is only now being realized. In fact, 50 percent of the fat mass of the brain is composed of these long-chain Omega–3 fats. No other organ in the body has such a concentration of Omega–3 fats. And since the greatest growth spurt for the brain occurs during the first two years of life, it's not surprising how important these Omega–3 fatty acids are for proper brain development. Human breast milk is rich in these types of fat. Just how important are these Omega–3 fats found in breast milk? One English study indicated that breast-fed children scored nearly eight points higher on IQ tests compared to children who were bottle-fed. This is why infant formula manufacturers are scrambling (at least in Europe and Japan) to try to incorporate these long-chain Omega–3 fatty acids, like EPA, into their products.

Dietary EPA is also strongly implicated in reducing heart disease, cancer, arthritis, and other chronic disease conditions in humans. Why? Because of its effect on a group of hormones called eicosanoids. Eicosanoids are described in far greater detail in *The Zone*, but simply stated, if you want to decrease the likelihood of developing chronic diseases, adequate amounts of EPA can help.

What are adequate amounts of EPA? Approximately 200 to 400 milligrams per day if you are in the Zone, much more if you aren't.

And the best source of EPA is cold-water fatty fish, like salmon, mackerel, and sardines. Eating fish is another Zone plus because fish represents a unique source of protein. Fish is the only source of protein that is low in Omega–6 essential fatty acids, and which provides relatively large amounts of long-chain Omega–3 fatty acids such as EPA. In the last eighty years, we have been consuming massive amounts of Omega–6 fatty acids while simultaneously reducing our intake of Omega–3 fatty acids. At the turn of the century, the ratio of Omega–6 to Omega–3 fatty acids was close to two to one. Now it's about twenty to one. One result of this shift in the essential fatty acid ratio is that we have created a massive eicosanoid imbalance, which is one of the key factors in the development of chronic disease. This is why eating fish has such a dramatic effect on the reduction of heart disease. First, eating fish means that you are probably eating adequate amounts of protein to help keep you in the Zone. Second, by eating fish you are consuming larger amounts of EPA. Third, you are decreasing your intake of Omega–6 fatty acids. Three very good reasons to eat fish.

However, there is a down side to eating fish. Fish are also great accumulators of chemically persistent toxins, like PCBs. These chemicals tend to be very resistant to being broken down by any species of life, and as a result accumulate at the end of the food chain. As a consequence fish oil can be rich in PCBs, even though PCB production was phased out decades ago. The solution to this dilemma is to supplement your diet with molecularly distilled fish oil. Molecular distillation is a high-tech process that removes PCBs from purified fish oil. Whether or not you like fish, I recommend molecularly distilled fish oils. They give you the EPA you need and peace of mind on the PCB issue.

The other essential supplement to the Zone Diet is vitamin E. Vitamin E was discovered in 1922 when it was found that a diet deficient in this vitamin was the cause of fetal death in pregnant rats and testicular atrophy in male rats. Vitamin E is not only a significant player in your reproductive system, but it plays a key role in virtually every aspect of human physiology. Unfortunately, it is simply impossible to obtain adequate levels of vitamin E through diet alone. As with fish oil, the data is compelling that increased supplementation with vitamin E will have a dramatic clinical effect on diseases ranging from heart disease to Alzheimer's and immune system disorders. I recommend taking a minimum of 100 International Units (IU) per day, with 400 IU as a reasonable upper limit for adults and 50 to 100 IU as a reasonable upper limit for children

The story of the manufacturing of vitamin E is a tale of our times. In the early days of vitamin E manufacturing, the raw material (which is still used), called distillate, was removed during the purification of soybean oil. This distillate was originally fed to cattle to further increase their milk production. Unfortunately, within a few months, thousands of cattle had died because it turned out this same distillate was also rich in herbicides and pesticides. Today the only way to manufacture natural vitamin E that is suitable for human consumption is to use molecular distillation to remove the fat-soluble herbicides and pesticides that contaminate the initial raw material that contains the vitamin E. To make natural vitamin E suitable for human consumption, you have to use the same high-tech process that also removes PCBs from fish oil.

SECOND TIER SUPPLEMENTS

Fish oil and vitamin E are essential supplements for the Zone Diet (and for any other diet, for that matter), but a second tier of vitamins and minerals can operate as an important and a very cheap insurance policy for anyone interested in his or her own health. This tier of supplements includes vitamin C and the mineral magnesium.

People often forget that the glory years of vitamin research were in the 1930s when several Nobel Prizes were awarded for discoveries in this field. In fact, the 1937 Nobel Prize in medicine was awarded to Albert Szent-Gyorgyi for his efforts in defining the structure of vitamin C.

Vitamin C is a water-soluble antioxidant. Most oxidation products in the body tend to be fat-soluble and therefore water-insoluble. The problem for the body is getting these water-insoluble oxidation products through the bloodstream to the liver so that they can be detoxified and excreted in the urine. This is where vitamin C comes in. Being water-soluble, it acts as the primary transporting agent to get rid of all the nasty oxidation products that are constantly being formed in your body. And if you don't have enough vitamin C, these oxidation products pile up and are stored in your fat cells, where they can cause trouble.

Fortunately vitamin C is plentiful, especially on the Zone Diet. Unlike vitamin E and purified fish oil, where supplementation is a must, fruits and vegetables tend to be rich in this vitamin. Not surprisingly, these are also key components of the Zone Diet. The best sources of vitamin C in fruits are kiwi, oranges, strawberries, and melons. Vegetable sources such as red peppers, broccoli, spinach, and mustard greens are also rich in vitamin C. Although megadoses are often touted, the best research indicates that a reasonable level for vitamin C supplementation is in the range of 500 to 1,000 milligrams per day. Because vitamin C is so inexpensive, this vitamin is a good recommendation even at these levels of supplementation.

The other supplement I highly recommended is the mineral magnesium. No mineral is as important as magnesium for the Zone Diet. It's the key mineral cofactor in the production of eicosanoids, and it is also a cofactor required for the proper function of more than 350 other enzymes. The latest research shows that adequate magnesium is critical for cardiovascular patients, which only makes it reasonable to assume that it is useful for the rest of us, especially since dietary surveys indicate that nearly 75 percent of Americans are deficient in this key mineral. Contained in chlorophyll, magnesium is found in every vegetable that is green, like spinach and peas. However, the richest naturally occurring sources of magnesium are nuts. Other sources that are relatively rich in magnesium are legumes, shrimp, crab, and, to a lesser extent, beef (cows represent the upper end of the food chain on land that begins with chlorophyll-containing grass). These foods are also the primary foods used in the Zone Diet. Perhaps not surprisingly, the foods that are poor in magnesium are starches, breads, and pasta, the new staples of the American diet. No wonder Americans are deficient in magnesium.

Store-bought magnesium supplements are difficult to take because magnesium tastes terrible, you need a lot of it, and it is poorly absorbed. So go the natural route first. Eat lots of nuts (especially those rich in monounsaturated fat like almonds and cashews), and other foods rich in magnesium. If you insist on taking store-bought supplements, the cheapest is milk of magnesia (but it tastes terrible). Capsule forms are very inexpensive because they are primarily magnesium oxide. Magnesium oxide, though it is not very soluble by itself, will become chelated (attached) to the amino acids formed during the breakdown of protein. This chelation process will facilitate the entry of magnesium into the bloodstream, but you have to take the supplement in the presence of protein for it to be effectively absorbed. Of course, you could buy magnesium that is already chelated, and take it on an empty stomach. However, you won't get a lot of magnesium in each capsule since the amino acid used to chelate the magnesium will take up much of the space and it's a lot more expensive. Regardless of the dosage form, try to take 250 milligrams of supplemental magnesium per day.

THIRD TIER SUPPLEMENTS

I think of the third tier of supplements as relatively inexpensive additional insurance policies. Their utility to an individual on the Zone Diet is limited compared to the benefits of the supplements recommended above, but third tier supplements represent peace of mind.

The first of these third tier supplements is beta carotene. Nowhere in the world of supplements is there more confusion than there is about beta carotene. Scientists always want to search for a "magic bullet" that can be put into a capsule as the essence of health. For many years beta carotene appeared to be a magic bullet. After all, many studies showed that higher blood levels of beta carotene were associated with lower risks of heart disease and cancer. The obvious conclusion was that beta carotene was the key factor in preventing both diseases, but it turned out that the scientists were looking at the trees (and a single tree, at that) instead of the forest.

No one thought for a minute that the bloodstream of healthy people contained a lot of beta carotene because they were eating a lot of fruit! After all, if you are consuming a lot of fruit, it is unlikely that you are eating a lot of high-density carbohydrates like starches and pasta. It wasn't that beta carotene had some mystical properties as researchers first thought, but simply because fruit eaters weren't consuming as many high-density carbohydrates. As a result, they were not making as much insulin as non–fruit eaters.

The mystique of beta carotene was recently diminished by two studies based on the magic bullet approach. One study focused on smokers and the other with asbestos workers; both are high-risk groups for cancer. Large research studies were undertaken to show that taking large amounts of beta carotene would prevent cancer. The trouble was that both studies indicated that the group taking beta carotene was actually developing cancer at higher rates! Had the magic bullet of beta carotene actually become a deadly dart? I don't think so, because the increase in cancer in these studies could have a simpler alternative explanation.

Beta carotene is a great antioxidant for fat-soluble free radicals. This simply means it picks up free radicals and stabilizes them before they can do some real damage. But unless removed from the body, a stabilized free radical is just trouble looking to strike. To get these free radicals out of your system, you need to have adequate levels of water-soluble antioxidants (like vitamin C) to take the fat-soluble free radical from beta carotene and transport it to the liver, where it can be metabolically emasculated and excreted. And that was the problem with the beta carotene studies: Neither added extra vitamin C to transport the beta carotene–stabilized free radicals to the liver for their final detoxification.

Is beta carotene really dangerous to your health? Of course not, and in fact it has great utility as long as the other part of the equation (vitamin C) is present at adequate levels. This is why vitamin C is *very* important as a supplement, and beta carotene is less important as a Zone supplement.

But before you go out and buy extra beta carotene supplements, try getting it from fruits like cantaloupe, and from vegetables like red peppers and spinach. And yes, carrots contain beta carotene, but unfortunately because of the structure of the carbohydrates in the carrot, they enter the bloodstream very rapidly and thus increase insulin levels, which can be worse for your health than the benefit gained by the increase in beta carotene.

Other supplements that I place into this third tier are vitamins B_3 (niacin) and B_6 (pridoxine), which are critical for the production of eicosanoids.

Lack of niacin was discovered as the cause of pellagra, which became a widespread epidemic in this country at the turn of the century when poorer populations subsisted on white flour, white rice, and sugar, products all devoid of niacin. (Not surprisingly these foods have once again become the staples of our country, but now in the form of pasta, bagels, and rice cakes.) Unlike most vitamins, niacin can be produced in the body through the conversion of the amino acid tryptophan into niacin. The process is not very efficient, but it does mean that if you are eating adequate levels of protein, you will probably avert an outright deficiency of niacin. The best source of niacin remains food, and particularly those foods that are integral to the Zone Diet, including lean meat, poultry, fish, eggs, cheese, and milk. And again, while whole grains are another good source, I don't recommend them because the higher density of carbohydrates in the grains will increase insulin levels, thus outweighing any benefit of increased niacin. If you are going to supplement with niacin, then 20 milligrams per day is a good dose. With vitamin B_6 (the second of the vitamin B pair), I recommend 5 to 10 milligrams per day. These amounts of B vitamins can also be found in any decent vitamin pill.

Folic acid is another vitamin that has received research attention because of its ability to reduce both neural tube defects in children and the levels of homocysteine, a risk factor for heart disease. The name *folic acid* comes from the Latin word for leaf because that is exactly where you find this vitamin: in leafy green vegetables. Although the RDA for this vitamin is 200 micrograms per day, the most recent research (especially on heart disease), indicates that it makes sense to take at least 500 to 1,000 micrograms per day. It turns out folic acid also works with vitamins B_3 and B_6 to reduce the levels of homocysteine, another example of synergy with other vitamins (like vitamin C and beta carotene) in the body.

Also in this same tier of useful supplements are the minerals calcium, zinc, selenium, and chromium.

You are told that calcium is necessary for strong bones, since 99 percent of the calcium in your body is in your bones. But it's also needed to control muscle contraction and nerve conduction. Dairy products, including cheese, are without a doubt the best sources of calcium. Our national fat phobia has made most dairy products persona non grata, forcing many women to go out and get calcium supplements. But dairy products aren't the only sources of calcium because broccoli, cauliflower, green leafy vegetables, and calcium-precipitated tofu also provide calcium, but the calcium in these foods is not nearly as absorbable as that found in dairy products.

Another important mineral to consider is zinc. Zinc plays a critical role in the proper functioning of your immune system and in the production of eicosanoids. Not surprisingly, good sources of zinc are the building blocks of the Zone Diet, including chicken, beef, fish, oatmeal, and nuts. If you are going to supplement with zinc, 15 milligrams per day should be sufficient. As with vitamins B_3 and B_6 you will probably find this amount of zinc in a typical vitamin-mineral supplement.

Selenium is an essential component of the enzyme known as glutathione peroxidase that reduces excess free radicals. This is why selenium supplementation is useful in cancer treatment and prevention.

Food sources higher up the food chain, such as seafood and beef, tend to be rich in selenium. Nuts are also rich in selenium. I advise a dose of 200 micrograms per day; L-selenomethionine is your best store-bought choice for maximum absorption of this supplement.

Finally, the mineral chromium is part of a biochemical complex known as glucose tolerance factor. This factor makes insulin more effective in driving blood glucose into cells for use. Therefore the more chromium you have, the less insulin you need to make. This is why chromium is called a potentiator of insulin action. Unfortunately, many supplement manufacturers have touted chromium as the only thing required to lose fat or gain muscle mass. Nothing can be further from the truth. To paraphrase President Clinton's 1992 campaign slogan, "It's the insulin, stupid." Your diet will have far greater effect on insulin than any supplement. If you choose to supplement your diet with chromium, I suggest taking approximately 200 micrograms per day.

EXOTIC AND NOT SO CHEAP SUPPLEMENTS

This last group of vitamins is interesting, but only if you have money to spare. It includes lycopene, lutein, CoQ_{10}, and oligoproanthocyanidins. All tend to be antioxidants. Two of the most interesting are the carotenoids lycopene and lutein. Lycopene has been associated with a decrease in prostate cancer and is found primarily in foods with red pigments, such as tomato and watermelon. Lutein, on the other hand, is associated with a decrease in macular degeneration (which causes an ever decreasing field of vision in the eye and leads to blindness). Where do you find lutein? In green leafy vegetables and red peppers. If you want to supplement your diet with these very expensive antioxidants, try 3 to 5 milligrams per day.

Another interesting antioxidant is CoQ_{10}. This is not really a vitamin, since the body can synthesize it, but the synthesis is usually very inefficient. CoQ_{10} functions like a souped-up vitamin E and may be the last line of defense for preventing the oxidation of low-density lipoproteins (LDL), which appears to be a major factor in the development of atherosclerosis. There is also evidence of its benefit in the treatment of congestive heart failure. I recommend 5 to 10 milligrams per day.

Finally, there are the overly hyped, but nonetheless potentially useful, antioxidants known as oligoproanthocyanidins (OPC), or polyphenolics. They are the antioxidants found in grapes and are part of the bioflavanoid family that works together with vitamin C. Since bioflavanoids have some solubility in both fats and water, they make a good shuttle system to help move stabilized free radicals from fat-soluble antioxidants, such as vitamin E and beta carotene, to water-soluble antioxidants, such as vitamin C, so that the free radical can be detoxified by the liver. A good recommendation is 5 to 10 milligrams per day.

My recommendations don't mean that other vitamins and minerals aren't important to human health, because they are. But if you are following the Zone Diet, you are probably getting adequate levels of these other micronutrients.

13

WHAT THE CRITICS SAY

Are there critics of the Zone Diet? You bet there are. And for the life of me, I don't know why. After all, the Zone Diet is not new, it's basically what your grandmother told you to eat. I believe a recent article on diets in the May 1997 issue of *Vogue* magazine hits on a potential reason for the uproar: "The Zone . . . is under constant attack by registered dietitians who would be washing floors if everyone followed the Zone."

It also seems as if many "critics" of the Zone Diet have never read any of my Zone books further than the jacket cover, and consequently have little understanding of the concept of hormonal control modulated through food. Therefore, let me summarize and debunk the various criticisms that have been leveled at the Zone Diet.

1. **"It's a high-protein diet."** This is a tired refrain that attempts to link the Zone Diet to the high-protein diets of the 1970s. These high-protein diets were exactly that—excessive in protein. The advocates of these diets said, "Eat all the protein you want, just don't eat any carbohydrate." Well, you can't eat all the protein you want because your body can only metabolize a certain amount of protein at any one meal. What's that maximum per meal? About the amount of low-fat protein you can put on the palm of your hand. And before you get too excited, that amount of protein also should be no thicker

than the palm of your hand. For most males this is about four ounces of low-fat protein, and for most females it is about three ounces of low-fat protein. Any more protein at a meal will be converted to fat, since your body can't store protein. Just make sure you get that amount of protein at each of your three meals per day. The typical American male will need about 100 grams of protein per day, whereas the typical American female will need about 75 grams per day. On a typical high-protein diet, a typical male might eat 150 or more grams of protein per day, an amount of protein that is simply too much except for world-class athletes.

Furthermore, high-protein diets are very low in carbohydrate, which generates an abnormal state called ketosis. Since you are consuming more carbohydrate than protein on the Zone Diet, it is impossible ever to be in ketosis.

Frankly, there is simply no relation between the Zone Diet and the typical high-protein diet. This is shown more clearly in Figure 13–1. As you can see from this figure, on a high-protein diet you would be consuming nearly 50 percent more protein than if you were on the Zone Diet. You would also be eating 50 percent more fat, and 250 percent *less* carbohydrate.

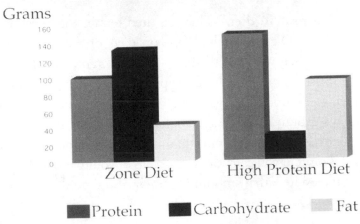

Zone Diet vs. High Protein Diet

Grams

Zone Diet	High Protein Diet	
■ Protein	■ Carbohydrate	■ Fat

So the Zone Diet is clearly a protein-adequate diet, not a high-protein diet, with enough carbohydrate to make it impossible to be in ketosis, but not enough carbohydrate to cause an overproduction of insulin.

2. **"A calorie is a calorie."** This is the basic mantra of most nutritionists. Weight gain and weight loss is simply a matter of calories in versus calories out. Unfortunately, this is not true for fat gain or fat loss. Gaining or losing body fat is controlled by levels of insulin. And the macronutrient makeup of a diet will have a dramatic impact on insulin levels.

   As an example, if "a calorie is a calorie," shouldn't anyone on a 1,000-calorie-per-day diet lose weight? And if "a calorie is a calorie," then the composition of the calories shouldn't matter. Right? Not necessarily. One study done more than forty years ago with overweight individuals in a hospital ward setting proves this critique wrong. If "a calorie is a calorie," then weight loss would have been the same regardless of the macronutrient composition of the diet. Yet the results don't support this theory (see Figure 13–2).

   In the study, when 90 percent of the 1,000 calories per day

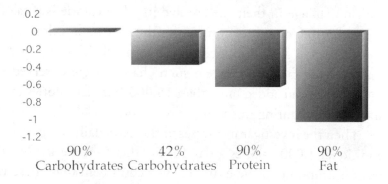

Is A Calorie A Calorie?

came from fat, weight loss was nearly one pound per day. This is because fat has no effect on insulin. When 90 percent of the 1,000 calories per day came from protein, weight loss was reduced to 0.6 pound per day. This is because protein has a slight stimulatory effect on insulin, but a far greater effect on the hormone glucagon that mobilizes stored carbohydrate from the liver to maintain blood sugar. When the 1,000 calories per day came from a mixed diet containing 42 percent carbohydrates (really the first published report of what has become the Zone Diet), the weight loss was reduced to about 0.4 pound per day.

Yet, when 90 percent of the 1,000 calories came from carbohydrates, the patients actually started to gain weight, even on a diet of only 1,000 calories per day! Obviously, a calorie is not a calorie when it comes to weight loss. This study is also the first published reference to what has been further refined to become the Zone Diet, because the protein-to-carbohydrate ratios were similar to those required to maintain insulin in its therapeutic zone—not too high, not too low.

The question of fat calories and weight gain was also addressed in research published in 1997 that studied the effect of adding extra fat calories to the diets of active runners. The study used athletes who ran more than thirty-five miles per week and who followed a standard diet that contained 16 percent of their calories as fat to maintain their weight at a constant level. For four weeks an extra 500 calories per day of fat were added to the runner's diet, with no change in their exercise habits. If "a calorie is a calorie," then after one month of consuming these extra fat calories, some change should have been observed in both their weight and percent of body fat. However, no such changes were observed even though they had added more than 15,000 extra fat calories to their standard diet during this four-week period.

Then the investigators increased the extra daily fat intake to an additional 1,000 calories a day for another four weeks. Now the fat consumption for these runners was equivalent to 42 percent of their calories (but their diets still maintained the same number of carbohydrate and protein calories). However, even after adding an extra 30,000 fat calories to their diet for another four weeks, there was still no change in their weight or their percent of body fat (actually they got slightly thinner).

Perhaps some nutritionist can explain to me why consuming these extra 45,000 calories of fat over an eight-week period did not increase the weight or percent of body fat in these athletes if "a calorie is a calorie"? Furthermore, the only statistically significant change was that their blood lipid profiles were significantly improved by consuming higher levels of fat, as shown in Figure 13–3. This result led the authors of the study to state that "the cardiovascular benefits of exercising by athletes may be negated by consuming a low-fat diet."

This is why the Zone Diet's focus on hormonal thinking is so different from caloric thinking.

The published medical research has shown that weight gain or weight loss is not simply a matter of fat calories in your diet. Hormonal thinking is based upon the role that excess insulin plays in making you fat and keeping you fat. And fat doesn't affect insulin.

Effects of Fat Content on Cardiovascular Risk Factors in Distance Runners

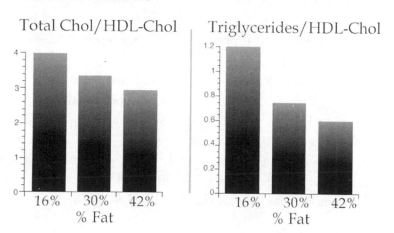

Total Chol/HDL-Chol   Triglycerides/HDL-Chol

% Fat   % Fat

from Leddy et al *Med Sci Sports Exerc* 29: 17-25 (1997)

3. **"The Zone Diet only works because it is a low-calorie diet."**
As research showed more than forty years ago, it is actually possible to gain weight on a low-calorie diet if it is rich in carbohydrates. The Zone Diet is a low-calorie diet that is hormonally correct. A low-calorie diet that generates high levels of insulin (i.e., a high-carbohydrate, low-fat diet) is not only hormonally incorrect, but it also represents outright deprivation. These diets are accompanied by constant hunger, fatigue, and irritability. Who wants that? The Zone Diet is very different because by keeping insulin in a tight zone, you can now access your stored energy (both fat and carbohydrate). You're not hungry on the Zone Diet because your blood sugar level is maintained by the hormone glucagon. You don't have any lack of energy because you are tapping into your stored body fat by keeping insulin levels under control. You don't have to put as many calories in your mouth if you can access your own stored body fat and stored carbohydrate. But this is only possible if you are keeping insulin in a zone.

Obviously, at some point you can lose too much body fat. Once you reach your desired weight, you don't add any more protein since that would make your protein consumption excessive. You don't add any more carbohydrate since that would increase insulin levels. What can you add to your diet that still has calories? It's fat. You start adding more monounsaturated fat to your diet like a caloric ballast to maintain your percent of body fat, since dietary fat has no effect on insulin. In fact, the extra fat will only improve your physical performance in the Zone.

4. **"You have to be fat to be making too much insulin."** It is true that overweight individuals (especially if they have an apple shape) are producing too much insulin. But research published in 1989 in the *New England Journal of Medicine* is quite clear in pointing out that individuals with normal weight can also be hyperinsulinemic, with a resulting increase in blood pressure.

If you are overweight, simply follow the Zone Diet to reduce insulin. If you are of normal weight and you don't want to become overweight, follow the Zone Diet. It's actually pretty simple.

5. **"There's no research to support the Zone Diet."** Actually I have already described the first published research for the prototype of the Zone Diet, which was published more than forty years ago, and another recent publication by independent investigators in 1996, which has confirmed that the Zone Diet can reduce insulin response. Furthermore, diets higher in fat and lower in carbohydrates improve the blood profiles of both Type II diabetic patients and postmenopausal women. In fact, the authors of the study on postmenopausal women stated that "it seems reasonable to question the wisdom of recommending that postmenopausal women consume low-fat, high-carbohydrate diets."

    Frankly, I am waiting for some research to appear to show that the Zone Diet doesn't work. Unfortunately, nutrition is often driven more by political agendas than by scientific facts.

6. **"The Zone Diet is too hard to follow."** If you have gotten this far in this book, then you know that statement is false. The Zone Diet is very similar to the diet your grandmother told you to eat, and all you have to do is simply balance your plate using your eyeball every time you eat.

7. **"It takes too much time to make meals on the Zone Diet."** It doesn't take long to prepare Zone-Perfect meals if you use the recipes in this book as a guide and template. And if you are really pressed for time, drive through a fast-food restaurant and create the appropriate protein-to-carbohydrate balance by throwing away any excess carbohydrate. Better yet, go to the salad bar at a local supermarket to get some fruits and vegetables, and then walk over to the deli to get some low-fat protein to balance it.

8. **"The Zone Diet is too expensive."** Yes, eating fresh fruits and vegetables instead of pasta and bagels is more expensive. But frozen fruits and vegetables are much cheaper and have more

nutrition. However, if you think the Zone Diet is expensive, then try being fat, lethargic, and prone to chronic disease as an alternative.

9. **"The Zone Diet is too radical."** Here I stand with your grandmother and the French. No one has ever accused the French of not eating well. And if the Zone Diet is radical, then everything your grandmother told you about a healthy diet is also suspect.

   But the final criticism of the Zone Diet is one that I must agree with. This charge is the following:

10. **"If I am right about the Zone Diet, then virtually every nutritional expert and the U.S. government are totally wrong."** This one might be a little over the top, because in reality there is no right or wrong diet for Americans. But there are hormonally correct diets. The definition of a hormonally correct diet is one that keeps insulin in a tight zone—not too high, not too low. And whatever diet you are following, if you are keeping insulin in that Zone, then keep doing it because it's working for your biochemistry. Frankly, if you are eating Pop Tarts three times a day, and you are maintaining your insulin levels, then keep eating the Pop Tarts—although I think that's an unlikely scenario.

The Zone Diet gives you the easy-to-follow hormonal rules that allow you to achieve your goal of lifetime insulin control, and with slight modifications to your current diet it can quickly become a Zone Diet. For individuals not having success on a high-carbohydrate diet, I suggest cutting back on the high-density carbohydrates (pasta, grains, and starches), adding a little extra low-fat protein, and adding a dash of monounsaturated fat. For individuals not having success on a high-protein diet, simply cut back on the protein, add more low-density carbohydrates (fruits and vegetables) and ease off on some of the excess fat. Presto, then everyone is following the Zone Diet, and what could be simpler than that?

⑭

THE FUTURE OF THE ZONE

I started to develop the Zone Diet over fifteen years ago as I came to realize that conventional nutritional "wisdom" was flawed and my own future (because of my family's poor cardiovascular history) hung in the balance. Today, there is a growing body of evidence that the Zone Diet has the potential to change the very core of our health-care system as we know it. Given the direction in which our health-care system is now evolving, it seems likely that you will ultimately bear the fiscal responsibility for your own health. The days of unlimited health care are over.

Why should the Zone Diet be especially important to you now? Because in five to ten years, I believe all health care in this country will be basically controlled by the insurance companies. And what do you think will happen when they discover that the earliest indication of a potential heart attack can be measured by your insulin levels? And then what happens if your insulin levels are elevated? You can bet that eventually your insurance company is going to put you on the Zone Diet to treat your excess insulin levels, or you are going to pay much more in insurance premiums. The Zone Diet is not a fad; it is a powerful technology that can save insurance companies billions of dollars by delaying the advent of chronic diseases, such as heart disease. And money makes things happen.

What would the overall lowering of insulin levels mean for this country? One result would be a tremendous increase in the general health of the nation, despite an aging population. Another would be a giant step forward in balancing the federal budget as costs for the treatment of chronic diseases (especially Type II diabetes) would be dramatically decreased. And finally, it would mean a return to common sense in our thinking about what constitutes good nutrition.

But more importantly for you, by using the Zone Diet, you have an exceptionally powerful food pharmacy available to help you avoid chronic disease while simultaneously increasing the quality of your life. This book, and others I wrote before it, teach you how to use that pharmacy to the best advantage.

At this point, you are probably asking yourself the following questions.

1. If it is understood at the research level that elevated insulin is the primary risk factor for heart disease, why hasn't the popular press told me about this?

2. If excess carbohydrates in the diet produce excess insulin, why does the popular press tell me to eat high-carbohydrate diets?

3. If eating high-carbohydrate diets is making me fatter, why does the same popular press tell me to eat even more carbohydrates?

My answer would be "I don't know." During the last fifteen years of advocating the benefits of a high-carbohydrate diet, nothing has seemed to work despite the best efforts of the government, nutritionists, and the popular press. Americans are more confused than ever about what they should eat. I think one reason may be that when you are taught to think calorically, it is very difficult to embrace hormonal thinking. This is especially true of most of the nutritional establishment, who have made their careers by believing in caloric thinking. This is also why so many of the myths of current nutrition refuse to die.

Here are a few more myths (that you hear all the time in the popular press) that guide our current nutritional policies. They are also wrong.

1. **"A diet high in saturated fat causes heart disease."** It does if you don't eat enough fiber. But when you correct for fiber intake (increased fruit and vegetable consumption), there is no relationship between heart disease and saturated fat. This is why Spaniards, who are eating more saturated fat and fewer grains, have seen their heart disease rates drop dramatically over the past twenty years.

2. **"A diet high in very saturated fat like lard increases cholesterol levels."** Lard is considered the most potent artery-clogging food known to man (at least in the popular press). Yet when you feed the primary fatty acid found in lard (stearic acid) to humans, there is no change in total cholesterol or even LDL cholesterol levels. It turns out that some saturated fat is neutral, and some saturated fat is bad. It's a lot more complicated than you have been led to believe.

3. **"Pasta is the ideal health food."** What you are not told is that excess consumption of pasta is associated with increased cancer risk. In fact, a growing body of evidence links increased insulin levels to cancer, just as increased insulin levels are linked to heart disease.

4. **"Complex carbohydrates decrease diabetes."** Not really true. It very much depends on the glycemic index of the carbohydrate. The slower the rate of entry of a carbohydrate into the bloodstream, the less likely you are to develop diabetes. And the carbohydrates with the lowest glycemic index are the ones recommended on the Zone Diet. But the Zone Diet is not about the glycemic index of carbohydrates, but the insulin index of a meal.

5. **"A high-carbohydrate diet rich in pasta, starch, and breads and low in protein prevents hypertension."** In reality, a higher pro-

tein intake coupled with an increase in fruits and vegetables reduces hypertension.

Despite the mass of myths, I still believe the hormonal truth will win in the end. And the implications of the Zone are not confined just to our country or to the developed world. Contrary to popular opinion, the three major causes of death in the undeveloped world are heart disease, cancer, and stroke—just as they are in the United States. Therefore, if the Zone Diet can reduce the chronic diseases that threaten to cripple our health-care system, the same benefits can be expected for health care worldwide.

This doesn't mean eating more animal protein, just more low-fat protein. And the cheapest, most renewable source of protein is soybeans. Simply grow more soybeans, isolate the protein, and fortify the most basic meals (usually consisting of bread, rice, or corn) with adequate levels of a vegetarian source of protein (i.e., isolated soy protein), and overnight world health will be improved.

But before you can change the world, you have to change yourself. All it takes is the commitment to understand hormonal thinking, and the ability to make Zone-Perfect meals. Now that you have read this book, you can begin the process.

Welcome to the Zone.

APPENDIX A

TECHNICAL SUPPORT

The Zone is constantly evolving based on new research, new insights, and continuing feedback from users of the Zone technology. As a consequence the best method of being updated on the Zone is through our web site at http://www.drsears.com. This web site should be used as an on-line Zone news center with updated medical research news, new Zone recipes, helpful Zone hints, and a community message board devoted to the Zone Diet.

If you don't have a computer, give us a call at 1-800-404-8171 for more information.

APPENDIX B

ZONE FOOD BLOCKS

The concept of Zone Food Blocks gives a straightforward method for constructing Zone meals. Listed below are the sizes of various blocks of protein, carbohydrate, and fat each consisting of one block. The protein blocks are for uncooked portions. Although favorable carbohydrates are usually low-glycemic carbohydrates, there are exceptions (like ice cream and potato chips) which are also high in fat.

I have rounded off the blocks to convenient sizes for easy memory. This list is by no means meant to be exhaustive. If you have a favorite food not listed, simply refer to Corinne Netzer's "Complete Book of Food Counts" (Dell Books) to expand the list.

Use of the Zone Food Blocks is easy. The first step is to determine the amount of protein you plan to eat at a meal. For most males this will be four blocks of protein, and for most females it will be three blocks. Then go to the protein section of the Zone Food Block guide and pick out the amount of protein you need for that number of blocks. This could be a single protein source or a combination of protein sources.

Then go to the carbohydrate section of the Zone Food Block guide, and pick out an equal number of carbohydrate blocks. Likewise, this could be a single carbohydrate source or a combination of several.

Finally go to the fat section of the Zone Food Block guide and

choose an equal number of fat blocks. The final ratio of protein, carbohydrate, and fat blocks in your meal should always be in 1:1:1.
Since you should also be consuming two one-block snacks (one in the
late afternoon and the other before retiring), this means the average
male should consume about fourteen blocks per day and the average
female eleven blocks per day. I personally recommend that every adult
consume at least eleven blocks per day.

PROTEIN BLOCKS (APPROXIMATELY 7 GRAMS PROTEIN PER BLOCK)

Meat and Poultry

Best Choices

Chicken breast, skinless	1 ounce
Chicken breast, deli-style	1½ ounces
Turkey breast, skinless	1 ounce
Turkey breast, deli-style	1½ ounces
Veal	1 ounce

Fair Choices

Beef, lean cuts	1 ounce
Beef, ground (10 to 15 percent fat)	1½ ounces
Canadian bacon, lean	1 ounce
Chicken, dark meat, skinless	1 ounce
Duck	1½ ounces
Corned beef, lean	1 ounce
Ham, lean	1 ounce
Ham, deli-style	1½ ounces
Lamb, lean	1 ounce
Pork, lean	1 ounce
Pork chop	1 ounce
Turkey, dark meat, skinless	1 ounce
Turkey bacon	3½ slices

Poor Choices

Bacon	3½ slices
Beef, fatty cuts	1 ounce
Beef, ground (less than 15 percent fat)	1½ ounces
Hot dog (pork or beef)	1 link
Hot dog (turkey or chicken)	1 link
Kielbasa	2 ounces
Liver, beef	1 ounce
Liver, chicken	1 ounce
Pepperoni	1 ounce
Salami	1 ounce

Fish and Seafood

Bass	1½ ounces
Bluefish	1½ ounces
Calamari	1½ ounces
Catfish	1½ ounces
Cod	1½ ounces
Clams	1½ ounces
Crabmeat	1½ ounces
Haddock	1½ ounces
Halibut	1½ ounces
Lobster	1½ ounces
Mackerel*	1½ ounces
Salmon*	1½ ounces
Sardine*	1 ounce
Scallops	1½ ounces
Snapper	1½ ounces
Swordfish	1½ ounces
Shrimp	1½ ounces
Trout	1½ ounces
Tuna (steak)	1½ ounces
Tuna, canned in water	1 ounce

(Source: *Rich in EPA)

Eggs

Best Choices

Egg whites	2
Egg substitute	¼ cup

Poor Choice

Whole egg	1

Protein-Rich Dairy

Best Choice

Cottage cheese, low fat	¼ cup

Fair Choices

Cheese, reduced fat	1 ounce
Mozzarella cheese, skim	1 ounce
Ricotta cheese, skim	2 ounces

Poor Choice

Hard cheeses	1 ounce

Vegetarian

Tofu, soft	3 ounces
Protein powder	⅓ ounce
Soy burgers	½ patty
Soy hot dog	1 link
Soy sausages	2 links

MIXED PROTEIN/CARBOHYDRATE (Contains one block of protein and one block of carbohydrate)

Milk, low fat (1 percent)	1 cup
Yogurt, plain	½ cup
Tempeh	1½ ounce

CARBOHYDRATE BLOCKS (APPROXIMATELY 9 GRAMS OF CARBOHYDRATE PER BLOCK)

Favorable Carbohydrates

Cooked Vegetables

Artichoke	1 medium
Asparagus	1 cup (12 spears)
Beans, green or wax	1 cup
Beans, black	¼ cup
Bok choy	3 cups
Broccoli	1¼ cups
Brussels sprouts	1½ cups
Cabbage	1⅓ cups
Cauliflower	2 cups
Chickpeas	¼ cup
Collard greens	2 cups
Eggplant	1½ cups
Kale	1 cup
Kidney beans	¼ cup
Leeks	1 cup
Lentils	¼ cup
Mushrooms (boiled)	1 cup
Onions (boiled)	½ cup
Okra, sliced	1 cup
Sauerkraut	1 cup
Spinach	1 cup
Swiss chard	1 cup
Turnip, mashed	1 cup
Turnip greens	1½ cups
Yellow squash	1 cup
Zucchini	1½ cups

Raw Vegetables

Alfalfa sprouts	11 cups
Bean sprouts	3 cups
Bamboo shoots	2 cups
Cabbage, shredded	3 cups
Cauliflower	2 cups
Celery, sliced	2½ cups
Cucumber	1
Cucumber, sliced	4 cups
Endive, chopped	7½ cups
Escarole, chopped	7½ cups
Green peppers	3
Green pepper, chopped	2¼ cups
Humus	¼ cup
Lettuce, iceberg	1½ heads
Lettuce, romaine, chopped	6 cups
Mushrooms, chopped	3 cups
Onion, chopped	1 cup
Radishes, sliced	2 cups
Salsa	½ cup
Snow peas	1 cup
Spinach	6 cups
Spinach salad (2 cups raw spinach, ¼ raw onion, ¼ raw mushrooms, and ¼ raw tomato)	1
Tomato	2
Tomato, chopped	1¼ cups
Tossed salad (2 cups shredded lettuce, ¼ raw green pepper, ¼ raw cucumber, and ¼ raw tomato)	1
Water chestnuts	⅓ cup

Fruits (fresh, frozen, or canned light)

Apple	½
Applesauce	¼ cup
Apricots	3
Blackberries	¾ cup
Blueberries	¾ cup
Cantaloupe	¼ melon
Cantaloupe, cubed	¾ cup
Cherries	¾ cup
Fruit cocktail	½ cup
Grapes	½ cup
Grapefruit	½
Honeydew melon, cubed	½ cup
Kiwi	1
Lemon	1
Lime	1
Nectarine	½
Orange	½
Orange, mandarin canned	⅓ cup
Peach	1
Peaches, canned	½ cup
Pear	½
Pineapple, cubed	½ cup
Plum	1
Raspberries	1 cup
Strawberries	1 cup
Tangerine	1
Watermelon	¾ cup

Grains

Oatmeal (slow cooking)**	⅓ cup (cooked)
Oatmeal (slow cooking)**	½ ounce dry

(Source: **contains GLA)

Unfavorable Carbohydrates (use in moderation)

Cooked Vegetables

Acorn squash	½ cup
Baked beans	⅛ cup
Beets, sliced	½ cup
Butternut squash	⅓ cup
Carrots, sliced	½ cup
Corn	¼ cup
French fries	5
Lima beans	¼ cup
Parsnip	⅓ cup
Peas	⅓ cup
Pinto beans	⅓ cup
Potato, baked	⅓ cup
Potato, boiled	⅓ cup
Potato, mashed	⅕ cup
Refined beans	¼ cup
Sweet potato, baked	⅓ cup
Sweet potato, mashed	⅕ cup

Fruits

Banana	⅓
Cranberries	¼ cup
Cranberry sauce	3 teaspoons
Dates	2 pieces
Fig	1 piece
Guava	½ cup
Kumquat	3
Mango, sliced	⅓ cup
Papaya, cubed	½ cup
Prunes (dried)	2
Raisins	1 tablespoon

Fruit Juices

Apple juice	⅓ cup
Apple cider	⅓ cup
Cranberry juice	¼ cup
Fruit punch	¼ cup
Grape juice	½ cup
Grapefruit juice	⅓ cup
Lemon juice	⅓ cup
Lemonade	⅓ cup
Orange juice	⅓ cup
Pineapple juice	¼ cup
Tomato juice	¾ cup
V–8 juice	¾ cup

Grains and Breads

Bagel (small)	¼
Barley	½ tablespoon
Biscuit	¼
Bread crumbs	½ ounce
Bread, whole grain	½ slice
Bread, white	½ slice
Breadstick	1
Buckwheat, dry	½ ounce
Bulgur wheat, dry	½ ounce
Carrot	1
Carrot, shredded	1 cup
Cereal, dry	½ ounce
Cornbread	1 square
Cornstarch	4 teaspoons
Couscous	½ ounce
Croissant, plain	¼
Crouton	½ ounce
Donut, plain	¼

English muffin	¼
Granola	½ ounce
Grits, cooked	⅓ cup
Melba toast	½ ounce
Millet	½ ounce
Muffin, blueberry	¼
Noodles, egg (cooked)	¼ cup
Pancake (four-inch)	½
Pasta, cooked	¼ cup
Pita bread	¼ pocket
Pita bread, mini	½ pocket
Popcorn, popped	2 cups
Rice, brown (cooked)	⅕ cup
Rice, white (cooked)	⅕ cup
Rice cake	1
Roll, bulky	¼
Roll, dinner	½ small
Roll, hamburger	¼
Taco shell	1
Tortilla, corn (six-inch)	1
Tortilla, flour (eight-inch)	½
Waffle	½

Others

Barbecue sauce	2 tablespoons
Candy bar	¼
Catsup	2 tablespoons
Cocktail sauce	2 tablespoons
Crackers (saltine)	4
Cracker (Graham)	1
Honey	½ tablespoon
Jam or jelly	2 teaspoons
Ice cream, regular	¼ cup
Ice cream, premium	⅙ cup

Molasses	2 teaspoons
Plum sauce	1½ tablespoons
Potato chips	½ ounce
Pretzels	½ ounce
Relish, pickle	4 teaspoons
Sugar, brown	1½ teaspoons
Sugar, granulated	2 teaspoons
Sugar, confectionery	1 tablespoon
Syrup, maple	2 teaspoons
Syrup, pancake	2 teaspoons
Teriyaki sauce	½ ounce
Tortilla chips	½ ounce

FAT (APPROXIMATELY 1½ GRAMS PER BLOCK)

Best Choices (rich in monounsaturated fat)

Almond butter	⅓ teaspoon
Almonds (slivered)	1 teaspoon
Almonds	3 teaspoons
Avocado	1 tablespoon
Canola oil	⅓ teaspoon
Guacamole	1 tablespoon
Macadamia nut	1
Olive oil and vinegar dressing	1 teaspoon
Olive oil	⅓ teaspoon
Peanut oil	⅓ teaspoon
Olives	3
Peanut butter, natural	½ teaspoon
Peanuts	6
Tahini	½ tablespoon

Fair Choices (low in saturated fat)

Mayonnaise, regular	⅓ teaspoon
Mayonnaise, light	1 teaspoon

Sesame oil   ½ teaspoon
Soybean oil   ⅓ teaspoon

Poor Choices (rich in saturated fat)

Bacon bits (imitation)   2 teaspoons
Butter   ⅓ teaspoon
Cream   ½ tablespoon
Cream cheese   1 teaspoon
Cream cheese, light   2 teaspoons
Lard   ⅓ teaspoon
Sour cream   ½ tablespoon
Sour cream, light   1 tablespoon
Vegetable shortening   ⅓ teaspoon

APPENDIX C

REFERENCES

Acherio A, Rimm EB, Giovannucci EL, Spegelman D, Stampfer M, and Willett WC. "Dietary fat and risk of coronary heart disease in men." Brit Med J 313: 84–90 (1996)

Addison RF, Zinck ME, Ackman RG, and Sipos JC. "Behavior of DDT, polychlorinated biphenyls and dieldrin at various stages of refining of marine oils for edible use." J Am Oil Chemists Soc 55: 391–394 (1978)

Addison RF. "Removal of organochlorine pesticides and polychlorinated biphenyls from marine oils during refining and hydrogenation for edible use." J Am Oil Chemists Soc 53: 192–194 (1974)

Allred JB. "Too much of a good thing? An over-emphasis on eating low-fat food may be contributing to the alarming increase in overweight amoug US adults." J Am Dietetic Assoc 95: 417–418 (1995)

Alpha-tocopherol Beta-carotene Cancer Prevention Study Group. "The effect of Vitamin E and Beta-carotene on the incidence of lung cancer and other cancers in male smokers." New Engl J Med 334:1150–1155 (1996)

American Heart Association. Heart and Stroke Facts: 1996 Statistical Supplement.

Appel LJ, Moore TJ, Obarzanek E, Vollmer WM, Svetkey LP, Sacks FM, Bray GA, Vogt TM, Cutler JA, Windauser MM, Lin P-H, and Karanja N. "A clinical trial of the effects of dietary patterns on blood pressure." N Engl J Med 336: 1117–1124 (1997)

Arsenian MA. "Magnesium and cardiovascular disease." Progress in Cardiovascular Diseases 35: 271–310 (1993)

Baggio E, Gandini R, Plancher AC, Passeri M, and Camosino G. "Italian multicenter study on the safety and efficacy of coenzyme Q10 as adjunctive therapy in heart failure." Molec Aspects Med 15: S287-S294 (1994)

Blayrock, RL. Excitotoxins. The taste that kills. Health Press. Santa Fe, NM (1994)

Campbell LV, Marmot PE, Dyer JA, Borkman M, and Storlien LH. "The high-monounsaturated fat diet as a practical alternative for non-insulin dependent diabetes mellitus." Diabetes Care 17: 177–182 (1994)

Crawford MA and Marsh DE. The Driving Force: Food, Evolution, and the Future. Harper and Row. London. (1989)

Crawford MA, Cunnane SC, and Harbige LS. "A new theory of evolution." In Essential Fatty Acids and Eicosanoids. Sinclair A and Gibson R eds. American Oil Chemists' Society Press. Champaign, IL (1993)

Daviglus ML, Stamler J, Orencia AJ, Dyer AR, Liu K, Greenland P, Walsh MK, Morris D, and Shekelle RB. "Fish consumption and the 30-year risk of fatal myocardial infarction." N Engl J Med 336: 1046–1053 (1997)

Denke MA and Grundy SM. "Effects of fats high in stearic acid on lipid and lipoprotein concentrations in men." Am J Clin Nutr 54: 1036–1040 (1991)

Despres JP, Lamarche B, Mauriege P, Cantin B, Dagenais GR, Moorjani S, and Lupen PJ. "Hyperinsulinemia as an independent risk factor for ischemic heart disease." N Engl J Med 334: 952–957 (1996)

Eades MA. The Doctor's Complete Guide to Vitamins and Minerals. Dell. New York, NY (1994)

Flatt JP. "Use and storage of carbohydrate and fat." Am J Clin Nutr 61: 952S–959S (1995)

Franceschi S, Favero A, Decarli D, Negri E, La Vecchia C, Ferraroni M, Russo A, Salvini S, Amadori D, Conti E, Montella M, and Giacosa A. "Intake of Macronutrients and risk of breast cancer." Lancet 347: 1351–1356 (1996)

Garg A, Bonanome A, Grundy SM, Zhang ZJ, and Unger RH. "Comparison of a high-carbohydrate diet with a high-monounsaturated fat diet in patients with non-insulin-dependent diabetes mellitus." N Engl J Med 319: 829–834 (1988)

Garg A, Grundy SM, and Koffler M. "Effect of high carbohydrate intake on hyperglycemia, islet function, and plasma lipoproteins in NIDDM." Diabetes Care 15: 1572–1580 (1992)

Garg A, Bantle JP, Henry RR, Coulston AM, Griven KA, Raatz SK, Brinkley L, Chen I, Grundy SM, Huet BA, and Reaven GM. "Effects of varying carbohydrate content of diet in patients with non-insulin-dependent diabetes mellitus." JAMA 271: 1421–1428 (1994)

Giovannucci E, Ascherio A, Rimm EB, Stampfer MJ, Colditz GA, and Willett WC. "Intake of carotenoids and retinol in relation to risk of prostate cancer." J Nat Canc Inst 87: 1767–1776 (1995)

Golay KL, Allaz AF, Morel Y, de Tonnac N, Tankova S, and Reaven G. "Similar weight loss with low- or high-carbohydrate diets." Am J Clin Nutr 63: 174–178 (1996)

Heini AF and Weinsier RL. "Divergent trends in obesity and fat intake patterns: an American paradox." Am J Med 102: 259–264 (1997)

Hillman H. Kitchen Science. Houghton Mifflin. Boston. (1989)

Hollenbeck C and Reaven GM. "Variations in insulin-stimulated glucose uptake in healthy individuals with normal glucose tolerance." J Clin Endocrin Metab 64: 1169–1173 (1987)

Jeppesen J, Schaaf P, Jones C, Zhou M-Y, Chen YD, and Reaven, GM. "Effects of low-fat, high-carbohydrate diets on risk factors for ischemic heart disease in postmenopausal women." Am J Clin Nutr 65: 1027–1033 (1997)

Katan MB, Grundy SM, and Willett WC. "Beyond low-fat diets." N Eng J Med 337: 563–567 (1997)

Kekwick A and Pawan GLS. "Calorie intake in relation to body-weight changes in the obese." Lancet ii: 155–161 (1956)

Kekwick A and Pawan GLS. "Metabolic study in human obesity with isocaloric diets high in fat, protein, or carbohydrate." Metabolism 6: 447–460 (1957)

Kern PA, Ong JM, Soffan B, and Carty J. "The effects of weight loss on the activity and expression of adipose-tissue lipoprotein lipase in very obese individuals." Metab 32: 52–56 (1990)

Laws A, King AC, Haskell WL, and Reaven GM. "Relationship of fasting plasma insulin concentration to high-density lipoprotein cholesterol and triglyceride concentrations in men." Arteriosclerosis and Thrombosis 11: 1636–1642 (1991)

Lieb CW. "The effect of an exclusive, long-continued meat diet." JAMA 87: 25–26 (1926)

Lieb CW. "The effects on human beings of a twelve-month exclusive meat diet." JAMA 93: 20–22 (1929)

Lands WEM. Fish and human health. Academic Press. Orlando, FL. (1986)

Lanting CI, Fidler V, Huisman M, Touwen BCL, and Boersma ER. "Neurological differences between 9-year-old children fed breast-milk or formula-milk as babies." Lancet 344: 1319–1322 (1994)

Leddy J, Horvath P, Rowland J, and Pendergast D. "Effect of a high or low fat diet on cardiovascular risk factors in male and female runners." Med Sci Sports Exerc 29: 17–25 (1997)

Lucas A, Morley R, Cole TJ, Lister G, and Leeson-Payne C. "Breast milk and subsequent intelligence quotient in children born preterm." Lancet 339: 261–264 (1992)

McCully KS. "Vascular pathology of homosystemia: implications for the pathogenesis of arteriosclerosis." Am J Pathol 56: 111–128 (1969)

McGee H. On Food and Cooking. MacMillan Publishing. New York. (1984)

Mohr A, Bowry VW, and Stocker R. "Dietary supplementation with coenzyme Q10 results in increased levels of ubiquninol–10 within circulating lipoproteins and increased resistance of human low-density lipoproteins to the initiation of lipid peroxidation." Biochem Biphys Acta 1126: 247–254 (1992)

Murray CJL and Lopez AD. "Mortality by cause for eight regions of the world." Lancet 349: 1269–1276 (1997)

Norman AW and Litwack G. Hormones. Academic Press. San Diego, CA (1987)

Nygard O, Nordehaug, JE, Refsum H, Ueland PM, Farstad M, and Vollset SE. "Plasma homocysteine levels and mortality in patients with coronary heart disease." New Engl J Med 337: 230–236 (1997)

Omenn GS, Goodman GE, Thornquist MD, Balmes J, Cullen MR, Glass A, Keogh JP, Meyskens, FL, Valanis R, Williams JH, Barnhart S, and Hammar S. "Effects of a combination of beta-carotene and vitamin A on lung cancer and cardiovascular disease." New Engl J Med 334: 1150–1155 (1996)

Parillo M, Rivellese AA, Ciardullo AV, Capaldo B, Giacco A, Genovese S, and Riccardi G. "A high-monounsaturated fat/low-carbohydrate diet improves peripheral insulin sensitivity in non-insulin-dependent diabetic patients." Metabol 41: 1373–1378 (1993)

Rasmussen OW, Thomsen C, Hansen KW, Vesterlund M, Winther E, and Hermansen K. "Effects on blood pressure, glucose, and lipid levels of a high-monounsaturated fat diet compared with a high-carbohydrate diet in non-insulin dependent diabetic subjects." Diabetes Care 16: 1565–1571 (1993)

Rimm EB, Stampfer MJ, Ascherio A, Giovannucci E, Colditz GA, and Willett WC. "Vitamin E consumption and risk of coronary heart disease in men." New Engl J Med 328: 1450–1456 (1993)

Roberts HJ. Aspartame. Is it Safe? Charles Press. Philadelphia, PA (1990)

Robertson RP, Gavarenski DJ, Porte D, and Bierman EL. "Inhibition of in vivo insulin secretion by prostaglandin E1." J Clin Invest 54: 310–315 (1974)

Robertson RP. "Prostaglandins, glucose homeostasis and diabetes mellitus." Ann Rev Med 43: 1–12 (1983)

Salmeron J, Manson JE, Stampfer MJ, Colditz GA, Wing AL, and Willett WC. "Dietary fiber, glycemic load, and risk of non-insulin-dependent diabetes mellitus in women." JAMA 277: 472–477 (1997)

Sears B. The Zone. Regan Books, NY (1995)

Sears B. Mastering the Zone. Regan Books, NY (1997)

Selhub J, Jacques PF, Bostom AG, D'Agostino RB, Wilson PWF, Belanger AJ, O'Leary DH, Wolf PA, Schaefer EJ, and Rosenberg IH. "Association between plasma homocysteine concentrations and extracranial carotid-artery stenosis." N Engl J Med 332: 286–291 (1995)

Serra-Majem L, Ribas L, Tresserras R, and Salleras L. "How could changes in diet explain changes in coronary heart disease mortality in Spain? The Spanish paradox." Amer J Clin Nutr 61: 1351S–1395S (1995)

Seddon JM, Ajani VA, Sperduto RD, Hiller R, Blair M, Burton TC, Farber MD, Gragoudas ES, Haller J, and Miller DT. "Dietary carotenoids, vitamins A, C, and E and age-related macular degeneration." JAMA 272: 1413–1420 (1994)

Stampfer MJ, Hennekens CH, Manson JE, Colditz GA, Rosner B, and Willett WC. "Vitamin E consumption and the risk of coronary disease in women." New Engl J Med 328: 1444–1449 (1993)

Stampfer MJ and Malinow MR. "Can lowering homocysteine levels reduce cardiovascular risk?" N Engl J Med 332:328–329 (1995)

Steinberg D, Parthasarathy S, Carew TE, Khoo JC, and Witztum JL. "Beyond cholesterol-modification of low-density lipoproteins that increase its atherogenicity." New Engl J Med 320: 915–924 (1989)

Wolever TMS, Jenkins DJA, Jenkins AL, and Josse RG. "The glycemic index: methodology and clinical implications." Am J Clin Nutr 54: 846–854 (1991)

Zavaroni I, Bonora E, Pagliara M, Dall'aglio E, Luchetti L, Buonanno G, Bonati PA, Bergonzani M, Gnudi L, Passeri M, and Reaven G. "Risk factors for coronary artery disease in healthy persons with hyperinsulinemia and normal glucose tolerance." N Engl J Med 320: 702–706 (1989)

INDEX

(Note on abbreviations: f.=female; m.=male)

Join the Revolution! Live Longer! Live Healthier!
Over 4 Million Zone Books Sold!

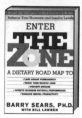

THE ZONE
The #1 *New York Times* bestseller. The dietary program that transformed the way America eats.

ISBN 0-06-039150-2 (hardcover)
ISBN 0-694-51555-8 (audio)
ISBN 0-694-52116-7 (audio-cd)

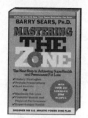

MASTERING THE ZONE
The next step to achieving Superhealth and permanent fat loss.

ISBN 0-06-039190-1 (hardcover)
ISBN 0-694-51777-1 (audio)

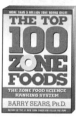

A WEEK IN THE ZONE
A quick course in the healthiest diet for you—7 days that will change your life forever.

ISBN 0-06-103083-X (paperback)

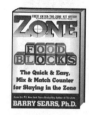

ZONE FOOD BLOCKS
Your guide to calculating food blocks for more than 12,000 items.

ISBN 0-06-039242-8 (hardcover)

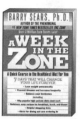

THE TOP 100 ZONE FOODS
A tour of the top 100 Zone foods, offering nutritional benefit summaries, delicious recipes, and Zone Food Block information.

ISBN 0-06-098894-0 (paperback)

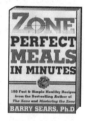

ZONE-PERFECT MEALS IN MINUTES
Features 150 fast and flavorful Zone recipes.

ISBN 0-06-039241-X (hardcover)

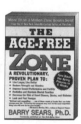

THE AGE-FREE ZONE
Formerly called *The Anti-Aging Zone*. A clinically proven plan to reverse the aging process.

ISBN 0-06-098832-0 (paperback)

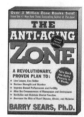

THE ANTI-AGING ZONE
A clinically proven plan to reverse the aging process.

ISBN 0-06-093305-4 (large print)
ISBN 0-694-51935-9 (audio)

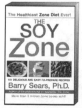

THE SOY ZONE
Dr. Barry Sears reveals how vegetarians and non-vegetarians alike can enjoy the healthiest Zone diet ever! Includes over 100 new and delicious recipes.

ISBN 0-06-093450-6 (paperback)

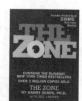

THE ZONE AUDIO COLLECTION

ISBN 0-694-51892-1 (cassette)

Visit the official website at www.drsears.com

 ReganBooks
An Imprint of HarperCollins*Publishers*
www.reganbooks.com

Available wherever books are sold, or call 1-800-331-3761 to order.

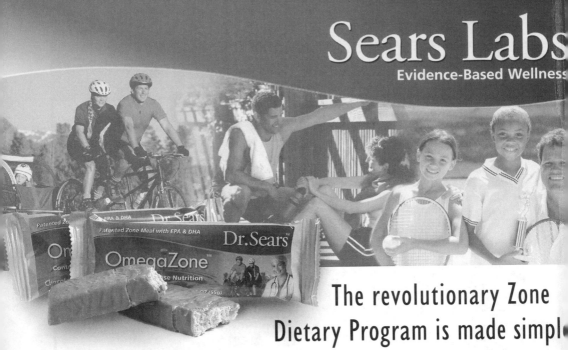
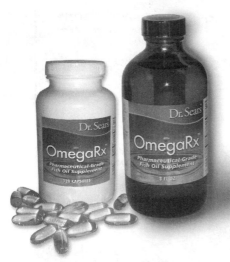